Occupational Therapy *for* People *with* Learning Disabilities

For Elsevier:

Commissioning Editor: *Rita Demetriou-Swanwick*
Development Editor: *Catherine Jackson*
Project Manager: *Anne Dickie/Hemamalini Rajendrababu*
Designer: *Stewart Larking*
Illustration Manager: *Merlyn Harvey*
Illustrator: *Jonathan Haste*

Occupational Therapy *for* People *with* Learning Disabilities

A PRACTICAL GUIDE

Jane Goodman MPhil DipCOT
Lecturer in Occupational Therapy, Occupational Therapy Programme, University of the West of England, Bristol

Jenni Hurst MSc DipCOT CertEd(FE)
Lecturer in Occupational Therapy, Occupational Therapy Programme, University of Plymouth, Devon

Christine Locke MEd DipCOT CertEd(FE)
Lecturer in Occupational Therapy, All Wales Part Time Occupational Therapy Programme, School of Healthcare Studies, Cardiff University, South Wales

Foreword by

Vincenzo Petruzziello

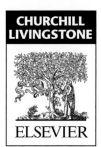

CHURCHILL LIVINGSTONE

ELSEVIER

Edinburgh London New York Oxford Philadelphia St Louis Sydney Toronto 2009

CHURCHILL
LIVINGSTONE
ELSEVIER

© 2009, Elsevier Limited. All rights reserved.

First published 2009

ISBN: 978-0-443-10299-8

British Library Cataloguing in Publication Data
A catalogue record for this book is available from the British Library.

Library of Congress Cataloging in Publication Data
A catalog record for this book is available from the Library of Congress.

Note
Knowledge and best practice in this field are constantly changing. As new research and experience broaden our knowledge, changes in practice, treatment and drug therapy may become necessary or appropriate. Readers are advised to check the most current information provided (i) on procedures featured or (ii) by the manufacturer of each product to be administered, to verify the recommended dose or formula, the method and duration of administration, and contraindications. It is the responsibility of the practitioner, relying on their own experience and knowledge of the patient, to make diagnoses, to determine dosages and the best treatment for each individual patient, and to take all appropriate safety precautions. To the fullest extent of the law, neither the Publisher nor the Editors assume any liability for any injury and/or damage to persons or property arising out of or related to any use of the material contained in this book.

The Publisher

Contents

Contributors

Sally Donati, MSc DipCOT
Head Occupational Therapist
Camden and Islington Learning Disabilities Service,
Camden and Islington NHS Trust, London

Jane Goodman, MPhil DipCOT
Lecturer in Occupational Therapy, Occupational Therapy
Programme, University of the West of England, Bristol

Christine Griffiths, Dip RCSLT
Head of Speech and Language Therapy, Directorate of
Learning Disability Services, Abertawe Bro Morgannwg
University Trust, South Wales

Jenni Hurst, MSc DipCOT CertEd(FE)
Lecturer in Occupational Therapy, Occupational Therapy
Programme, University of Plymouth, Devon

Edwin Jones, PhD BA Hons
Service Development Consultant, Special Projects Team
Abertawe Bro Morgannwg University Trust, South Wales

Angela Kelsall, MA DipCOT DipSE
Occupational Therapist, Vale of Glamorgan, Community
Support Team, South Wales

Christine Locke, MEd DipCOT CertEd(FE)
Lecturer in Occupational Therapy, All Wales Part Time
Occupational Therapy Programme
School of Healthcare Studies, Cardiff University, South
Wales

Rhonwen Parry, BSc DClin Psych C Psychol
Consultant Clinical Psychologist/Head of Psychology,
Directorate of Learning Disability Services, Abertawe Bro
Morgannwg University Trust, South Wales

Vanessa Townsend, DipCOT
Deputy Head Occupational Therapist, Directorate of
Learning Disability Services
Abertawe Bro Morgannwg University Trust,
South Wales

Case illustration contributors

Elisabeth Martins, DipCOT
Clinical Risk Manager, Health and Social Services, Jersey
General Hospital, West Wing, Peter Krill House, St Helier,
Jersey

Dot Palastanga, MA MCSP Cert.Ed.(HE)
Lecturer, Cardiff University, All Wales Part Time Occupational Therapy, Cardiff (retired September 2007)

Advising on occupational therapy student perspectives

Barbara Strobel
Lynnette Bush
Polly Burrows

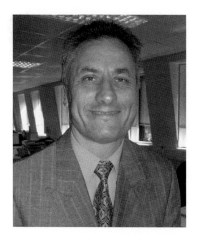

As a person that uses learning disability services I can see that there are lots of ways of looking at what the occupational therapist can do for people with learning disabilities. This book tells people what occupational therapy is, what they do and how they can help people. After speaking to someone who has had occupational therapy I can see they help people do the things they want to do and it makes them feel better and happier.

I think this book will help occupational therapists and students to talk about things that they do when at work. The writers have looked at different things that occupational therapists do; how they can help people as parents, how they can help people live healthy lives. Occupational therapists can help people and make things easier around the home, in their job and when having a good time.

I feel it is very important that people with learning disabilities are listened to, given enough time, not looked down on and treated with respect as people.

Vincenzo Petruzziello
Peterborough

"What occupational therapy text can you recommend for my placement in a learning disabilities team?" **Student OT**

"What do student occupational therapists need to know about learning disabilities?" **Student OT**

"I'd like to know about the role of OT within the learning disability specialty with up to date case studies and approaches and interventions." **Student OT**

"I am going to my first post in a learning disabilities team. What useful texts could I read to prepare for this new field?" **New practitioner**

Student occupational therapists, as any student, need access to a range of learning resources to enable them to become competent practitioners in their chosen field. Student and novice occupational therapists have consistently asked questions similar to those above and these have motivated us to write a text that goes some way towards meeting their needs.

As therapists it is vital to keep abreast of current thinking about the unique philosophies and core skills of occupational therapy and our contribution to changes in provision and new initiatives when working with people with learning disabilities.

In this book, we have attempted to intertwine the developing philosophies of occupational therapy, with the historical and current services for people with learning disabilities. The focus is on the role of occupation in supporting and enabling people with learning disabilities to enjoy a fulfilling quality of life within their social environment. The service user voice is acknowledged throughout the book.

There is an increasing evidence base about aspects of occupational therapy in this field, both in occupational therapy journals and through the work of the College of Occupational Therapists Specialist Section; People with Learning Disabilities. However, historically there is a paucity of specific texts relating to the role of the occupational therapist. Therefore influences on thinking and practice of the new practitioner often come from trusted colleagues and by trial and error. Whilst these approaches to learning have many merits they also leave gaps in the specific evidence shared across the profession to support, underpin, motivate and promote occupational therapy

practice in this field. As a result, outcomes of intervention may take longer to achieve or be less effective and therapists and service users may lose motivation.

In writing this book we have sought to redress the balance by recognizing the experience of valued colleagues and putting their work into print for others to share. The book therefore contains perspectives on different aspects of occupational therapy practice in this field. Inevitably the final version is not the book we envisaged at the outset and there have been many changes of direction on the way. However, our goal remains the same, which is to inspire current and future occupational therapists about this rewarding area of work.

As editors of this text we have between us a wide range of experience as practitioners, researchers and teachers in the field of learning disabilities. We have come together to share our expertise in the promotion of the role of the occupational therapist. We especially aim to offer students and new practitioners a theoretical and practical resource to help guide their practice.

The process of working together and coordinating the input from other contributors has been both interesting and enlightening and we have also learnt much from this experience. As first time editors there has been a lot to learn and many challenges and changes along the way. However, it has been a very positive opportunity to combine our experience and interest for the client group and occupational therapy for the benefit of both. We aim to encourage and motivate students and therapists alike to further follow up links and references to challenge and enhance their learning and practice.

Because the book covers a diverse range of subjects, continuity is maintained throughout with each chapter structured as follows:

- Overview
- Learning outcomes
- Detailed content and knowledge base
- Reader activities
- Case scenarios with reflective questions
- Summary
- Recommended further reading and resources
- References

Case scenarios are used to enhance the topics for each chapter. Details of how the cases were followed up and possible answers or discussion points are presented in appendices at the end of each chapter.

The book first introduces the philosophy of practice for occupational therapists focusing on occupation and its potential to benefit an individual's health and wellbeing. Interwoven in this introductory chapter is the role of occupation in the lives of people with learning disability.

The book is then divided into four sections: Section 1 discusses the underpinning knowledge base for the rest of the book. It takes the reader through the occupational needs of people with learning disabilities, historical perspectives, the occupational therapy process, communication skills. The role of the occupational therapist in health promotion is also considered here.

Section 2 focuses on specific occupational performance areas in relation to client needs considering activities of daily living, work and leisure.

The importance of the influence of life changes on occupational performance is covered in Section 3, presenting transitions, parenting, loss and bereavement, the older adult and life changes.

The final section focuses on wider aspects of service provision including user participation and service user networks as well as providing a conclusion.

Whilst the book is aimed at occupational therapy students and novice therapists it will also provide an introduction for other health and social care students who wish to gain knowledge of occupational therapy in this field. Readers should view the book as an overview of key perspectives to prompt debate, and question the issues that impact on the lives of people with learning disability and hence the role of the occupational therapist.

Acknowledgements

The three of us would like to thank those who have helped and supported us through the process of planning, writing and editing this book. This includes our families and friends whose perseverance at keeping us going has been commendable.

We would like to thank all our colleagues at Cardiff University, University of Plymouth and the University of West of England who have given us support and encouragement just by listening to us, discussing and suggesting ideas.

In particular we thank Jayne Cox, Resource Room Manager and Linda Pires, Library Assistant, Cardiff University, All Wales Part Time Occupational Therapy Programme for their support throughout and especially through the final editing phase. Also Fiona Douglas, Elaine Chamberlain, Gina McKellar Susanna Robinson, and Stella Birch. We especially thank Barbara Strobel, Lynnette Bush and Polly Burrows for their reading and advice on the chapters from the student perspective.

Finally we would like to thank Catherine Jackson, Development Editor, for her support and belief that she would eventually receive a completed book to publish.

Introduction

Jane Goodman • Jenni Hurst • Christine Locke

Overview

This introductory chapter provides a rationale and explores the key concerns that underpin this book. It starts with the purpose and style of the book, followed by definitions and terminology used in learning disability services, and concludes with influences on people's lives. The main concerns for occupational therapists and the underpinning principles for their practice in this field are covered. The chapter draws on historical perspectives to inform current practice and considers future trends and new challenges for working in the field. Useful resources are provided at the end of the chapter.

Why this book is needed

Occupational therapy for people with learning disabilities is a diverse and interesting field of work. It is also an area of work that is undergoing significant change in relation to service philosophies, contexts for practice and attitudes towards people with learning disabilities. For students and new practitioners to the field the complexities surrounding the client group, service provision and the role of the occupational therapist can seem daunting.

Practice placements, voluntary work opportunities and university modules provide good experiences of the range of work involved and may help to allay some of the fears and misunderstandings about what is required to work in this area. However, typically, undergraduate occupational therapy students and people who are new to this area have many concerns about the needs and demands of the client group and fears about how they should and could relate their occupational therapy knowledge into practice. There are many texts about working with people with learning disabilities, but none that focus specifically on the philosophies of occupation. A textbook, therefore, that offers the theory and practice of occupational therapy and influence on health and well-being for this client group is long overdue.

The book offers a starting point from which to develop your practice and take on new roles. It challenges you to continue to consider how significant influences can be relevant in your current and future work with people with learning disabilities.

Purpose

The purpose of the book is to provide the reader with an introduction to theoretical, practical and philosophical underpinnings of occupational therapy in the field of learning disabilities. Relevant influences (both historical and current) will be explored from the perspectives of occupational therapists and other professionals. Existing sources of evidence are given as a basis for presenting ideas for working in the field and to engage the reader in using evidence to influence their thinking and everyday experiences. Examples of good practice, research and new ideas are presented to demonstrate ways of working.

Style of the book

While the style of the contributors varies the editors have provided a unified approach and provided consistency with each chapter and section following the same pattern. Within the book you will find a diverse range of material providing examples of research, practical application, underpinning theory and challenges to consider your practice differently. The four sections of the book each focus on a theme relevant to occupational therapy for people with learning disabilities. An overview of each section provides the reader with the flavour of what it contains. Links between the various chapters are made throughout and readers are referred to further reading and resources.

People with learning disabilities

Terminology

People with learning disabilities are a diverse group of people with diverse needs. Northfield (2004) describes the term learning disabilities as a convenient label useful when discussing or planning services for people. He makes the point that a label does not give an indication of the individuality of the person and that a person with a learning disability should be considered as a person first. In the Valuing People White Paper (DoH 2001) it is clearly stated that 'people with learning disabilities are people first' and that the focus is on people's abilities and the support they need to be able to fulfil their needs and wishes. This idea is central to this text and throughout we attempt to engage the reader with the service user voice and most importantly to consider the idea that people with learning disabilities have the same human needs and wishes as other human beings.

As occupational therapists, considering your own human needs and values can be a starting point from which to consider the needs of people that you work with. Enabling them to have both the opportunity to identify their own occupational needs and to experience new occupations will help them to satisfy these needs. These ideas are explored further in Chapter 1.

In your practice you may also come across 'people with learning difficulties' the term preferred by People First, the international organization that advocates for and with people with learning disabilities (Northfield 2004). This term is also used in other services, for example to describe specific learning problems in children. The DoH (2001) clearly distinguishes between the two terms and states that '"Learning disability" does not include all those that have a "learning difficulty" which is more broadly defined in education legislation (p. 14). In this text we have therefore used the terms 'people with a learning disability' or 'people with learning disabilities' throughout.

It is also relevant here to mention that the focus of this book is on adults with learning disabilities. The role of the occupational therapist with children with a learning disability will be within children's services first and foremost. However, issues of transition from children's to adult services will be considered in Chapter 9.

Definitions of learning disability

Defining what is meant by the term 'people with learning disabilities' and deciding whether or not a person has a learning disability are complex areas of concern. Other texts already give comprehensive information to answer these questions (Gates 2003, Carnaby 2004). However, it is helpful to consider the various stances that have been taken so that the reader can follow up in more detail if required.

Gates & Wilberforce (2003) provide an overview that considers defining learning disability first by testing intellectual ability, second by exploring legislative definitions, and lastly by looking at social competence as a measure of a person's ability to cope in society. Each of these approaches has its limitations and benefits; readers are advised to look at how the client group is identified within practice settings for the purpose of referral to occupational therapy or the community learning disabilities teams for example. These approaches clearly influence the definition of learning disabilities used by the Department of Health (2001):

Learning disability includes the presence of:

- A significantly reduced ability to understand new or complex information, to learn new skills (impaired intelligence), with

- a reduced ability to cope independently (impaired social functioning), which started before adulthood, with a lasting effect on development (DoH 2001, p.14).

A wide range of needs are included within this definition and people may also have other sensory or physical impairments as well as those presented by their learning disability. In assessing whether or not a person has a learning disability one should therefore consider a range of aspects including social functioning, communication skills and their intelligence quotient (IQ).

Occupational therapists may contribute to decisions about whether an individual is accepted into your service. Information about the nature of their learning disability will be one of the considerations that help you judge the likely impact of the person's learning disability on their occupational performance (COT 2003).

Historical perspectives

Historical attitudes towards people with learning disabilities and policies of segregation have had a huge effect on the way that services have been developed and on the lives of individuals. The impact of historical attitudes and practices still has significance today and has influenced decisions about how current services are organized. The closure of long-stay institutions, resettlement to the community and the development of community learning disabilities teams are just some of the changes that have affected people's lives. More recently, the advocacy movement, the Disabled Persons (Independent Living) Bill (Parliament 2006) and the Valuing People White Paper (DOH 2001) have given a voice to people with learning disabilities at a national level so that they can begin to overcome some of the barriers to leading an ordinary life that have prevailed in the past. In Chapter 2 you are introduced to some of the main influences on both the individual and the way that services are organized. For occupational therapists, being aware of service issues and policies that have and continue to affect people's lives will enable them to put the needs of clients into context and to practise in a way that is up to date and evidence based.

Current perspectives

The four principles contained within the Valuing People White Paper (DoH 2001) provide a good starting point for those interested in considering approaches to working with people with learning disabilities. The challenge for occupational therapists and others working in the field is to incorporate these principles into their practice alongside their own personal and professional values.

Rights

People with learning disabilities are citizens too (DoH 2001) p. 23.

This principle is devoted to the premise that people with learning disabilities have the same legal and civil rights as others. This includes the right to the range of opportunities within education, work, family and community life. Central to this principle is the need for active support to have a voice and opinions heard at all levels of society. Some of these issues are explored further in Section 1, Chapter 1, Perspectives on occupational needs of people with learning disability; Chapter 2, Historical perspectives – the lives of people with learning disabilities and the influence of occupational therapy and Chapter 4, The interface between communication and community living. The potential of opportunity for service user participation and research is also discussed in Chapter 13, More than having a say – user participation in learning disability services.

Independence

All this can be done… by believing that people with learning disabilities can move on and be independent (DoH 2001) p. 23.

This principle is based on the idea familiar to occupational therapists that people have the capacity to learn and become independent in areas of their lives that are important to them. For people with learning disabilities past political and social influences have often meant low expectations of the individual resulting in lack of opportunities for developing skills that would enable a greater degree of independence. In the context of the White Paper (DoH 2001) independence does not mean that the person has to do everything without support. For occupational therapists enabling people to become more independent and to develop the right level of support to do this is central to our role. The recent Disabled Persons (Independent Living) Bill

(Parliament 2006) brings to the fore again the issues of rights to independence for people with disabilities supporting 'choice, freedom, dignity, control and substantive opportunities' (p. 1) for disabled people in all aspects of their lives. The right to an assessment of need (including support need) provides useful evidence and a resource for occupational therapists to use to support their work in this field (Parliament 2006). Chapter 3 and the chapters in Section 3 of this book give more detailed information about the role of the occupational therapist in enabling independence for people with learning disabilities.

Choice

> People with learning disabilities have been saying for a long time that we can speak up for ourselves (DoH 2001) p. 24.

This principle relates to the need for people with learning disabilities to have a real say in decisions about their lives and to be able to advocate for others who may be less able to voice their personal choices. Occupational therapists are committed to client-centred practice and this includes finding ways to enable people to make informed choices about the things that are important to them in their lives. This may sometimes include advocating their wishes to others or providing support to enable them to speak for themselves. Some of these issues are addressed in Chapter 13, which looks at how service users can be fully involved in service evaluation and research. The chapters in Section 3 consider choices at particular life stages and circumstances.

Inclusion

> People with learning disabilities can lead just as good a life (DoH 2001) p. 24.

Inclusion means enabling people with learning disabilities to do the ordinary things in society that everyone else does such as going to work, looking after their families and making use of community facilities. It also means enabling people to '...make use of mainstream services and be fully included in the local community' (p. 24). Inclusion is a central theme of client-centred practice and occupational therapy philosophy for example '...contributing to the social and economic fabric of their communities...'

(Law et al 1999). Occupational therapists working with people with learning disabilities have a significant role in supporting people to use mainstream services. They have a role in developing links across service boundaries such as with primary care services and in accessing resources in local communities with and on behalf of their clients. Again this may involve advocacy roles at times. Issues of inclusion are explored in a number of sections in this book but you may find it helpful to look at Sections 2 and 3 to see how these issues can be addressed through occupation for different client needs.

Occupational therapy for people with learning disabilities

Occupational therapists are concerned with 'the nature of a client's occupational identity' as well as the person's 'occupational performance' (Duncan 2006). Occupational therapy for people with learning disabilities can be considered from the perspective of the *person* – with learning disabilities, their carers, the occupational therapist and the inter-professional team, the *environment* – including the context for life and practice and service philosophies and values, *occupations and roles* – the use of meaningful occupations and occupational roles for occupational therapists and people with learning disabilities (Law et al 1996, Stewart et al 2003).

Considering the current philosophies for people with learning disabilities challenges occupational therapists to place the client at the centre of their interventions and consider their needs in an holistic way. By this we mean considering the person as an individual with individual needs, values and interests and also considering them as occupational beings with the capacity to influence their health and wellbeing through the doing of valued occupations. The ideas that people with learning disabilities have the same occupational needs and need to be viewed as valued individuals as the rest of society are explored throughout the books, suggesting that occupational therapists can draw on knowledge of human needs and consider this in relation to the meeting needs of people with learning disabilities through occupation.

In 2003 the College of Occupational Therapists' specialist section for people with learning disabilities introduced four principles for education and practice in this field. These principles (shown below) provide occupational therapists with a guide to the outcome of interventions for the individual that incorporate both occupational therapy and learning disability service philosophies.

Principles for practice

1. Occupational therapists working in learning disability services provide a service for people whose primary reason for referral relates to the effect of their learning disability upon their occupational performance.

2. People with learning disabilities need to be enabled to have choice and influence over their occupational therapy interventions.

3. People with learning disabilities have the right to access generic health and social care.

4. Occupational therapy services should be provided in partnership with the person with learning disabilities, his or her carers and all relevant agencies (COT 2003).

An audit of these principles is ongoing to evaluate how occupational therapists have been able to implement them and to identify areas of good practice in providing a service to people with learning disabilities. Incorporating these principles and values into occupational therapy services is considered to be important in both organization and delivery of services. Occupational therapists are therefore challenged to consider the range of strategies at their disposal to link theory to practice in a specialist area of work.

Occupational therapists have access to a broad knowledge base and a wide range of tools to enable them to put into practice their core philosophies and principles.

Using models of practice and the occupational therapy process to frame practice will help to ensure that the above principles and philosophies of occupation are interwoven throughout interventions and guide clinical reasoning. Nelson & Jepson-Thomas (2003 pp. 132–134) use the term 'therapeutic occupational synthesis' to describe the design of 'therapeutic occupational form in collaboration with the recipient of occupational therapy services'. They suggest that this concept involves using occupational therapy models of practice to guide clinical reasoning. They use the term synthesis to describe the complex consideration of many simultaneous factors about occupations and their contexts (occupational form) and the individual's development and experience (developmental structure). The outcome of occupational synthesis is '…an occupational form that provides a person with the just-right challenge to the developmental structure' (p. 132).

For people with learning disabilities where delayed developmental processes may be compounded by low expectation and limited experiences, occupational therapists have a significant role in enabling occupation (Townsend 1999). For people with learning disabilities this may mean enabling them to continue with valued occupations that they are currently doing or have recently stopped due to illness or injury. However, there is also a significant role in providing opportunities to try new occupations and experiences due to past deprivation. Taking into consideration environmental influences on the individual may be particularly relevant in relation to social and institutional contexts as historically these have presented barriers to people's independence and occupational health. In order to use tools and strategies for practice in this field, therapists must also build into their interventions time to get to know the individual through a range of communication skills and relationship building.

Looking to the future

This book covers historical, current and emerging perspectives and roles for occupational therapists when working with people with learning disabilities. Inevitably, as ideas and philosophies grow and as people with learning disabilities have more involvement in the services that they receive then the role of the occupational therapist will change. Although the Valuing People White Paper is clear in its principles there is still a long way to go to achieve these principles in practice for all people with learning disabilities. Consequently, occupational therapists and all other stakeholders in supporting people with learning disabilities (including the people themselves) have a part to play in continuing to review their roles and practices and to evaluate them against current and future service principles. Some emerging areas of work for occupational therapists are presented in this book, e.g. parenting, health promotion and transitions. Occupational therapists have taken a role in aspects such as work, education and independence over a longer period of time but these should continue to be reviewed in the light of current service philosophies. There will also be new areas of work and roles not yet taken on by the occupational therapist.

This is an exciting time to be involved in learning disability services and an opportunity to reflect on our core values as occupational therapists and continue to develop client-centred services with and for people with learning disabilities.

Summary

This chapter has given an introduction to the key concerns of occupational therapists when working with people with learning disabilities. It acknowledges the historical and current perspectives that influence the lives of people with learning disabilities and practice in the field and presents an outline of terminology and definitions used with this client group.

The reasons for writing the book are given along with its contents and key purposes for this text. Readers are reminded of the unique role of the occupational therapist in focusing on occupational performance and identity and how this role may be implemented within the current contexts for practice and service principles. Contributors provide different views and perspectives on occupational therapy practice in the field today and readers are challenged to consider their examples in relation to their own current and future practice.

Useful resources

British Institute of Learning Disabilities (BILD) website: www.bild.org.uk (accessed 14 March 2008)

Kramer P, Hinojosa J, Brasic Royeen C 2003 Perspectives in human occupation: participation in life. Philadelphia, Lippincott, Williams & Wilkins

Valuing People website: www. valuingpeople.gov.uk (accessed 14 March 2008)

www.bristollearningdifficulties.nhs.uk (accessed 14 March 2008)

www.publications.parliament.uk (accessed 14 March 2008)

References

Carnaby S (ed.) 2004 Learning disability today. Brighton, Brighton Pavilion

College of Occupational Therapists 2003 Principles for education and practice: occupational therapy services for adults with a learning disability. London, College of Occupational Therapists

Department of Health 2001 Valuing people: a new strategy for learning disability for the 21st century. London, HMSO

Duncan EAS (ed.) 2006 Foundations for Practice in Occupational Therapy, 4th Ed. London, Elsevier Churchill Livingstone

Gates B (ed.) 2003 Learning disabilities: toward inclusion, 4th edn. London, Churchill Livingstone

Gates B, Wilberforce D 2003 The nature of learning disabilities. In: Gates B (ed.) Learning disabilities: toward inclusion, 4th edn. London, Churchill Livingstone

Law M, Cooper B, Strong S et al 1996 The person–environment– occupation model: a transactive approach to occupational performance. Canadian Journal of Occupational Therapy 63(1):9–23

Law M, Polatajko H, Baptiste S, Townsend E 1999 Core concepts of occupational therapy. In: Townsend E (ed.) Enabling occupation: an occupational therapy perspective. Ottawa, Ontario, CAOT, pp 29–56

Nelson D, Jepson-Thomas 2003 Occupational form, occupational performance and a conceptual framework for therapeutic occupation. In: Kramer P, Hinojosa J, Brasic Royeen C Perspectives in human occupation: participation in life. Philadelphia, Lippincott, Williams & Wilkins, pp 132–134

Northfield J 2004 Factsheet – what is learning disability? Kidderminster, British Institute of Learning Disabilities

Stewart D, Letts L, Law M et al 2003 The person–environment– occupation model. In: Crepeau EB, Cohn ES, Schell BAB (eds) Willard & Spackman's occupational therapy. Philadelphia, Lippincott Williams & Wilkins, pp 227–233

Townsend E (ed.) 1999 Enabling occupation: an occupational therapy perspective. Ottawa, Ontario, CAOT

UK Parliament 2006 Lord Ashley of Stoke Disabled People's (Independent Living) Bill, Bill 122. London, Authority of the House of Lords

Section **One**

The chapters in this section explore the influence of occupation on the lives of people with learning disabilities. They also emphasize how recognizing the importance of the historical context, communication and health needs is essential if people with learning disability are going to have the opportunity for live productive and healthy lives in the community. Chapter 1 explores the influence of occupational needs and considers the human rights of people with a learning disability. In Chapter 2 the relevance of understanding the historical perspectives of the changes in service provision is highlighted. This is of particular importance for new professionals as a significant number of service users have experienced previous service provision including living within an institutional setting for most of their lives.

Chapter 3 explores the application of the occupational therapy process and the use of meaningful occupation as a practical approach to working with service users. For Chapter 4 introduces the reader to the importance of communication when working with people with a learning disability and highlights how essential this is to ensure occupational participation. This section ends by exploring how occupation can contribute to promoting the health of people with a learning disability in Chapter 5.

The reader activities in all the chapters gives the opportunity to reflect on your understanding of the importance of occupation, communication and promoting health through participation with meaningful activity.

1

Perspectives on occupational needs of people with learning disability

Jenni Hurst • Jane Goodman • Christine Locke

Overview

As occupational therapists work across the spectrum of learning disability this book explores the occupational challenges that are met when promoting access to meaningful occupation as part of a balanced lifestyle. This first chapter discusses the current context for practice to meet the occupational needs for people with learning disabilities. It does not assume that the occupational needs of people with learning disabilities are different from the rest of the population but acknowledges that they can have difficulties experiencing occupations that give purpose and meaning to their daily lives (Heason et al 2001). It is from this starting point of lack of opportunity that occupational therapists often enter into a therapeutic relationship with an individual who has a learning disability. The client-centred philosophies that underpin occupational therapy practice reflect the change in approach posited in the learning disability White Paper, Valuing People A New Strategy for Learning Disability for the 21st Century (Sumsion 2006, DoH 2001a). Never has there been greater opportunity for people with learning disabilities to achieve greater self-determination and control over their lives.

It is important that occupational therapists incorporate a human needs approach to identifying occupational needs for people with learning disabilities. The belief that people with learning disabilities have the same human needs as all human beings is reflected in the current context for practice where the focus is on the individual's rights, choice, inclusion and participation in ordinary life as experienced by other members of society (DoH 2001a). Occupational therapists working in a multidisciplinary team need to be able to raise awareness of how they incorporate occupation and its value within the context of current service delivery. They will then be able to promote client-centred practice and work within an occupational framework that is relevant to people with learning disabilities.

Learning Outcomes

By the end of the chapter you will be able to:

- Explore the occupational needs of a person with a learning disability

- Be able to justify the importance of occupation within the context of service provision.

The service users' voice

To understand the occupational needs of people with a learning disability you first need to listen to their perspective. For people with a learning disability the main change in the strategic development of service provision occurred when services users were involved in the development of the strategy that underpinned the Valuing People White Paper. This resulted in the production of 'Nothing About Us Without Us' (DoH 2001b) by a Service Users Advisory Group, which included representatives from People First, MENCAP, Change and Speaking up. This document signified a change in attitude as it was the first time that people with learning disabilities were recognized by the UK government as being able to make a contribution to service configuration. Their ideas, needs and aspirations are embedded in the White Paper and give a clear message to the occupational therapist when working with clients to identify their occupational needs.

All service providers are expected to include people with learning disabilities in the planning and provider processes. It was emphasized that this should not be just one token individual but a representative group of people who can support each other to facilitate change. This has resulted in the formation of a National Advisory Group and a range of funded projects including the Valuing People website and the MENCAP telephone support service (refer to useful resources at the end of this chapter).

Other issues addressed in the document related to an individuals human rights by making specific statements of the changes needed. The Independence Section covers the changes needed in day care provision and ways of supporting people into paid employment. It focuses on how people could be supported in paid employment and how staff supporting them needed to be educated (e.g. disability advisors knew nothing about people with learning disability). They also wanted independent advice about benefits and the opportunity to participate in the direct payments scheme. One area highlighted is that people with learning disability have difficulty in participating fully in their community because of their problems accessing public transport.

When discussing where they lived service users gave clear messages about residential care. They asked for services that promoted their independence and that residential homes and long-stay hospital provision should be closed. Respite care needed to meet the needs of the users as well as providing a rest for their carers. The Healthcare Commission has now recommended closure of all NHS residential provision for people with learning disability because of poor standards of provision and care (Healthcare Commission 2007). Parenting and need for good support services was another area of concern highlighted, which is discussed further in Chapter 10.

As well as independence the document deals with issues about the qualifications of the support staff that work with people with learning disabilities and their integration into the health and social care service provision rather than having a separate service. Issues relating to self advocacy and human rights are also identified with clear recommendations given. People with learning disabilities were able, given the opportunity, to articulate their own needs as human beings and demonstrated that they required services that acknowledged and respected their human rights and they required support to gain these through:

- Self advocacy – speaking up for themselves
- Citizen advocacy – people who get to know someone with a learning disability so that they can help get their wishes understood and heard
- Short-term, issue based or crisis advocacy – where people are (usually) paid to speak up for someone about a particular issue, or when they are in a crisis.

The principles of including service users are explored in depth in Chapter 13. The short-term crisis issues can arise at times of transition, when people with a learning disability, in line with the rest of us, can experience occupational dysfunction and disruption (Worden 2003). An occupational therapist can often find that they meet a new service user at this time. Chapter 11 explores loss and bereavement and the implications for people with a learning disability.

Having established their needs, people with learning disability now need to establish their rights to service provision in the climate of increasing service demand in the rest of the population. The introduction of the White Paper set the strategy and established Partnership Boards (DoH 2001a). However, this does not guarantee any specific rights within the UK legislative framework.

Person-centred planning

To understand how to view current service philosophies from an occupational perspective you need to understand how these needs can be met for people with learning disabilities through one of the key principles of the Valuing People White Paper (DoH 2001a). The role of health and social care professionals in putting these principles into place through person-centred planning is to help people with a learning disability to identify and meet their own individual needs. Sanderson (2003) suggests that the shift of services for people with learning disabilities to encompass planning systems focusing on the strengths as well as the problems or needs that challenge an individual, has made us think about how to involve the individual in their own plan. It is important to reflect on what the plans should contain and how to identify and meet a broader range of needs that influence all aspects of the person's life. Sanderson (2003 p. 370) offers two questions which can gather the information needed and these are:

- Who are you, and who are we in your life?
- What can we do together to achieve a better life for you now, and in the future?

Reflecting on the above two questions may have highlighted those people who are closest to you and who would give some indication of your occupational preference, which you may or may not agree with. As part of person-centred planning the occupational therapist can approach these questions from the perspective of purposeful or meaningful occupation. Assessing the occupational needs and aspirations of the person with learning disability will be at the centre of the occupational intervention and involve those who are closest to the individual. Consider now the Case illustration in Box 1.1. and how this might be different for someone such as Tony.

Reader activity

- Who would be important to speak to about Tony's occupations?

Box 1.1

Case illustration: Tony

Tony's mother, who is in her 70s, contacted the CLDT as she was finding it increasingly difficult to manage Tony's behaviour at home and subsequently a referral was made to an occupational therapist for assessment. Tony is 28 years old and is her youngest child, her two older children having left home several years ago but visiting once a month. Tony has always been willing to help out at home and often took great pride in doing the chores for his mother. Recently, he has been unwilling to help his mother with the cleaning and refuses to go shopping. He has attended a day centre for the last 3 years and staff there report that he particularly enjoyed the creative classes, and swimming with a small group of friends. However, since his support worker has left he has become increasingly withdrawn and refuses to participate. There have also been a number of verbal outbursts, particularly with one of his friends and they are now not talking to each other.

From the perspective of his mother and staff at the day centre the issues were his change in behaviour within his routine occupations. Through establishing rapport with Tony and observation of his occupations both at home and at the day centre, the occupational therapist established that from Tony's perspective he was bored with doing the things he had always done and was wanting to do something else and have his own flat like his brother and sister. Although he was aware of how his mother relied on him he also didn't want to keep 'working' for his mother, but was sorry he shouted at her. The planning process identified the issues for Tony. This required implementing clear support strategies from those closest to him and the MDT to enable Tony to fulfil his occupational preferences and to support his mother through this.

- How might Tony be helped to establish his own preferences for meaningful occupation?

The White Paper (DoH 2001a) required Learning Disability Partnership Boards to implement person-centred planning to increase 'the extent to which supports were tailored to the needs and aspirations of people with learning disabilities' (Robertson et al 2005 p. i). National UK implementation is taking longer as demonstrated by an evaluation study commissioned by the Department of Health in 2001 (Robertson et al 2005). The authors aimed among other aspects to evaluate the impact of person-centred plans on 'the life experiences of people with learning disabilities' (p. i). At the end of the study, there was a clear indication that person-centred plans had had positive benefits, in particular for community participation, contact with friends and family and choice. However, the study indicated several disadvantages, such as person-centred planning having no impact on those domains linked to quality of life (i.e. more inclusive social networks and employment). It found that some groups, especially those with more complex difficulties, for example people with additional mental health problems, autistic spectrum disorders or those with restricted mobility, were less likely to have a plan. The report concluded that the overall experiences of the implementation of person-centred planning reflected inequalities in 'the extent to which people are likely to receive a person-centred plan and, if they do, the level of benefits they can expect' (p. iv). The report reflects similar inequalities can be found in the general life experiences of people with learning disabilities. This emphasizes the challenge to professionals in the implementation of principles into practice. Person-centred planning is the current name for the process that promotes inclusion of people with learning disability into their communities and it will continue to evolve. In fact '... person-centred planning may be best considered as an evolutionary step in the long-standing trend towards the increasing individualization of supports and services.' (Robertson et al 2005 p. iii.)

Occupation as a primary human need

Exploring the idea that human beings have needs that if satisfied will lead to better health and well-being is not unfamiliar to occupational therapists. Duncan (2006 p. 6) suggests that 'Each person wants to participate effectively in life and to remain healthy and happy. To achieve these goals a person needs a degree of personal competence in a range of culturally accepted, useful and meaningful occupations.' To enable this to happen for people with learning disabilities requires us to consider both the current context for practice and what we can do as occupational therapists to work within the practice context in the best interests of the individual. The occupational therapist's focus is on identifying and meeting the occupational needs of the individual or group. With people who have profound and multiple disabilities, there is a need to understand how an individual's ability may impact on their capacity to fully engage with occupations and therapeutic activities presented to them. The importance of the context (environment) and how this impinges on human needs, has to be considered within the context of cultural influences on the individual's occupation. People with learning disabilities are not only vulnerable to occupational deprivation but also to the fact that this can be reinforced by cultural expectation. Watson (2006) developed the discussion about 'being' which has considerable influence on a person with a learning disability. The stigma attached to a learning disability can vary considerably depending on the cultural influences around. Some cultures view people with a learning disability as a perpetual child and offer experiences which reinforce this image. For example, consider the stereotypical image of a middle-aged woman with a learning disability wearing white ankle socks and sandals. Whilst culture is about far more than a fashion statement about white ankle socks, in today's western society dress has a different significance to other cultures.

Some families may wish to maintain a culture of normality, which denies the person with learning disability development experiences that would make everyone's life easier. Alternatively, other parents may wish to encourage their child to reach their 'full' potential and provide a structured learning experience, which leaves little time for leisure and fun. Occupational therapists need to take time to see the service user within the complexity of the family and other aspects of their occupational form to ensure that the client-centred care they offer will be acceptable to those supporting the service user. Heason et al (2001) remind professionals that they should avoid cultural stereotyping. Iwama (2006) illustrates this by an example of the integration of cultures when people move countries.

Your client may possess an Indian surname and have all the physical characteristics of a person originating from South Asia but may speak English with a cockney accent, prefer to eat Schezchuan food and groove to the sound of hip hop and American R&B.' (Chapter 1 p. 9).

To ignore the influence of culture is to deny the lived experience of the service user and display the cultural competence that enables occupational therapists to fully engage with a service users 'being' (Watson 2006). Take a moment to consider if the culture you have grown up in has influenced the person you are today.

Reader activity

Reflect on the following questions:

- Did your family have rules on what you could or could not do and are these still relevant to you today?
- Have you decided that you will never become your mother/father?
- Were you envious of your friends or they of you and if so what were the reasons?
- In what way does your culture enhance and support you?

Occupation in context

Current service philosophies are based on humanistic and human needs approaches, which invite professionals to consider the individual's needs and rights to participate in society on an equal footing with others (Gates 2003). These are worthy principles on which to base occupational therapy services particularly as in the past services for people with learning disabilities did not often reflect or meet the range of needs important to human growth and development. Nor did they recognize the potential for people with learning disabilities to engage in meaningful occupations that would enable them to develop skills and competencies in the community. As occupational therapists consider that the ability to engage in occupation is a basic human need to underpin and guide their practice it is helpful to explore how this ethos can be put into place when working with people with learning disabilities. It is sometimes easy to forget when working in a new field that existing knowledge about occupations, occupational needs and our view of humans as occupational beings is still applicable. Considering and reflecting on human needs is one way of enabling client-centred practices that are central to the occupational therapists' role (Sumsion 2006).

Occupational science and learning disabilities

The rest of this chapter will explore how occupational science can inform occupational therapists involved in current services for people with learning disabilities. There is a clear role for occupational therapists to understand and focus on occupational needs and to assist the service user to identify them. Danielsen (2005) defines human needs as essentials that humans need in order to live and achieve well-being. He proposes that if we focus just on those needs that have to be met in order to survive such as food, shelter, etc. this may limit our view of human beings to just existing as biological creatures (p. 3). In order to develop this view we need to consider the potential for human beings to grow and develop. Wilcock (1998) uses the term 'need' to mean '...the mechanism by which unconscious biological requirements that alerts the conscious state to the existence of some kind of disequilibrium.' (p. 117). She focuses on the human need for occupation and proposes that humans have occupational needs that go beyond needs of other organisms in that they need to establish a sense of identity and autonomy. The categories offered relate needs to having '...a three-way role in maintaining the stability and health of the organism through occupation' (Wilcock 1998 p.117). The three roles of needs are:

- to warn and protect
- to prevent disorder and prompt use of human capacities
- to reward use of capacities such as meaning and satisfaction.

Wilcock (1998) also defines what is meant by occupational needs proposing that '...the biological need to engage in occupations is a major characteristic of humans aimed at species' survival and individual health.' (p. 89). Her categories of need reflect the functions of occupation:

- meeting bodily needs of sustenance, self care and shelter (subsistence, physical nurturance, physiological needs)

- skills development and social structures to gain safety and security (safety and security, protection)
- maintain health through balanced exercise of personal capacities
- individual and social development for species growth.

Wilson & Wilcock (2005) completed a quantitative study with first-year occupational therapy students to explore the understanding of the meanings of occupation, health and well-being. When analysing their replies to the question on occupational balance they found this was achieved by very few students. Unsurprisingly people, time and money factors were identified as the main factors which impeded occupational balance. Consider the following reader activity to identify occupational balance in your life.

Reader activity

- What occupations do you currently use to promote occupational balance?
- How articulate do you need to be to ensure that you have time for yourself?
- Do those around you appreciate the effort that is involved in balancing your occupations (i.e. home life, studying, leisure, work)?
- How would you define occupational balance to others?

By exploring if you have the 'elusive' occupational balance and defining what it is, you can now begin to explore how you can support people with a learning disability to make choices about their own lifestyle.

Choosing purposeful, meaningful and valued occupations

The introductory chapter of this book briefly considered how choice can be introduced into the lives of people with learning disabilities. This involves individuals having a real say in decisions about their lives and being able to advocate for others, who may be less able to voice their personal choices. The idea that all human beings have the capacity to make choices is central to humanistic philosophy and that all individuals have influence and choices over their

behaviour, is the cornerstone of client-centred practice (Parker 2006).

Melton (1998), interpreting the narratives of service users, demonstrated that cookery could be both purposeful because of the basic human need for food and meaningful with the introduction of a creative or fun element. Sumsion (2006) suggests that meaningful choice is possible when the person has been provided with all the necessary information by the therapist. For an occupational therapist working with people with mild learning disability this is possible using appropriate communication, as is discussed in Chapter 4. Just who has the right to make complex choices and the capacity to choose will emerge through the implementation of the Mental Capacity Act 2005 (Department of Constitutional Affairs 2005). Therefore, while the concept of choice can be seen simplistically as everyone having the right to make choices, this can be very difficult when working with people with little or no verbal skill. People with profound and multiple impairments may also have lacked the opportunity to engage in meaningful occupations. For people with a learning disability, their human needs are often fulfilled (i.e. food, warmth). However, their occupational need or choice (i.e. opportunity of occupational choice), in terms of cultural values, may be lacking when measured against the following criteria:

- Be socially acceptable
- Enhances dignity
- Has a positive or negative effect on other people
- Is age appropriate
- Promotes independence and self-esteem.

The occupational therapist therefore needs to be aware of values when accepting a referral to consider ways that they might introduce tasters of opportunity to enable the person to make informed decisions. Opportunity tasters also offer experiences to widen the occupational opportunities horizon. Heason et al (2001) highlight the importance of considering the likelihood of the risk event occurring and the consequences for both the service user and the member of staff. It is important to remember that we all take risks as part of our adaptation to changes in demand, both in an occupation and in the environment. Through informed choice and good risk assessment of occupational performance risk can be minimized.

Reader activity

- First, make a list of all the occupations in which you could reasonably claim to be proficient. Remember that for you these can be purposeful occupations such as cleaning the bath or boiling an egg. Equally, they may be creative occupations, for example painting or decorating a room.
- Now make a list of all the taster occupations you would like to engage in if only you had the time, money or perceived skill.
- Choosing one of the taster occupations, reflect on what risks are inherent in that occupation for you.

You have just demonstrated your ability to reflect on your own abilities and to make choices about other possible opportunities. Schkade & Schultz (2003) offer occupational adaptation as an approach, in which they define occupation as actively involving the person in a way that is meaningful to them. They believe that there must be a product involved but this could be tangible or intangible. The occupation is therefore adaptable to change as the person responds to the experience and this will fluctuate across the lifespan. The influences of gender, class or other social factors all have a bearing on the choice of occupational pursuits. Indeed some occupations that are usually not valued can increase in significance at times of stress. This can also be a gender-related activity, i.e. students often report clean kitchen floors or completed piles of ironing when an assignment is due. For people with a learning disability it is important to explore what meaning they attribute to an occupation. A good example of this is to decide how you determine whether certain occupations are valued economically or socially. Many people with a learning disability are encouraged to undertake voluntary work as a route to employment. Volunteering is chosen by many people who have been unemployed, which can be construed as a valued route to employment. All volunteers give their time willingly but do expect that their contribution is valued by the organization that they 'work' for. Now consider the example of June in Box 1.2 and her experience of voluntary work.

June's engagement in her occupation continued long after it had ceased to be meaningful because she did not know that she had the right to disengage. Take a minute to reflect how you learnt to engage

Box 1.2

Case illustration: June

June had mild learning disability and was found a voluntary job at a restaurant 5 years ago by the local college. When she completed the college course the funding ended. June however, continued to go to the local restaurant every Wednesday and spent the lunchtime washing the dishes. When June moved to new accommodation with her partner, she was referred to an occupational therapist. June had told her care manager that she could not use her new cooker and so could not cook meals. As June was used to only heating up ready meals she wanted to be able to cook fresh food.

During the occupational therapy intervention, June told the occupational therapist how she hated her 'work' as the restaurant staff 'were not very nice to her and did not even give her lunch'. What emerged from the narrative was the simple fact that June did not understand the concept of voluntary work. It was clear that June did not value her 'work' so after the explanation from the occupational therapist on what being a volunteer actually meant she exercised her right to choose and left. With support, she selected a more meaningful occupation, which was a microwave cookery course at the local college.

in productive occupations and how you make that judgement.

Relationship building and occupation

An occupational therapist, working with people with a learning disability, especially when a person has profound and multiple disabilities, will want to consider how relationship building impacts on intervention. To establish what is meaningful for a new service user can take time, as the importance of relationship building is essential to the focus for therapeutic intervention with any client (Duncan 2006). However, it is worth giving special attention to relationship building as there are some significant differences that the occupational therapist should be aware of when attempting to build a relationship in this field. A person with a learning disability is usually not ill when referred and the occupational therapist is involved in habilitation rather than rehabilitation. Unless the prime reason for referral is an ongoing or sudden health deterioration, the occupational therapist will be looking to build a relationship over a longer period of time. It is important to be able to allow time where necessary to overcome some of the barriers to communication that may arise and not to expect an instant result. A newcomer to this field may find that communication issues are the first barrier to overcome and it is worth spending time both to find out about common communication issues and strategies to overcome them, as discussed in Chapter 4. When considering occupational engagement with a service user it is important to recognize that the relationship building may be prolonged and it can therefore, be difficult to decide at what point assessment ends and intervention starts. This can also involve finding out about specific needs of the individual from those who know them best such as family or carer. During this time, you may also need to build relationships with keyworkers who will advocate for the client's needs and support and maintain the selected occupation. Consider how staff supported Richard (Box 1.3) to develop his occupational choices.

Taking time to listen to all concerned and remaining client-centred is a challenge for occupational therapists working in learning disability services. Building relationships and effective communication cannot be rushed, which can mean that the service moves at a different pace to a busy acute setting, with more time to engage in selecting meaningful occupation.

The need to be creative

Being creative can apply to both the occupational therapist and the service users. The White Paper states: 'Each individual should have the support and opportunity to be the person he or she wants to be' (DoH 2001a). With the changes in the NHS and the move to the community's occupational therapists have lost some of the resources which enabled them to work closely with clients using creative media (Sadlo 2004). An important concept to consider when working with people with a learning disability is the excitement and increase in self esteem that humans gain from engaging in and learning new skills. Melton (1998) found evidence of this in a study exploring how people with a learning disability evaluated their experience of cooking with an occupational therapist. There was an increase in their perceived ability and confidence that illustrated how cooking was a creative and meaningful experience; including how to recognize when spaghetti was cooked by 'throwing it at the wall'.

Individuals who are creatively involved in an occupation will often not be aware of time passing. This concept has been described as flow and has been linked to happiness (Csikszentmihalyi 1992). Occupational science is interested in exploring this idea and identifying how meaningful occupation promotes the 'flow' experience. Sometimes simple repetitive activity that may be seen by support workers as 'too easy' can totally absorb a person with a learning disability. For example, when they sit and complete a simple puzzle several times the support worker then considers that they have the potential to complete a complex one. The service user is expressing their own occupational choice, albeit one that may be linked to a developmental stage rather than one that is age appropriate.

 Box 1.3

Case illustration: Richard

Richard is a young man with cerebral palsy and mild learning disability who wanted to manage his own environment in his bedroom. Unfortunately, this bid for independence resulted in a high level of breakages with cups, his television and CD player all being damaged. Support staff solved the problem by taking all the controls away and banning drinks in his bedroom, which amounted to occupational deprivation. When this difficulty was highlighted during person-centred planning a referral to an occupational therapist introduced a different approach. A range of solutions to stabilize equipment and introduce more robust electronic controls, plus some choice in drinks containers allowed Richard more control over his environment so he was happy to delegate the task of loading selected CD's into his player.
Staff could then withdraw and not feel that they were responsible or that Richard was at risk if left alone.

An occupational therapist participating in a research study expressed herself clearly when asked about her creative approach:

> going with the flow... empowering people to think... by saying to clients... well I think you've got some ideas of your own of how you can get over that problem... and I see that as a creative process (Schmid 2004 p. 84).

It is important to remember this so as to ensure that the context of occupation, which provides meaning, is unique to the individual (Ikiugu 2005). As illustrated by Tony's situation (refer to Box 1.1), boredom can impinge on the lives of people with learning disability and lack of occupational choice and opportunity can result in occupational deprivation. Long (2004) recognizes that boredom can fit into two categories. First, there is boredom arising from activity that lacks meaning. This aspect of occupation was considered by the contributors to Nothing About Us Without Us (DoH 2001b p7), when they referred to the difficulties encountered in day centres. 'We should get rid of the day centres and start to employ people with learning difficulties in proper paid jobs not just cheap labour jobs'. Boredom can also occur because of lack of opportunities and service users may have no stimulation in their lives, resulting in considerable time spent asleep. Occupational therapists through assessment consider all aspects of a services user's occupational form to ensure a balance of occupations.

The impact of boredom raises another important area for occupational therapists working with people with profound and multiple learning disabilities to consider, which is how to identify if a service user is occupied when little awareness or feedback from the service user is available. Collins (2001) explores the importance of an individual's self-awareness of their own human identity and how the link between this awareness and processing allows us to develop into occupational beings. Looking at the complex factors that contribute to this developmental process helps to make sense of how sensory deprivation can limit engagement in occupation. The role of the occupational therapist in promoting sensory integration is explored in more depth in Chapter 6 – Activities of Daily Living (ADL) for Individuals with a Learning Disability: Using a Sensory Integrative Approach.

Occupational science also examines the concept of meaningfulness in relation to occupation and this has importance in the learning disability field especially if there is limited opportunity for real choice. Ikiugu (2005) highlights several areas to be considered when working with people who because of their learning disability have limited life experience of a range of occupations.

- Meaningfulness is unique to the individual
- Our sense of meaningfulness is strongly linked to our sense of our own identity
- Meaningful occupations increase a person's sense of well-being.

The challenge for the occupational therapist is how to make the selected occupation client-centered and therefore meaningful to the service user.

Summary

This chapter has discussed how people with learning disabilities are themselves striving to change old attitudes and to build new ideas into current and future legislative framework to support individuals to meet their needs. This has resulted in the establishment of support networks, through which they can continue to lobby for the recognition that they have the same needs as others in society.

At present, occupational therapists working in learning disability services need to adapt the occupational science evidence from other specialist areas to support their practice. This will enable them to convince other members of the multidisciplinary team that occupational performance can be enhanced by working with service users within an occupation framework. They can also use evidence from the field of positive psychology and health promotion that supports the view that we need to understand how to maintain and develop positive qualities as human beings in order to lead satisfying and optimistic lives. Occupation can enhance satisfaction with our lives, optimism for the future and engagement in positive life experiences in the present, and is important for our health both as individuals and as members of society. Finally, the chapter has provided you with an opportunity to reflect on your own attitudes to culture and occupation and to your experiences of purposeful and meaningful occupation. The chapter has highlighted how you can apply your own existing knowledge of occupation and transfer this to service users in present day learning disability services.

Box 1.4

Case illustration: Penny

Penny has been referred to occupational therapy for assessment. She has lived as a joint tenant with two other individuals with learning disabilities since resettlement from a large institution 7 years ago. Penny has a profound learning disability, has non-verbal communication, is dependent for most aspects of self-care and uses a wheelchair with a supported seating system. She has developed weakness in her right arm and hand over the last 3 weeks, reducing her ability to feed herself and pick up objects. The support staff at home are concerned about her health as she is often distressed and they have not taken her out for the last 2 weeks. Prior to this staff had supported Penny to access local community, facilities, including local shops, and a music group, which she attended once a week. She also uses a local resource centre that provides a sensory environment and staff reported she particularly enjoys this session. The house manager has requested advice on activities within the home.

Reader activity

How might you address Penny's occupational needs and preferences?

Useful resources

CHANGE: http://www. changepeople.co.uk (accessed 27 February 2008)

MENCAP: http://www.mencap.org. uk (accessed 27 February 2008)

People first: http://www. peoplefirstltd.com (accessed 27 February 2008)

Speaking up: http://www.speakingup. org and http://www.oneforus.com (both accessed 27 February 2008)

References

Collins M 2001 Who is occupied? Consiousness, self awareness and the process of human adaptation. Journal of Occupational Science 8(1):25–32

Csikszentmihalyi M 1992 Flow: the psychology of happiness. London, Rider

Danielsen G 2005 Meeting human needs, preventing violence: applying human needs theory to conflict in Sri Lanka University of Salvador Buenos Aires. Online. Available: http:// filebox.vt.edu/users/tcaruso/ NVC%20Research%20Files/NVC %20and%20Violence%20Preventio n/Danielsen2005.pdf on 5/11/07

Department of Constitutional Affairs 2005 Mental Capacity Act. London, Office of public sector information

Department of Health 2001a Valuing people: a new strategy for learning disability for the 21st century. London, DoH

Department of Health 2001b Nothing about us without us. London, DoH Publications

Duncan E (ed.) 2006 Foundations for practice in occupational therapy, 4th edn. Edinburgh, Churchill Livingstone

Gates B (ed.) 2003 Learning disabilities: towards inclusion. Edinburgh, Churchill Livingstone

Heason C, Stracey L, Rey D 2001 Valuing occupation for people who have a learning disability. In: Thompson J, Pickering S (eds) Meeting the health needs of people who have a learning disability. Edinburgh, Ballière Tindall

Healthcare Commission 2007. Online. Available from www. healthcarecommission.org.uk/ reviewsandinspections/reviews/ learningdisabilities

Ikiugu MN 2005 Meaningfulness of occupation as an occupational – trajectory attractor. Journal of Occupational Science 12(2): 102–109

Iwama M 2006 The Kawa Model: culturally relevant occupational therapy. Churchill Livingstone, Edinburgh

Long C 2004 On watching paint dry: an explanation of boredom. In: Molineux M (ed.) Occupation for occupational therapists. London, Blackwell, pp 78–89

Melton J 1998 How do clients with learning disabilities evaluate their experience of cooking with the occupational therapist? British Journal of Occupational Therapy 61(3):106–110

Parker D 2006 The client centred frame of reference. In: Duncan E (ed.) Foundations for Practice in occupational therapy, 4th edn. Edinburgh, Churchill Livingstone, pp 193–215

Robertson J, Emerson E, Hatton C et al 2005 The impact of person centred planning. Institute for Health Research, Lancaster University

Sadlo G 2004 Creativity and occupation. In: Molineux M (ed.) Occupation for occupational therapists. London, Blackwell, pp 90–100

Sanderson H 2003 Person centred planning. In: Gates B (ed.)

Learning disabilities: towards inclusion. Edinburgh, Churchill Livingstone, pp 369–389

Schkade S, Schultz S 2003 Occupational adaption. In: Kramer P, Hinojosa J, Royeen CB (eds) Perspectives in human occupation: participation in life. Baltimore, Lippincott, Williams & Wilkins, pp 181–221

Schmid T 2004 Meanings of creativity with occupational therapy practice. Australian Occupational Therapy Journal 51:80–88

Sumsion Q 2006 Client-centred practice in occupational therapy. Edinburgh, Churchhill Livingstone

Watson RM 2006 Being before doing: the cultural identity (essence) of occupational therapy. Australian

Occupational Therapy Journal 53(3):151–158

Wilcock A 1998 An occupational perspective of health. Thorofare, Slack

Wilson L, Wilcock A 2005 Occupational balance: what tips the scales for new students? British Journal of Occupational Therapy 68(7):319–323

Worden JW 3 (ed.) 2003 Grief counseling and grief therapy: a handbook for the mental health practitioner. Hove, Brunner Routledge

Wright J 2004 Occupation and flow. In: Molineux M (ed.) Occupation for occupational therapists. London, Blackwell, pp 66–77

Appendix 1.1 Case illustration: Penny, possible answers

By applying the categories of need suggested by Wilcocks(1998), the occupational therapist can explore the issues for Penny in relation to the interruption to her occupations, her needs and preferences.

1. Meeting bodily needs of sustenance, self-care and shelter.

Penny has been relatively independent in self-care, feeding herself until recently. Her wheelchair and supported seating system would need to be reviewed to ensure that both comfort and pressure relief are optimized but also to see whether a change in posture has affected her upper limb function for both self-care occupations and creative occupations of exploration in the sensory and music sessions.

2. Skills development and social structures to gain safety and security (safety and security, protection).

There may be issues of safety and security for Penny and the support staff in her home and/or community, which have restricted Penny to the home and deprived her of social occupation. A risk assessment in terms of manual handling, transfers, transport to and from her previous chosen social outlets would therefore be carried out and interventions in strategies and adaptations identified and applied to minimize the risk(s).

3. Maintain health through balanced exercise of personal capacities.

Her distress may be caused by a number of reasons including discomfort, change of staff or a medical condition. The priority for the MDT and occupational therapist would be to establish the cause of her upper limb weakness through referral to a doctor to identify or eliminate any medical reason. A hand assessment may help to establish interventions to facilitate regaining her independence for feeding and other activities. Assessment and intervention to establish Penny's food preferences and opportunity to make choice is also another area to be considered.

4. Individual and social development for species growth.

The occupations that Penny had previously enjoyed included the creative activity of music, sensory exploration and the social occupation of shopping. Taster opportunities can be used to establish rapport with both Penny and the support staff and identify her key methods of non-verbal communication. In this way the occupational therapist can explore Penny's preferences to regain or adapt skills in previous or new occupations within the home or community.

Historical perspectives

The lives of people with learning disabilities and the influence of occupational therapy

Jane Goodman • Jenni Hurst • Christine Locke

Overview

The historical background for people with learning disabilities has influenced the way in which they are perceived by and contribute to modern society. For occupational therapists and other health and social care professions working in this field, this is significant, as it determines how and why we work with people with learning disabilities. This chapter first explores three broad areas of the historical background and influences in the field and then intertwines them with occupational therapy history. These are:

- Individual perspectives
- Philosophical perspectives
- Service context.

The starting point for any history of people with learning disability is with the person themself who can provide a valuable perspective. Existing histories of the lives of people with learning disabilities have focused on political, social and philosophical accounts but more recently have drawn on the lived experiences of people themselves. Relating some of the wider history of how current services are organized will help new practitioners understand that some of the individuals with whom they work will have experienced very different services than are on offer today. It must also be remembered that the individual's situation does not stand alone but is integrated inevitably with family and societal experiences and thus the histories of individuals will be shared with others and those with whom they have come into contact with. Inevitably, they will also be influenced by philosophical and historical events so that the history of the individual becomes intertwined with other facets of the historical story. This chapter seeks to incorporate some of the more recent literature in an attempt to '… learn what things went on all those years and they learn to change: they listen and learn.' (Cooper 1997 in Brigham et al 2000 p. 23). New practitioners in this field today may have little experience of the institutional settings that have influenced the practice of their more senior colleagues. Exploring the historical perspective of provision and services for people with learning disabilities enables us to understand the relevance and implications of present-day service needs. Major developments and perspectives in the 20th century up to the present day will be explored as they cover the lifespan of people with whom current occupational therapists will come into contact. This period has also seen the inception and growth of occupational therapy as a profession. Relevant earlier influences are identified to show how they have shaped recent thinking. Case studies and reflective questions are used to consider the impact of differing historical perspectives on the lives of individuals and the changing role of the occupational therapist. Finally, a summary addresses the key historical influences and their potential to link with aspects of current and future practice.

Learning Outcomes

By the end of this chapter, the reader will be able to:

- Explore the historical development of services for people with learning disabilities from an individual perspective
- Identify key historical and philosophical influences on learning disability services
- Consider the impact of these influences on the emerging role of the occupational therapist
- Consider lessons to be learnt from history that can influence current practice.

Individual perspectives

My story and a lot more will help people with a learning difficulty, and I hope it will learn them to tell their story of what happened to them. Other people too can learn from it like the people who came to our workshop in Kent [for practitioners]' (Mabel Cooper 1997 in Brigham et al 2000 p. 23).

Mabel's story is fully recounted in the book *Forgotten Lives: Exploring the History of Learning Disability* (Atkinson et al 1997). Whilst it is not the history of all people with learning disabilities it does reflect many of the significant events that have been similar experiences for those people who were brought up in institutional settings and the impact that this has had on their lives. Cooper & Atkinson (2000)

 Box 2.1

Jackson 2000

'.... it seems clear that any history of learning disability must make the lives and experiences of people central. Indeed, the experiences of people with learning difficulties constitute a critical starting point for any history' (Jackson 2000 pp. xi–xii).

describe the experiences of women and children who find themselves, for reasons of illegitimacy or being poor or unmarried, within the institutional setting as 'excluded from everyday life' and as a result children in particular were '... excluded from their own life stories'. (p. 18)

The history of people with learning disabilities 'remains an emerging field of study' and there are many sources of evidence that the historian may draw on to relate this history (Atherton 2003). Inevitably, different sources of evidence will provide different historical perspectives. Existing histories of the lives of people with learning disabilities have focused on political, social and philosophical accounts and more recently drawn on the lived experiences of people themselves. Jackson (2000) suggests that it is only by making a full and informed analysis of the past that in the present we can start to develop a future that learns from past lessons and is free from 'stigma and prejudice' (Box 2.1).

Those individuals that have managed to research their history have found painful reminders of the stigmas and attitudes that influenced their life path. Atkinson (2000 p. 24) makes the point that enabling people with learning disabilities to research their own history and to tell their story can help them to '... understand and reflect on the individual and social circumstances which have shaped (their) own experiences, and to see them in a wider historical context'. The individual histories of people with learning disabilities make compelling reading and can offer significant insights and challenges for anyone working in this field (Oswin 1991, Atkinson et al 1997, Stuart 2002, Stalker & Connors 2005, Llewellyn & McConnell 2005). Atherton (2003 p. 42) acknowledges this: 'For a great number of years the history of people with learning disabilities was that empty jigsaw board. This group had an invisible presence within society, indistinct from other social groups'. Consider the following reader activity on how you form and express your own life story:

Reader activity

- Reflect back on your earliest memories – what can you remember and what type of feeling do you attribute to those memories?
- What type of objects do you have that help you remember the past? Do you have them on view and easy to reach or are they tucked away somewhere?
- What people are significant to how you view your past?
- Do you share your memories of your past with anyone?

For individuals living in institutions, despite gradual improvements, the disadvantages of custodial care remained. The impact of being taken away from family and friends often resulted in loss of individuality, lack of control, freedom and choice, combined with segregation into male and female sections. Social networks were restricted and the lack of space and dignity left people vulnerable to abuse. Although the move into the community opened up other opportunities it did not necessarily widen the social networks. However, it would be wrong to paint a totally bleak picture of institutional care as Madge and Joan's life course narrative illustrates (see Box 2.2). For many there were numerous positive aspects; for example, a known, safe environment and friendships, which were often lost on transfer into the community.

For some people their personal stories have been more influenced either by their experiences of transition from institutional to community living or by always living in a family or community environment. Historically, institutional care has played a significant part in how services were organized and it is easy to forget that not all people with a learning disability have come through this system. These other histories should not be forgotten as they too will influence the lives of the individual concerned and the role that occupational therapy can play. Learning disability teams can receive referrals for individuals who have lived within the family unit and who are identified only when a crisis occurs. This may be due to the death of a surviving parent (Oswin 1991). This crisis has implications for the person with a learning

Box 2.2

Case illustration: Madge and Joan

As an occupational therapis it is sometimes difficult to grasp how other people could believe that they have the right to control friendship. Staff interpreted social role valorization to mean the resettlement should encourage links with the immediate community rather than recognizing the importance of existing friendships. Madge was currently living in a residential hostel when she told the occupational therapist who was working with her about Joan who used to be her special friend before the hospital was closed down. She said that Joan had been very old and she was sad that she had probably died and she had not been able to stay in contact. The occupational therapist recognized Joan from her description and knew she was still living in another local town. While still maintaining confidentiality it was possible to establish contact and the occupational therapist arranged a visit to an older but very sprightly Joan. The delight of these two old friends at meeting after 10 years left the therapist and staff acknowledging the value of friendship. Madge still did not find the restrictions of living in a residential hostel any easier, but her regular visits to Joan and being able to have her return the visits established a pleasurable meaningful occupation back into her life.

disability who may encounter services, as illustrated later in this chapter with Den (case illustration), when they are well into middle age.

Individual life histories have been significantly influenced by societal and political agendas in the late 19th and early 20th centuries. The formation and closure of institutions and decisions taken about how people should be cared for have meant the loss of past and recent personal histories for many individuals. Lack of records or access to people who remember their history have added to this loss. For this reason it is important to consider the impact of historical influences on the lives of individuals with a learning disability as well as the development of present day service provision. To understand how learning disability services have been shaped by historical influences you need to consider some of the key underpinning philosophies that have shaped service delivery and therefore people's lives.

Key historical perspectives

The lack of parents' ability to support their children to attend school is one of the reasons given for admission to the colony (Carpenter 2002).

Custodial care

Segregation from mainstream society has been a feature of how people with learning disabilities have been treated in the late 19th century and for a significant part of the 20th century. In the development of institutional care, the voice of the individual with learning disabilities or their carers was given minimal attention. The focus was very much on the societal and decision-maker's role in deciding what was good for the individual, group and for society in general. The political and social agendas in the early 1900s were in tune with the view that people be segregated from society for their own good and that of the community (Carpenter 2002, Atherton 2003). The emphasis was on being part of a separate self-sufficient community with no need to be part of society.

The legislation at that time, including The Mental Deficiency Acts 1912 and 1913, outlined the concepts of 'certification' and detention in an institution under guardianship. Under this legislation, individuals were segregated within institutional environments and the ethos was towards the educability of those classified under The Mental Deficiency Act 1913. Mental deficiency was not enough for certification to be applied using this Act, although if there was no one to care for a child this was often the only criterion used. The removal of children from their local community into institutions replaced the family roles in terms of educational, medical and social custodial care. This is shown clearly by the reported attitude towards children who were admitted to Stoke Park Colony in 1911 (Carpenter 2002). These children were deemed susceptible due to their mental defect, to perceived poor influence, irregular attendance at school and moral defectiveness. A poor home environment was considered a key factor in children being influenced by society into 'vicious habits' and parents came under criticism for taking '... no trouble to enforce their children's attendance at school'. The lack of parents' ability to support their children to attend school is one of the reasons given for admission to the colony (Carpenter 2002).

Education and training

With the advent of the industrial revolution and the reorganization of society into large towns and cities, the need to develop abstract skills such as reading and writing in order to master the new technology and commercial processes highlighted those individuals who were of an educationally low competence. Although The Lunatic Asylums Act 1853 and The Idiots Act 1886 laid the foundation for the authorities to focus on provisions of care, education and training within special asylums, these concepts did not result in change in the institutions until the later part of the 19th century. However, this view influenced the development of a strong work ethic within the institutions in the belief that almost all individuals with training could do useful work under supervision. Consequently, most institutional care had a strong reliance on its inmates to support the general running of the community through work in the laundry, kitchens, on the farm or in sheltered workshops doing sewing, woodwork, etc. Ultimately, this led to the expectation that people put in an institution were trained to complete simple tasks and could then return to their own community when they had acquired useful skills.

The change from the view of potential for education to lifelong dependent custodial care cannot be attributed to only one reason. However, the eugenics movement and the development of a standardized instrument to measure intelligence did contribute to this change. Significantly, between the two World Wars the number of individuals committed increased sevenfold, thus increasing the size of institutions. These concepts applied to both children and adults and remained in place until The Mental Health Act 1959.

Legislative changes over the decades

The post-war years and advent of the National Health Service (NHS) in 1948 consolidated the emergence of the medical model and changes in perception of responsibility. However, there was little change for people with learning disabilities and they continued to be categorized by the assessment of the permanence of the disability, the identification of the need for treatment and lifelong custodial care (Thomas & Woods 2004 pp. 12–14). Studies in the 1950s challenged the supposition of permanent defect as measured by an IQ test and the lack of rehabilitation facilities within the institutions (Malin et al 1980).

These studies showed that the introduction of specific training and sheltered employment in an institution resulted in improved potential for learning industrial tasks. This led to the identification of the association between stimulating environments and performance (Clarke & Clark 1987). Most institutions provided some kind of day services for their residents in the form of workshops, educational activities, entertainment and rehabilitation (Manners et al 2003). At this time occupational therapy services within the institutions often had managerial responsibility for the majority of day services which were provided by nursing and care staff or supported from external agencies such as adult education.

Outcry about the poor physical conditions and permanent detention of patients rather than opportunity for rehabilitation resulted in the introduction of The Mental Health Act 1959. This legislation effectively retained the establishment of large institutions, despite studies which showed improved skill levels following training and introduction into stimulating environments (Clarke & Clark 1987). The legislation, however, did remove the 'compulsory' aspect of detention and the stigma of certification found in The Mental Health Act (1913), by introducing 'informal admissions' and creating categories of 'mentally disordered'. It continued to include people with a learning disability within the label of mental illness.

Concepts of community care

Segregation and institutional care are not the only significant influences in the 20th century. The focus on work and education within the institutions continued and developed until the 1970s and 1980s. In the 1970s changes in attitudes towards people with learning disabilities led to a move away from institutional care to the concept of community care and changes to how services should be delivered. This was evident in the language and approach to defining people with learning disabilities and the focus of education and training in both work and life skills.

The present-day concept of community based services was first suggested in the White Paper 'Better Services for the Mentally Handicapped' (DHSS 1971) which advocated reducing the number of hospital beds while expanding community services. The recommendations included alternatives to large institutions by substituting them with local authority establishments and later the implementation of models of supported living. The cornerstone of the White Paper was for both adults and children, of whatever level of ability, to develop their skills through educational and training methods. There were, however, no guidelines on the process of how to achieve this. Principles for service provision were developed locally to support community living, such as the All Wales Strategy (Welsh Office 1983) three principles to support community living:

1. People with a mental handicap have a right to ordinary patterns of life within the community.

2. People with a mental handicap have a right to be treated as individuals.

3. People with a mental handicap have a right to additional help from the communities in which they live and from professional services in order to enable them to develop their maximum potential as individuals (Welsh Office 1983:2.1).

Supporting the move from institution into the community

The White Paper 'Better Services for the Mentally Handicapped' (1971) paved the way for the closure of hospitals, resettlement into the community and development of community services. Although it was seen as a positive change and an ideal to move away from the disadvantages of institutional care, it must be remembered that the transition from hospital to community care was not easy. For people who had lived all their lives in an institution the transition proved difficult and challenging to their well-being (see Box 2.3). Whilst the environment may have changed, the experience of change and transition still had an impact on people with a learning disability, which is discussed further in Chapter 9.

Resettlement into the community

Although community care policies can be traced back to the 1954–1957 Royal Commission on Mental Illness and Mental Deficiency, progress on closing large institutions was slow. Even into the late 1980s and early 1990s resettlement was still not taking place and various reports found that community care practice was limited (Values into Action 1992). The introduction of the NHS and Community Care Act (DoH 1990) nearly two decades later outlined that within

Box 2.3

Case illustration: a story of resettlement

Janet is now 48 years old. From the age of 12 years she had lived in large institutions and had no contact with her family. For the 7 years leading up to resettlement she lived on a locked, mixed ward environment with 20 others, all of whom had some challenging behaviour. She has profound learning difficulty, no speech but can vocalize a number of sounds. For the majority of the day she was in the ward day room and paced for most of the time. She did walk around the grounds of the hospital with two staff but as she could run off very quickly outings were limited by available staffing levels. Dependent for all aspects of personal activities of daily living Janet also has obsessive behaviours, including biting her fingers and gouging her face. She had no friendships or acknowledged relationships with others on the ward as they avoided her due to her aggressive behaviour. Her only initiated form of physical contact was to approach people from behind and hit them. She was underweight and although could finger feed tended to miss meals due to her disruptive behaviour with other ward residents. Her sleep pattern was poor and she had both constipation and menstruation problems.

Through the resettlement process Janet was resettled in a house with one other woman from the same ward. Working with MDT the occupational therapist worked with support staff prior to resettlement to orientate her to new surroundings by using joint sessions, graded to improve communication with the other women and staff. The Community Learning Disability Team (CLDT) nurse liaised with primary care services to resolve Janet's health problems. Augmenting communication strategies and responses by staff resulted in a reduction of aggressive outbursts. Risk assessments were carried out for aspects of care including travelling in a car, road safety and kitchen assessments as well as self-care activities. A feeding assessment in a quiet room identified that Janet could use a fork or spoon without any problems. She soon started to gain weight. On resettlement into the community, the occupational therapist continued interventions with Janet and staff until she established independence in dressing and feeding herself and accessing community facilities.

the learning disabilities sector the authorities should work together to assess needs and provide appropriate support for clients living in the community. It highlighted that appropriate support should be available in the community to ensure admission to long-stay institutions was not necessary. It also acknowledged that the majority of people with a learning disability have always lived in their local community with their parents and families. This Act accelerated the resettlement of the remaining people living in long-stay institutions into the community. The NHS continued to provide residential accommodation for those with physical handicaps or behavioural problems that required special medical, nursing or other care. Social Services retained responsibility for provision of day services, hostels, respite and group homes as well as a range of support services for people with learning disabilities. At this time some occupational therapists continued to work in day centres.

The introduction of the NHS and Community Care Act 1990 did pave the way for effectively supporting the resettlement processes. However, the development of the resettlement processes varied according to local service perspectives and resources. The closure process of a hospital service involves many challenges in terms of preparation of people to move to the community, staff training and development, identification and provision of accommodation, purchase and growth of new services whilst retaining existing services to support those not yet resettled (Values into Action 1992).

For the individual the resettlement process or any process of change depends on services taking a careful and resourced approach to moving people into new environments. Research carried out by Values into Action (1992) found that there were tensions between taking a slow approach and finding appropriate community accommodation and a faster approach where the most appropriate service may not be chosen, resulting in unsatisfactory resettlement for the client (Values into Action 1992).

Resettlement teams

Resettlement teams were set up to ensure a managed and organized process with minimum trauma and maximum respect for the individual. Resettlement teams were to work independently of service providers, in the best interests of clients waiting to be resettled and having the power to develop services that best met client needs (Values into Action 1994).

They were multi-disciplinary teams that included occupational therapists from health and social services backgrounds with experience of hospital and community based services. Their remit was to set up services to assess individual needs and abilities for resettlement, identify and design new services to meet residential needs in the community and promote ways of implementing service user needs.

There was wide national variation as to the type of services developed in the community and ways of preparing people for the changes to their lives. Use of existing services in the community in setting up completely new services reflected the range of resources available and local approaches to resettlement. The ideal that was pursued was that 'Closing the mental handicap hospitals is not just about people moving back into the community, but about the community being the site of quality support and care services' (Values into Action 1994). In effect, some supported living services reflected aspects of the institutions from which people had moved rather than fully embracing this goal.

Community Learning Disabilities Teams

Community Learning Disabilities Teams (CLDT) were first developed in the 1970s following the recommendations of the National Development Team for the Mentally Handicapped (DHSS 1978). Part of this requirement was the development of Community Mental Handicap Teams (CMHT), now known as CLDT. Their aim was to provide a coordinated and planned local service for people with learning disabilities. Teams were to develop their own way of working, being able to respond flexibly to local situations. They would focus mainly on meeting the needs of people with learning disabilities served by the NHS. (Simon 1981).

They were multi-disciplinary in nature with core members usually being community nurses and social workers and coordinated by a consultant psychiatrist. Varying other team members, including occupational therapists, were also part of the team, though often on a part-time basis. The teams' three main roles were defined as: coordinating service delivery; providing direct services to people and their families; and a 'gate-keeper' role in raising awareness of available resources and access to them (Mansell 1990).

By the mid 1980s CLDTs were well established and most had succeeded to some degree in providing and developing the local services required to support people who had always lived in the community and later those who would be resettled from the institutions. There is agreement in the literature of the time that teams were carrying out diverse roles aimed at improving local situations and varied in the number and type of professions involved (Mansell 1990). Working in community teams required professionals to adopt different working patterns in order to work closely with colleagues from different backgrounds, respond to referrals for a wide range of client needs in a community setting and to take on new roles in service development. In effect, teams developed in diverse ways across the UK and there is still variance in the nature of their provision across different locations (Jenkins et al 2003).

Day services

During the latter part of the 20th century 'community care' was defined essentially in terms of training centres, sheltered workshops, special classes and schools rather than community home based service provision. The need for a joint approach by the NHS and Social Services for care provision of the 'mental handicap field' became implicit in planning services. With the closure of hospitals came re-provision of day services. This was often by setting up specialist provision by health services in conjunction with social services to meet needs in sheltered workshop settings and to enable people to use community facilities.

In the late 1970s and 1980s the National Development Group (Department of Health and Social Security 1978) provided the principles for day services for mentally handicapped people. In 1986–1987, the Social Services Inspectorate (SSI) carried out a national review of 150 local authority day services. They discovered variable types of service often built on existing services and inheriting '... provision, staff, attitudes and expectations' (SSI 1989) and wide ranging client needs including those with profound and physical disabilities. They recommended that day services should become part of a 'cohesive pattern of services' and take into account the rights and needs of people with a mental handicap.

In the community, Adult Training Centres (ATCs) provided a range of day support for those who lived at home, with the original ethos of training for work and sheltered workshop provision, usually on a long-term basis (Williams 1995). In the late 1980s many of these centres were renamed Resource and Activity Centres, reflecting more emphasis on lifelong learning, making use of activities and using resources that could enable more integration into local communities. A range of activities were provided by the Resource and Activity Centres including social contact, advice, assessment and intervention and work related activities and to meet a wide range of client needs.

The 1980s also saw great strides forward in the philosophies of day services with the growth of the self-advocacy movement, links with ordinary services in the community and identifying individual needs for personal development (Williams 1995). The ideas contained within the Social Services Inspectorate 1989 report paved the way for more integrated services provided by a range of providers. These increasingly in the late 1990s included health and social care and independent organizations commissioned by statutory authorities.

This chapter will now consider in more detail how philosophical perspectives have and continue to shape the lives of individuals with a learning disability.

Philosophical perspectives

The underpinning philosophy of current learning disabilities services is fundamental to how society deals with those who fall outside the perceived 'norm'. As discussed previously, the provision of care for people with mental health and learning disability involved keeping them safe and protecting society. This was achieved by using both what would now be considered either humane or inhumane methods (Atherton 2003). At all times this resulted in others making what they considered to be the best choices for individuals who in society had deemed incapable of making their own choices or in some way had offended against the 'norm'. The interpretation of society's values was therefore left to untrained and sometimes unenlightened individuals who worked within a custodial framework.

Medical model versus social model

The creation of the National Health Service (NHS) in 1948 strengthened the emergence of the medical model. Doctors established the position that enabled them to prescribe treatments whilst the role of all other staff was seen as supporting them in their medical practice. During this time two advances occurred: first, scientific advances that increased understanding and therefore the treatment of disease; and second, the realization that clean water and adequate disposal of waste were effective public health measures that when linked to improved living conditions could prolong lives and prevent disease (Orme et al 2007). After the introduction of good basic public health measures in the United Kingdom a change in the political climate increased the dominance of the medical model, with patients expecting medication to solve health issues (Thomas & Woods 2004). Additionally, with the discovery of the damaging effect of certain health behaviours (smoking, for example), individuals began to be held responsible for their own 'unhealthy behaviour'. For people with learning disabilities in institutional care the impact of the medical model was to focus on aspects of individuals' health and behaviour that could be changed for the benefit of the wider community, often without their consent.

Proponents of the social model challenged this view and argued that individuals and their families should be viewed from a wider perspective and the influence of this can be seen in Saving Lives: Our Healthier Nation (Secretary of State for Health 1999). The alternative was to consider how the institution influenced the individual's ability to contribute fully to society and to start to create enabling environments based on meeting individual needs and wishes. Ill health was perceived as being influenced by society and the way that it treated those who were disabled and vulnerable to poverty, poor housing and social exclusion. In the current political climate, there is less division between the health and social aspects of an individual's life course. Services aim to provide seamless access across service boundaries to meet both health and social needs. Occupational therapists with their health and social care colleagues have a part to play in enabling access to generic and specialist services that best meet people's needs.

Normalization/social role valorization

One of the major influences on learning disabilities service provision was the emergence of the philosophical perspective initially referred to as 'normalization'. Significant differences in the underpinning ideology of normalization developed by Nirje (1972) and Wolfensberger (1972) are examined by Szivos (1992). Nirje (1972) focused on providing the 'handicapped adult with the range of conditions and experience of life that will support his self confidence and feelings of adulthood'. Wolfensberger aimed to disperse people with learning disability 'throughout the community as a prerequisite for reduced visibility, appropriate role models and increasingly appropriate behaviour' (Szivos 1992 p. 115).

The ideological concepts underpinning both began to encourage a shift in attitudes towards people with learning disabilities in terms of recognizing their human right to be treated as equals in society. The principles of normalization are based on the idea that everyone has the right to experience both family and community life including routines of leisure and work activities. Nirje's aim was to enable people to experience normal patterns of life, thus enabling them to experience developmental stages and increase their self-confidence. Normalization does not directly make people change to become different people based on service planners' ideas of what constitutes normal. Rather, it propounds allowing people to experience and contribute to ordinary life experiences that you or I might value in our lives. However, Dally (1992) noted that within normalization there are elements which are notably conservative and authoritarian and have an emphasis on conformity.

In response to criticisms of the use of the word 'normal' and because of the difficulties in interpretation in practice, Wolfensberger (1983) used the term 'social role valorization' (SRV). This changed the emphasis from what is 'normal' to what is 'socially valued'. However, even though this is the philosophy that underpins present day legislation and service provision, difficulties still exist in the interpretation and implementation of this concept (Race 2002). Applying social role valorization in learning disabilities services challenged staff and service providers to change long-standing beliefs, attitudes and working practices in favour of more inclusive methods. The change took time and patience for many people to both understand what the change involved and to believe that it is the right direction. During the early 1980s there was a huge emphasis on staff training and development in SRV principles both from a theoretical perspective and in changing practices to incorporate principles into the lives of people with learning disabilities.

Box 2.4

Five Service Accomplishments (O'Brien & Tyne 1981, O'Brien 1988 cited in Emerson 1992 pp.13–15)

- Community presence: ensuring service users have the same access in their neighbourhoods to schools, work places, shops, facilities and churches as ordinary people.
- Respect: develop and maintain positive reputations for people who use the service by ensuring choice of activities, locations, forms of dress and use of language to promote positive perceptions of people with disabilities.
- Community participation: ensuring participation in the community by supporting service users' natural relationships with families, neighbours and co-workers; widening networks.
- Competence: developing skills and attributes that are functional and meaningful and reduce dependency. Developing personal characteristics that others value in the community and relationships.
- Choice: ensuring that service users are supported to make choices about their lives, understand their situation and options and act appropriately on decisions such as who to live with or what type of work to do.

O'Brien & Tyne (1981), cited in Emerson (1993), presented a model of provision of care that identified service accomplishments (based on implementing normalization principles), which, if achieved, would improve individual lifestyle or quality of life. The Five Service Accomplishments (see Box 2.4) outline practical strategies for setting up services that are built on individual choice, active participation and development of the individual's skills and competencies. The influence of these ideas reflected in the White Paper, Valuing People (DoH 2001a) and modern day service delivery.

Service responses to the new ideology

The more recent policy documents and legislation introduced at the beginning of the 21st century have set the scene for people with learning disability to live independently or with minimal support in the community. The main driver for this change is the introduction of the White Paper exclusively for people with learning disabilities, Valuing People: a new strategy for learning disabilities for the 21st century (DoH 2001a). This was the first real political agenda to both identify and resource implementation as defined outcomes for service provision within the United Kingdom. The White Paper identifies principles of choice, participation, inclusion and rights for people with learning disabilities across all aspects of their lives.

Choice and participation

The White Paper Valuing People (DoH 2001a) acknowledges the principles of choice and participation as being the basis of service provision for people with learning disabilities. How we make choices is fundamental to everyday living, from choosing to get up in the morning and deciding what to wear, or more complex choices such as changing our job or starting or ending a relationship. For individuals with learning disability the opportunity for making choices has been historically limited by other people's view of perceived inability to make competent choices or by organizational factors that imposed control and restricted choice. There was growing recognition that people with mild, moderate, severe or profound learning disabilities (with possibly physical and/or sensory impairments) were excluded from decision making and choice at all levels of society.

In Valuing People (DoH 2001a), continuation of care management is considered central to any formal mechanism for working with individuals with learning disabilities. However, the service systems '... must be responsive to person-centred planning and have the capacity to deliver the kinds of individualized services likely to emerge from the process' (DoH 2001a p. 4.20). The person-centred approach, which is fundamental to occupational therapy, is based on humanistic principles that any planning process starts with the individual and not with the services that exist. Person-centred planning enables the individual to identify what the individual wants, needs and chooses and, through the care management process, individualized services are provided in terms of housing, leisure, education and employment (an example

of this process is discussed in relation to work in Chapter 7). The individual is supported to draw up a community care plan about what they would like to do with their lives and consider the support they will need to achieve this. This process is often referred to as a circle of care with all those (both multi-disciplinary and multi-agency) involved with the individual providing support, facilitation and resources for the individual's needs (i.e. a care package). For some individuals this may involve inclusive communication (discussed in Chapter 4), supported employment (discussed in Chapter 7) or active support (discussed in Chapter 13). However, one of the difficulties of the person-centred approach is the dynamic of who holds the balance of 'power' through this process and particularly in areas of risk (Thomas & Woods pp. 159–160). With little or no information, communication or superficial relationship with the individual, assumptions are often made by professionals or by others, either through assessments or from working with the individual. There is continuing debate about the issues of capacity and consent in this area and the legal status of the individual to make a decision or not. Difficulties can occur for support staff in giving opportunities of risk taking and tensions can arise between how to support choice and decision making in terms of perceived risk within the legal obligations of maintaining protection and care.

The impact of applying SRV principles for staff who work with individuals with a learning disability has been to challenge their beliefs, attitudes and working methods. Embracing SRV principles meant increasing their inclusion in staff training courses at all service levels including underpinning organizational management, service design, quality assurance, deinstitutionalization and supported living. Whether based in the community or within institutions, occupational therapists were involved jointly with other members of the CLDT in formulating and carrying out induction and continuing training for community support staff. Occupational therapists were particularly involved in working with support staff in relation to identifying and enabling meaningful occupations using a person-centred approach. Whilst the principles of SRV and O'Brien & Tyne's five service accomplishments have been incorporated into present day services within the context of community living and especially within supported accommodation, there is still a challenge to ensure choice and participation in practice.

Inclusion and rights

Inclusion and rights are broad terms that encompass how we expect to be part of a community, access facilities for work, education, leisure and activities of daily living and establish friendships and relationships.

> *People with a learning disability have the right to as full and independent a life as the rest of the community. Co-ordinated planning should occur, aiming for the achievement of independence, competence, normal relationships, involvement with the community and respect. p1. All Wales Strategy (Welsh Office 1983).*

The right to access health care is an example of how rights and inclusion have proved to be difficult for people with a learning disability. Valuing People (DoH 2001a) highlighted areas of need that were not being fully met by community learning disability teams and, particularly with regard to health needs of clients. For those in institutions their health care needs were managed within the institutions. The move from institutional care to community living increased the need to identify and provide for the general health needs of people with a learning disability across their life span. This raises issues about the importance of effective inter-professional working to break down barriers to clients receiving assessment and intervention from appropriate services. People with learning disabilities have the right to access generic health and social care (National Association of Occupational Therapists Working with People with Learning Disabilities 2003) and to be supported through the processes of:

- Assessment and intervention of change in health status related to life stages
- health action plans
- inpatient status – including discharge planning.

The World Health Organization has increasingly drawn attention to health problems within a global context and worked to redefine disability (Wilcock 2005). People with learning disabilities are also acknowledged within the new National Service Frameworks being produced to introduce professionals to the standards set for different conditions. An example of this is the National Service Framework for Older People, which is discussed in more detail in Chapter 12.

Social inclusion embraces the idea of developing social networks through establishing circles of support or friendships within family, cultural and leisure outlets. The concept of biopsychosocial models in the 21st century has increased the emphasis on health and wellness rather than illness and on social inclusion rather than segregation. The introduction and gradual implementation of the Disability Discrimination Act 1995 and legislation such as the Human Rights Act 1998 give the opportunity for the individual, their families and other non-governmental organizations to challenge the existing medical and social practices. Another major move has been towards shifting the power base to support individuals with learning disability to take on responsibilities as citizens and to participate in political debate. The establishment of the principles of advocacy and empowerment has led to a strong self advocacy movement in which the voice of people with a learning disability is increasingly being heard in decision making processes.

Rights and advocacy

Community presence (O'Brien & Tyne 1981) for people with a learning disability introduces the concept that if people have rights to ordinary things then they also have rights to be able to speak for themselves. For individuals with learning disabilities there has been a need to be empowered to take on the right to speak for themselves. Empowerment is related to how an individual takes control and gains power in their own life. The aim of empowerment is closely linked to the advocacy process through which an individual or group can participate and make choices. This is illustrated in Box 2.5: Empowerment hypotheses suggested by Du Bois & Miley (1999). Advocacy support that incorporates empowerment has been developed in different ways, including:

- Voluntary advocacy agencies – that offer one to one sessions (i.e. citizen advocacy) involving people who support an individual with learning disability who does not have family or friends
- Group advocacy – large or small groups of people working together for a similar cause towards common goals
- Self advocacy – developed by the organization People First. The individual can work either individually or in a self advocacy group to make real, informed choices.

Box 2.5

Empowerment hypotheses suggested by Du Bois & Miley (1999)

Level of awareness is a key issue in empowerment; information is necessary for change to occur:

- Empowerment is a collaborative process, with professionals and participants from excluded populations working together as partners
- The empowering process views the participant as competent and capable, given access to resources and opportunities
- People must participate in their own empowerment; goals, means and outcomes must be self-defined
- Participants must perceive themselves as causal agents able to effect change
- Informal social networks are a significant source of support for mediating stress and increasing one's competence and sense of control.

A demonstration of how the principles of advocacy have developed is the inclusion of people with a learning disability in the production of Valuing People including 'Nothing about us without us' (DoH 2001b), along with the White Paper (DoH 2001a). Initially these ideas resulted in a major challenge for service providers, as staff had to allow, enable and believe that people with a learning disability have the right and capacity to do this. This change of role from the prevalent caring role to a facilitative, enabling role challenged existing cultures. The move from the hospital to the community did not always result in the principles of advocacy being applied as recent investigations have demonstrated (Commission for Healthcare Audit and Inspection 2006). There are still barriers to how advocacy is implemented for an individual within the care management and assessment processes as advocacy support and resources are often unavailable or limited.

This is not a definitive overview of all of the issues concerning service provision for people with learning disabilities. Many other factors have affected the histories of people with learning disability. What can be missed by focusing on the historical and present day changes are the parallel changes in services for people with mental health or physical disabilities. Wilcock (2002), in her exploration of the development of occupational therapy, highlights the changes that occurred in the journey from 'prescription to self health.' However, further exploration of the philosophies, policies and legislation can help identify the changes over the last century and how people with learning disability have journeyed from mainly custodial institutionalization to the community care services of today. For further reading, please refer to the recommended reading at the end of the chapter and Appendix 2.2 Legislation and policies.

Learning disability – occupational therapy philosophy and practice

Occupational therapy philosophy has historically recognized the influence of occupation on an individual's health and well-being whilst the influence of institutional and community care on occupation has not always been acknowledged (Wilcock 2002). The emergence of occupational therapy as a profession in the UK started before the First World War and focused firstly on working in mental health then physical health and only latterly in 'mental handicap' settings (Wilcock 2002). The implementation of the medical model and the pressure of government targets on hospitals led to faster discharge. Occupational therapists found they had less patient contact, resulting in less emphasis on rehabilitation and the importance of occupation. In line with attitudes of the time, the occupational therapy training and support for those who wished to work with this client group historically valued the more physical aspects of the role. Therefore, it was hard for the first occupational therapists in learning disabilities to establish the need for occupational therapy in the institution. There were, however, already key philosophical and practical attitudes within the institutions such as the work ethic and educational input that made a good basis on occupational therapists which could build their professional role and start to look at the individual's needs with regard to occupation.

During the 1980s and 1990s occupational therapy philosophy was challenged in the need to 'fit' with the medical model by the realization of the importance of holistic client-centred approaches already formulating and developing in terms of identifying occupational behaviour. The development of a paradigm which emphasized occupation enabled the profession to return to its humanistic roots and develop the social study of human occupation (Kielhofner 2004).

Occupational therapy in the institution

Occupational therapy for people with learning disabilities began within the institutional settings in the early part of the 20th century. The ethos of self sufficiency in some ways supported the basis for occupational therapy at that time as workshops and industrial units within the hospitals were eventually to come under the auspices of occupational therapy services. This continued until the introduction of resettlement into the community in the 1980s.

In the early days, the lone occupational therapist worked to increase daytime occupations and teach skills usually in creative or educational activities. Occupational therapy services grew in many institutions to incorporate woodwork, industrial therapy, educational activity, creative skills such as rug making, gardening. As well as keeping people occupied, these activities also contributed to the running costs of the institutions. By the early 1980s occupational therapy was an established part of institutional life and occupational therapists had begun to work with the whole range of people with learning disabilities including those with multiple disabilities and challenging behaviour who were more difficult to engage in meaningful occupation.

Occupational therapy progressed from initially being directed by doctors to the 'blanket referral' of all the patients on a ward, to a professional who assessed people's ability and used group work or individual activities as appropriate to meet needs. This gave the opportunity for the development of new skills, albeit to do with survival in the institutional setting rather than focused on rehabilitation. The philosophical challenges to the occupational therapy profession at this time also paralleled the move towards deinstitutionalization adopted in the 1970s and 1980s with emphasis on policies and management for health care and home based services in the community. The decision to close institutions in the 1980s meant that occupational therapists developed assessments to identify strengths and abilities to prepare individuals for a more independent life in the community (Wilcock 2002). These were

Box 2.6

Occupational therapy assessments toward resettlement

- Interpersonal and social skills
- Daily living activities (i.e. housework, cooking)
- Management of personal needs (i.e. hygiene, dressing, washing)
- Vocational assessments
- Leisure inventory
- Cognitive (i.e. numeracy, money skills)
- Risk (i.e. road safety, manual handling, personal safety)
- Assessment of equipment and adaptations, environmental factors.

related to the individual's activities of self care, leisure and productivity needs, a summary of which is presented in Box 2.6. For insight into the pioneers of the profession and the role they played in demonstrating the use of activity for people in institutions, further recommended reading is the history of the emerging profession of occupational therapy by Ann Wilcock in *Occupation for Health* Volume 2 (Wilcock 2002).

Occupational therapy role and resettlement

Fundamental to the process of resettlement and community care management was the concept of assessing and creating a care package responsive to both the needs of the individual and the carer. Programmes of intervention were developed to prepare the individual for community living and to offer opportunities within sheltered environments to develop and use these skills.

The role of the occupational therapist working in learning disability services has changed considerably from the lone therapist working within the institution. During the resettlement process it was recognized that occupational therapists could contribute to the assessment of needs and abilities of the individual and also the assessment of environments for their capacity to enable meaningful occupation as people were moved to homes in the community. The emergence of community multidisciplinary teams resulted in a reconfiguration of services with most occupational therapists working in a specialist role. Occupational therapists contributed to practical outcomes as members of the multidisciplinary team in enabling people with learning disabilities through person-centred planning. Assessments and interventions were not only of needs in relation to community skills, but also on compatibility of moving into new accommodation with others. The occupational therapist could act as a facilitator or advocate role in these circumstances to ensure that individuals are able to participate at the level they wish. These principles were explored in the document 'An Ordinary Life' (Kings Fund 1980) and occupational therapists alongside other staff were able to implement the idea of establishing ordinary homes within the community, to access ordinary facilities and to widen occupational opportunities.

However, the resettlement process was often long and decisions about who should be resettled first, who with and how they should best be accommodated in the community needed considered negotiation. In many instances, the first to be resettled were the more able and they usually were resettled into small group homes staffed by nursing staff. For those with more complex needs and physical disabilities the occupational therapist's role in the resettlement process involved environmental assessment to identify equipment and resources for adapting housing or working with architects' plans for new homes.

Occupational therapy training role

With the introduction of SRV occupational therapists found themselves contributing to training courses. The training was essential to enable staff moving to the community to understand how to incorporate underlying SRV principles into management design of new services, measuring quality and counteracting the negative aspects of institutional life. Occupational therapists, whether based in the community or within institutions, were involved with other members of the multidisciplinary team in formulating and jointly carrying out induction and continual training for community support staff. This training role gave an opportunity to emphasize the philosophy of occupational therapy and the unique way in which occupational therapists use occupation to assess, analyse, adapt and grade activities (such as those summarized in Box 2.7). The fundamental skill of the occupational therapist is the ability to use occupations to develop a whole range of therapeutic

Box 2.7

Occupational therapy training for support staff

Identifying community living skills and needs of clients (e.g. SRV)

This also involved training support staff working to identify environmental, communication and motivation factors that influence learning in relation to SRV and skills such as:

- The acquisition and use of practical skills (i.e. dressing)
- Problem-solving skills (i.e. road crossing, cooking)
- Dealing with challenging and inappropriate behaviour (i.e. self injurious behaviour, aggression)
- Assessment techniques (i.e. risk assessments, manual handling)
- Skills teaching (i.e. task analysis, systematic analysis, precision teaching)
- Communication strategies, (i.e. verbal and non-verbal)
- Engaging and fostering participation in daily living activities (i.e. identifying motivational factors)
- Use of equipment and adaptation.

experience for the client and to promote their ability to learn and master a skill. The importance of individualized, structured routines and programmes incorporates skill teaching in everyday life to maintain or acquire new skills has long been recognized. The role of the occupational therapist is one that enables and facilitates the individuals towards independence in community living, with appropriate support. In doing this the occupational therapist had and still has to be aware of the variable factors and pass onto support staff how pacing of the activity and environmental factors could influence successful learning.

Occupational therapy role and community living

The needs of people with a learning disability who lived in the community were mainly met by their families. Those more able individuals were able to access adult training centres run by social services departments. These centres provided both opportunity for productive occupations and productive roles for people with a learning disability. Occupational therapists developing their role within the multidisciplinary team would contribute to Individual Programme Planning meetings and work with individuals to experience opportunities and develop skills that they needed to participate in the community.

The role of the occupational therapist was changing from running predominantly group and therapeutic based interventions within large institutions, day centres or adult training centres or special needs units to more community based individual interventions. Curry (1988) investigated the roles and time management of occupational therapists and concluded that over a year there was a significant change illustrating the move from hospital into the community to a more 'specific and normal environment'. The occupational therapist developed assessment and intervention skills that enabled individualized learning strategies for the individual both in the community and for those being resettled from large institutions. Llewellyn (1991) identified 'adaptive daily living skills' to include eating, bathing, dressing, communication, mobility and community living skills. Pimental & Ryan (1996), in a study comparing USA and Australian occupational therapy community interventions with people with learning disabilities, identified two specific categories as 'remedial and adaptive living skills'.

The move into the community gave occupational therapists opportunities to work with service users in their own homes. Melton (1998) asked service users for their opinions on the experiences they had preparing food with an occupational therapist. She notes how the 'occupational therapist exposed the client to a range of possibilities ... the client was then able to make an active choice about organizing the occupation into his or her use of time' (Melton 1998 p. 109). The range of community occupational therapy interventions is summarized in Box 2.8.

Interpreting SRV

Whilst the ideas underpinning SRV helped introduce people with learning disabilities to an increasingly independent life in the community, there were still some difficulties in interpretation. Occupational

---

Box 2.8

Occupational therapy – community interventions

Occupation towards quality of life in relation to:

- Personal growth accomplishments
- Physical independence
- Transportation/physical accessibility
- Social and community involvement
- Leisure activities
- Personal and family relationships
- Employment/economic independence.

---

therapists working with people who had moved to community homes could encounter staff who interpreted normalization as 'do as I do'. In one instance, provision of adapted cutlery to help someone with poor grip was rejected on their behalf by staff who decided that to be 'normal' the service user had to use an ordinary knife and fork. Before the introduction of the Manual Handling Operations Regulations 1992, staff also risked their own health and safety in lifting service users (Tarling 1992) by claiming that for people with multiple and profound learning disability being hoisted would be a frightening experience. Careful planning and introduction of this experience to become part of that service user's occupational form required the therapist to complete a detailed occupational performance analysis and be able to understand, promote and work within the regulations.

This highlights one of the difficulties that face occupational therapists working in community residential situations: they are often reliant on the quality and effectiveness of staff who will carry out interventions on a daily basis with clients. Support staff in these situations are busy people and whilst they respond well to professionals they need to understand the 'reasons why' they need to support a planned intervention. Ultimately, occupational therapists are employed to provide a service for people with a learning disability. In order to do this they need to work closely with carers, understand their perspective and work together to overcome barriers to interventions being carried out with individual service users. This is explored further in Chapter 14. It is important that any intervention planned with the person with a learning disability reflects a client-centred approach.

Learning from history

There are many barriers that have been and continue to be drawn between people with learning disabilities and the rest of the population. Jackson (2000) argues that boundaries need to be crossed in order to move forward. The challenge is how these can be resolved for the benefit of the individual and society. One way of crossing boundaries is to ensure that our approach to exploring the history of learning disabilities attempts to integrate different stories at many different levels and values what historical evidence can contribute to current practice. Evaluating historical perspectives in relation to individual life stories helps to raise awareness of the impact of history on the people we work with and to understand the relevance of current service philosophies. Key factors that have had an impact on people's lives are summarized below and the reader is invited to reflect on these in relation to the Case illustration: Den (Box 2.10).

The history of people with learning disabilities can be considered from different angles: individual, service provision, family, professional, political, social, etc. However, considering these aspects in context is only part of the picture, it is also significant to draw on the experiences of the individual and compare similarities and differences to the experiences of the professional. The reason for this is that it provides a framework in which philosophies, attitudes and developments can be viewed. For occupational therapists this means reviewing our own philosophical underpinnings to ensure that they enable us to work in line with current philosophies for people with learning disabilities. The emergence of occupational science to underpin the research base of occupational therapy and the importance of meaningful occupation is increasingly recognized as a major contributor to the health and wellness of the individual and society (Wilcock 2002). Occupational therapists are also committed to promoting a client-centred approach to enable the individual to have the opportunity to make healthy occupational choices (Sumsion 2005). As verbal communication is not possible for some people with a learning disability, Chapter 4 offers other approaches to communication to establish a clear client-centred approach. Applying these principles to learning disabilities was outlined in the document, 'Occupational therapy services for

Box 2.9

Principles of occupational therapy services for adults with learning disabilities

- Principle 1: Occupational therapists working in learning disability services provide a service for people whose primary reason for referral relates to the effect of their learning disability upon their occupational performance p. 3–4.
- Principle 2: People with learning disabilities need to be enabled to have choice and influence over their occupational therapy intervention p. 5–6.
- Principle 3: People with learning disabilities have the right to access generic health and social care p. 7–8.
- Principle 4: OT services should be provided in partnership with the person with his or her carers and all relevant agencies p. 9–10.
  National Association of Occupational Therapists Working with People with Learning Disabilities: 11/2003.

adults with learning disabilities' (National Association of Occupational Therapists Working with People with Learning Disabilities 2003) summarized in Box 2.9.

People with learning disability want to be part of their community, but they can be vulnerable and be subject to the stresses that many people experience when living alone. Improvement in services does not mean that listening to the voices of people with learning disability is any less important today. The opportunity is set for people with a learning disability to be fully represented and heard in the community. An example of this in the electronic age is the establishment of a Valuing People website, www.valuingpeople.gov.uk, which provides resources and is a useful way for professionals to keep up to date with client directed initiatives. Voluntary agencies and charities that support people with learning disabilities have also changed since the publication of Valuing People. Current website addresses can be found in the resources sections in the relevant chapters in this book.

Summary

This chapter has considered the historical background to working with people with learning disabilities as a basis for reflecting on current service provision and raising awareness of historical influences. From the individual perspective, the chapter has identified the historical journey that many people with learning disabilities have experienced. The ability to carry out self care tasks, have a productive day-time occupation and have time for leisure pursuits is something that most individuals aspire to, including people with a learning disability. Enabling this to happen, whilst being aware of the impact of past barriers, is a challenge for occupational therapists working in this field today.

The chapter has introduced you to the main historical influences, the changes that have occurred in learning disability services, and the impact of philosophical debate on changing service provision. Despite many changes in the lives of people with learning disabilities as regards community living there are still challenges to ensure choice, participation and opportunities for social inclusion.

The chapter has also considered the emerging and changing role of the occupational therapist working in what was in the early days an under-funded service. It has considered how occupational therapists, by considering individual life histories in relation to service philosophies, can use a client-centred approach with people with learning disabilities. This does mean that today's service providers have to be imaginative if they are going to increase the opportunities for the health and wellness of service users and to overcome historical barriers. They can strive to make meaningful occupation available for the service users they work with.

Box 2.10

Case illustration: Den

Den has recently been admitted to an acute ward at the local hospital with pneumonia. He is a 50-year-old man who lives with his mother in an adapted bungalow. Den uses a wheelchair for mobility but prior to admission was able to transfer from the wheelchair to bed and armchair with minimal assistance and prompting. He did, however, need physical assistance to dress and maintain his self care. He has some speech. He attends a day centre 3 days a week where he is popular with staff and other clients. Although Den is still weak following treatment, the hospital now considers him ready for discharge. Prior to admission a number of issues were raised by members of the CLDT as there were signs of neglect and physical abuse. Subsequently his mother has recently been diagnosed with Alzheimer's disease and has been referred to the Older Adult Team. Following a discharge plan Den is to be placed in a nursing home as a temporary measure. His Case Manager had referred him to the occupational therapist on the CLDT for assessment.

Reader activity

The White Paper Valuing People: a new strategy for learning disabilities for the 21st century (DoH 2001) identifies four service principles for people with learning disabilities across all aspects of their lives. How can the occupational therapist contribute to maintaining these principles for Den in his present situation?

Further reading

Atherton H 2003 A history of learning disabilities. In: Gates B (ed.) Learning disabilities toward inclusion, 4th edn. London, Elsevier, pp 41–60

Booth T 1990 Better lives: changing services for people with learning difficulties. Sheffield, Joint unit for Social Services Research

Brown S, Wistow G (eds) 1990 The roles and tasks of community mental handicap teams. Aldershot, Avebury, Avebury studies of care in the community

Carpenter P 2002 A history of Brentry. Bristol, Friends of Glenside Museum

Emerson E 1993 What is normalisation. In: Brown H,

Smith H (eds) Normalisation: a reader for the nineties. London, Tavistock Routledge

Malin N (ed.) 1995 Services for people with learning disabilities. London, Routledge

Race DG (ed.) 2002 The historical context. In Learning disability – a social approach. London, Routledge

Wilcock A 2005 The culture and context for promoting health through occupational therapy. In: Scriven A (ed.)

Health promoting practice: the contribution of nurses and allied health professionals. Basingstoke, Palgrave Macmillan

Williams P 1995 Residential and day services. In: Malin N (ed.) Services for people with learning disabilities. London, Routledge

Useful resources

British Institute of Learning Disabilities www.bild.org.uk (accessed 27 February 2008)

Foundation for People with Learning Disabilities http://www. learningdisabilities.org.uk (accessed 27 February 2008)

Valuing People website has information and useful links: www. valuingpeople.gov.uk (accessed 27 February 2008)

References

Atherton H 2003 A history of learning disabilities. In: Gates B (ed.) Learning disabilities toward inclusion, 4th edn. London, Elsevier, pp 41–60

Atkinson D, Jackson M, Walmsley J (eds) 1997 Forgotten lives: exploring the history of learning disability. Kidderminster, BILD Publications

Atkinson D 2000 Parallel stories. In: Brigham L, Atkinson D et al (eds) 2000 Crossing boundaries: change and continuity in the history of learning disabilities. Kidderminster, BILD Publications

Brigham L, Atkinson D et al (eds) 2000 Crossing boundaries: change and continuity in the history of learning disabilities. Kidderminster, BILD Publications

Carpenter P 2002 The national institutions for persons requiring care and control: Stoke Park Colony, Stapleton Bristol A 1911 description reproduced and arranged with further photographs and commentary. Bristol, Friends of Glenside Museum

Clarke ADB, Clark AM 1987 Research on mental handicap 1957–1987 a selective review.

Journal of Mental Deficiency Research 31:317–328

Commission for Healthcare Audit and Inspection 2006 Joint investigation into services for people with learning disabilities at Cornwall Partnership NHS Trust. Healthcare Commission, Commission for Social Care Inspection, Cornwall NHS Trust

Cooper M, Atkinson D 2000 Parallel stories. In: Brigham L, Atkinson D et al (eds) Crossing boundaries: change and continuity in the history of learning disabilities. Kidderminster, BILD Publications

Curry M 1988 The occupational therapist for people with a mental handicap. British Journal of Occupational Therapy 51(7): 239–241

Dally G 1992 Social welfare ideologies. In: Brown H, Smith H (eds) Normalisation: a reader for the nineties. London, Routledge

Department of Health and Social Security 1971 White Paper, Better services for mentally handicapped. London, HMSO

Department of Health and Social Security 1978 Development Team for the Mentally Handicapped. First Report: 1976–77. London, HMSO

Department of Health 1990 The NHS and Community Care Act. London, HMSO

Department of Health 2001a White Paper Valuing people: a new strategy for learning disabilities for the 21st century. London, HMSO

Department of Health 2001b Nothing about us without us. London, HMSO

Du Bois B, Miley KK 1999 Social work: an empowering profession, 3rd edn. Boston, Allyn & Bacon

Emerson E 1993 What is normalisation? In: Brown H, Smith H (eds) Normalisation: a reader for the nineties. London, Tavistock Routledge

Jackson M 2000 In: Brigham L, Atkinson D et al (eds) Introduction Chapter; Crossing boundaries: change and continuity in the history of learning disabilities. Kidderminster, BILD Publications

Jenkins R, Mansell I, Northway R 2003 Specialist learning disability services in the UK. In: Gates B (ed.) Learning disabilities; toward inclusion, 4th edn. Edinburgh, Churchill Livingstone

Kielhofner G 2004 Conceptual foundations of occupational therapy, 3rd edn. Philadelphia, FA Davis

Kings Fund Centre 1980 An ordinary life: comprehensive locally based residential services for mentally handicapped people. London, Kings Fund Centre

Llewellyn G 1991 Occupational therapy treatment goals for adults with developmental disabilities. Australian Occupational Therapy Journal 38(1):233–236

Llewellyn G, McConnell D 2005 You have to prove yourself all the time. In: Grant G, Goward P, Richardson M, Ramcharan P (eds) Learning disability: a life cycle approach to valuing people. Maidenhead, Open University Press

Malin N, Race D, Jones G 1980 Services for the mentally handicapped in Britain. London, Croom Helm

Manners R, Stevens G, Chaplin E 2003 Art, drama and music therapies. In: Gates B (ed.) 2003 Learning disabilities: towards inclusion, 4th edn. Edinburgh, Churchill Livingstone

Mansell J 1990 The natural history of the community mental handicap team. In: Brown S, Wistow G (eds) The roles and tasks of community mental handicap teams. Avebury, Aldershot, Avebury Studies of Care in the Community

Melton J 1998 How do clients with learning disabilities evaluate their experience of cooking with the occupational therapist? British Journal of Occupational Therapy 61(3):106–110

National Association of Occupational Therapists Working with People with Learning Disabilities 2003 Occupational therapy services for adults with learning disabilities. London, College of Occupational Therapists

Nirje B 1972 The right to self determination. In: Wolfensberger W (ed.) The principle of normalisation in human services. Toronto, National Institute of Mental Retardation, p 181

O'Brien J, Tyne A 1981 The principles of normalisation: a foundation for effective services. London, The Campaign for Mentally Handicapped People

Orme J, Powell J, Taylor P, Grey M 2007 Public health for the 21st century, 2nd edn. Maidenhead, Open University Press

Oswin 1991 Am I allowed to cry? A study of bereavement amongst people who have learning difficulties. London, Souvenir Press

Pimentel S, Ryan S 1996 Working with clients with learning disabilities and multiple physical handicaps: A comparison between hospital and community based therapists. British Journal of Occupational Therapy 59(7): 313–318

Race DG 2002 The historical context. In: Race DG (ed.) Learning disability – a social approach. London, Routledge

Secretary of State for Health 1999 Saving lives – our healthier nation. London, The Stationery Office

Simon GB 1981 Local services for mentally handicapped people. British Institute for Mental Handicap, Kidderminster. In: Brown S, Wistow G (eds) 1990 The roles and tasks of community mental handicap teams. Avebury, Aldershot, Avebury Studies of Care in the Community

Social Services Inspectorate 1989 Inspection of day services for people with a mental handicap. London, HMSO

Stalker K, Connors C 2005 Children with learning disabilities talking about their everyday lives. In: Grant G, Goward P, Richardson M, Ramcharan P (eds) Learning disability: a life cycle approach to valuing people. Maidenhead, Open University Press

Stuart M 2002 Not quite sisters: women with learning difficulties living in convent homes. Kidderminster, BILD Publications

Sumsion T 2005 Promoting health through client centred occupational therapy practice. In: Scriven A (ed.) Health promoting practice: the contribution of nurses and allied health professionals. Basingstoke, Palgrave Macmillan

Szivos S 1992 The limits to integration? In: Brown H, Smith H (eds) Normalisation: a reader for the nineties. London, Routledge

Tarling C 1992 Developing safe handling policies. Nursing Standard Aug 12 6(47):33–36

Thomas D, Woods H 2004 Working with people with learning disabilities; theory and practice. London, Jessica Kingsley Publishers

Towell D 1988 An ordinary life in practice developing comprehensive community based services for people with learning disabilities. London, King Edwards Hospital Fund for London

Values Into Action 1992 When the eagles fly: a report on the resettlement of people with learning difficulties from long-stay institutions. London, VIA

Values Into Action 1994 Still to be settled: strategies for the resettlement of people from mental handicap hospitals. London, VIA

Welsh Office 1983 The All Wales strategy for the development of services for mentally handicapped people. Cardiff, Welsh Office

Wilcock A 2002 Occupation for health Volume 2: a journey from prescription to self health. London, College of Occupational Therapists

Wilcock A 2005 The culture and context for promoting health through occupational therapy. In: Scriven A (ed.) Health promoting practice: the contribution of nurses and allied health professionals. Basingstoke, Palgrave Macmillan

Williams P 1995 Residential and day services. In: Malin N (ed.) Services for people with learning disabilities. London, Routledge

Wolfensberger W 1972 The principle of normalisation in human services. Toronto, National Institute of Mental Retardation

Wolfensberger 1983 Social role valorisation: a proposed new term for the principle of normalisation. Mental Retardation 21(6): 234–239

Appendix 2.1 Case illustration: Den, possible answers

Question

The White Paper Valuing People: a new strategy for learning disabilities for the 21st Century (DoH 2001). identifies four service principles for people with learning disabilities across all aspects of their lives. How can the occupational therapist contribute to maintaining these principles for Den in his present situation?

Choice

All of us need to experience a sense of autonomy and control in our lives. Both Den and his mother have experienced changes to health and have gone through a process of crisis in which control or choice has been limited. Until recently, Den and his mother had managed without any involvement with statutory services other than attending the day centre. Due to the nature of the situation the Case Manager and occupational therapist will need to work closely with colleagues within the NHS Trust, including medical, therapists and ward, staff through the discharge planning process. Person-centred planning should involve both the individual and family or carers. Care management should aim to streamline the assessment process to meet the needs of an individual with learning disability. An assessment of Den's abilities and needs with regard to activities of daily living prior to discharge is vital, including assessment of transfers, wheelchair mobility and communication needs. The community based occupational therapist can liaise with his/her colleague in the hospital to ensure duplication does not occur.

Participation?

Ensuring that the client is part of the whole process may involve other risk assessments as well as visiting the proposed nursing home setting. Using a client-centred approach ensures that Den is involved in all aspects of his discharge process. Home visits can identify difficulties with transfers, as in Den's case, such as the bathroom and limited room to manoeuvre in his mother's bungalow. During the visit to the nursing home Den was pleased when he identified that he would have more space to move around in his wheelchair and also a bedroom to himself. He also enjoyed being with other people. Through the assessment process with the occupational therapist and physiotherapist he draw up a list of goals for himself. A referral for a powered indoor wheelchair was made, which he was successful in obtaining. He liaised with his case manager to identify a long-term goal to live in a supported housing scheme with other individuals.

Inclusion?

For an individual such as Den there are difficulties in establishing inclusion during change in both health status and social status. For the occupational therapist as a member of the CLDT, effective communication is important in inter-professional working to identify those barriers to clients receiving appropriate support and services within the community. For this reason occupational therapy assessment and intervention especially in health and social settings can establish the needs of the individual. In Den's case he was referred during inpatient status – and the service priority was discharge planning. From Den's point of view this was his priority as well but he needed support to identify and communicate his preferences while on the ward. The second priority was to re-establish access to both services and resources within the community. Discharge planning involved liaising with nursing home staff regarding transfers, hoisting and supporting Den in activities of daily living. For his long-term goal his case manager drew up a community care plan (i.e. a care package) based on Den's short and long-term goals. Den ultimately moved into his own accommodation sharing with one other person. The occupational therapist was involved in identifying suitable accommodation, environmental assessments such as transport to and from the day centre and location of shops, risk assessments on manual handling issues while in the wheelchair, hoisting, self care needs. Provision of equipment included the supply of hoist and bath aids as well as a special bed, and he was involved in training staff in their use.

Rights

The issues of capacity and consent should be addressed with all individuals in this area and acknowledgement of the legal status of the individual to make a decision or not. The MDT liaised with Den's mother with regard to him going into a nursing home setting as a short-term solution. They lived in a small one bedroom bungalow and as she has found it increasingly difficult to manage Den she has agreed to this. However, this had not been discussed with Den. It was agreed that a joint visit to the ward with Den's mother, social worker and the occupational therapist would address this issue and introduce the idea of going to a nursing home. Although initially Den was not keen on the suggested move he agreed to visit the nursing home with the occupational therapist and physiotherapist. From this visit he agreed to the move.

Appendix 2.2 Legislation and policies

Apart from the legislation referred to in the chapter there are other reports, white papers and acts that also apply. Some of these will apply to the whole population and some only to different countries in the United Kingdom (UK). It is therefore important to ensure that you are using the legislation that applies to the part of the UK in which your client resides. Most laws which concern people with learning disabilities, also apply to other members of the population.

The chronological list below gives you titles of relevant documents; remember that only an Act of Parliament is enshrined in the law. Commissioned reports and government papers are not legally enforceable. These are not inclusive of all legislation relevant for service users with a learning disability and legislation from the 1970s and 1980s should also be referred to.

- The Lunatic Asylums Act 1853 and the Idiots Act 1886
- Warnock Report Special Educational Needs (HMSO 1978)
- Welsh Office 1983 The All Wales Strategy for the Development of Services for Mentally Handicapped People
- The Children Act 1989
- Education Act 1981

- The NHS and Community Care Act 1990 Part III
- The Manual Handling Operations Regulations 1992
- The Education Act 1993
- The Disability Discrimination Act 1995
- The Disability Rights Commission (1999) implements the DDA
- The Community Care (Direct Payments Act) 1996
- The Human Rights Act 1998
- Review of Services for People with a Learning Disability 1999 Scotland
- Saving Lives: Our Healthier Nation (Secretary of State for Health) 1999
- The Health Act 2000
- The Carers and Disabled Children Act 2000
- White Paper (England) 2001: Valuing People: A New Strategy for Learning Disability for the 21st Century
- Fulfilling the Promise Welsh Strategy 2001
- The Learning and Skills Bill 2001
- The Commission for Care Standards 2002
- Mental Incapacity Act 2005/2007.

Occupations and the occupational therapy process

Jane Goodman • Christine Locke

Overview

This chapter will consider how occupational therapists can meet the principle of providing a service for people whose learning disability impacts on their occupational performance (COT 2003). It will take into account other factors that may significantly influence the individual's ability to engage in and perform meaningful occupations. For many individuals with a learning disability their level of occupational performance and behaviour may be attributed to their learning disability before other factors are fully considered.

The structure of the chapter is based on the occupational therapy process to present underpinning areas of concern for occupational therapists, followed by an exploration of key influencing factors at each stage of the process. To explore the process this chapter will use the American Practice framework domain and process (Youngstrom et al 2002) as a guiding framework to enable application for this client group. Case illustrations are used to illustrate some of the issues that can arise when working with people with a learning disability and the intervention

and management implications for the occupational therapist.

Learning Outcomes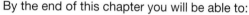

By the end of this chapter you will be able to:
- Consider the factors that influence referral of people with learning disabilities to occupational therapists
- Explore the role of occupation as central to implementing an occupational therapy process
- Apply an occupational therapy process for meeting challenges to occupational performance for people with learning disabilities.

Occupational therapy process

Most health and social care professions use a problem-solving or decision-making process to help them to structure their interventions in an organized way; occupational therapy is no different in this respect. Although the stages of the process may be similar for all professions (referral to discharge), for occupational therapists the purpose is to ensure that people are enabled to engage in daily life occupations that are meaningful and valuable to them (Youngstrom et al 2002). The challenge for occupational therapists is to ensure that occupation remains central while addressing specific issues and support systems related to people with learning disabilities and to consider the individual's needs in the environment or context in which the person operates (Strong et al 1999).

The American occupational therapy practice framework defines seven areas of occupation: activities of daily living, instrumental activities of daily living, education, work, play, leisure and social participation (Youngstrom et al 2002). Other authors use different divisions: most commonly self care, leisure and productivity (Law et al 2005). Kielhofner (2002) uses the terms work, play and activities of daily living. To structure this chapter we have used the terms activities of daily living (ADL), productivity and leisure, whilst being mindful of other aspects that fall within these categories.

The outcome of occupational therapy interventions is described as occupational performance and is the result of interactions between the individual, the occupations they carry out and the environment in which they take place. Occupational performance has been defined as 'the ability to carry out activities of daily life' (Youngstrom et al 2002) or to complete those occupational forms that have importance in our lives (Forsyth & Kielhofner 2006) including occupations in ADL, leisure and productivity. People with learning disabilities are referred to occupational therapy for support in occupations in one or more of these domains.

Occupation and occupational therapy for learning disabilities

Mosey (1981) believes that 'a profession's domain of concern consists of those areas of human experience in which practitioners of the profession offer assistance to others' (p. 51).

For occupational therapists, key occupational areas are often presented as ADL, productivity and leisure. Embedded in the occupational therapy ethos of occupation and its influence on well-being, they may be considered as primary occupations essential for maintaining occupational balance and health.

Occupation can be defined as 'activities...of every day life, named, organized, and given value and meaning by individuals and a culture. Occupation is everything people do to occupy themselves, including looking after themselves...enjoying life...and contributing to the social and economic fabric of their communities...' (Law et al 1997, p. 34). Although occupations in themselves are acknowledged as having

a remedial potential for health and well-being, any activity within the occupations of ADL, productivity or leisure needs to be considered within the context of the individual and the environment. Youngstrom et al (2002) view occupations as both a 'means' and an 'end'. Occupation is used within therapy interventions as a means of changing performance. As an 'end product' of the therapeutic process the client makes the achievement by fully engaging in meaningful occupations.

People with learning disabilities have not always had the opportunities to realize the benefits of occupations in their lives for reasons explored earlier (Chapters 1 and 2). The challenge for occupational therapists is how to enable occupation for people with learning disabilities while overcoming historical barriers to occupational satisfaction inherent in this field of work.

The impact of the environment on a person's ability to perform their desired occupations is a significant consideration when working with people with learning disabilities. Although the context for carrying out occupations may provide opportunities and resources to support their success, there may also be environmental demands and constraints that limit ability to perform successfully. The constraints of past residential environments may mean that many people with learning disabilities have been limited in their occupational choices. Current community environments equally may inhibit people from participating fully in their community due to the low expectations and prejudices of those around them.

Activities of daily living (ADL)

Kielhofner (2002) refers to activities of daily living as 'the typical tasks that are needed for self maintenance and self care' and includes items such as grooming, and housework. Youngstrom et al (2002) divide activities of daily living into two areas:

1. ADL (self care) activities that are to do with caring for one's own body.

2. Instrumental activities of daily living (IADL), which involve the individual interacting with the environment or other people, such as caring for others, financial management, meal preparation, etc.

Being able to manage or being supported to manage ADL may provide the basis for enabling individuals to participate in other occupations and be accepted within society (e.g. maintenance of health, cleanliness, demonstration of personal preferences/identity in dress, etc.). ADL is the one area consistently recognized by other professionals and occupational therapists as central to their role and is also the occupational area most frequently referred for occupational therapy assessment. However, whilst important, one should not forget its interrelationship with other occupational areas that may have greater importance for the individual.

The ADL needs for people within the learning disability spectrum are varied, for example the individual with a mild or moderate learning disability can be fully independent while someone with a profound learning and physical disability is fully dependent. An individual may be able to dress and groom but be unable to maintain routines or have poor awareness of personal hygiene without prompting. The following Box 3.1 Case Illustration: Alan, illustrates the complexity of issues that can be referred for an occupational therapy assessment.

Alan's situation illustrates that both physical and social environmental risk factors can have an impact on the individual's ability to manage ADL. In the bathroom for instance, the room layout, levels of assistance needed for transfers and support for bathing or showering may need consideration as

Box 3.1

Case Illustration: Alan

For the last 2 years Alan, who is 37 years old, has shared a house with two other men. Alan has frequent, complex, partial epileptic seizures and is monitored by the community nurse. Although able to walk around inside the house, he relies on his support workers to push his wheelchair to get around in the community. He has moderate learning disabilities and has been referred for an occupational therapy assessment for issues of safety in the bathroom, transferring on and off the toilet and using the shower. He has increasingly become dependent on his support workers for most of his activities including assisting him in his self-care activities i.e. shaving, bathing, washing and eating. Antagonism has also arisen from the other two tenants because of the increased attention he is getting from staff.

well as the teaching of new skills to carry out familiar tasks. The issue of changed levels of support for Alan has arisen because of an episode of ill health and change of familiar staff. His relationship with the other members of the household has also deteriorated, and he is perceived by them to be not doing things he used to be able to. The social environment (i.e. including new support staff) will have an impact in ADL as learning new techniques, accepting support with personal occupations or even being referred for help in these areas is a sensitive subject. Whatever the reason for the referral, ADL is a personal area that, depending on the nature of the issues, will need handling with sensitivity to consider the needs of the individual. Using the following questions reflect on what it might feel like to be referred to an occupational therapist for help with issues in ADL.

Reader activity

- What would an occupational therapist need to know before agreeing to accept the referral?
- How would you feel if you had to discuss sensitive issues with a stranger?
- Who would you want to support or advocate for you?

People with learning disabilities have limited opportunity to develop roles in supporting others (IADL) or if they do they are often not given credit for it (refer to Chapter 11: Loss and bereavement). Occupational therapists should therefore take into consideration the impact of self-care issues on the person's ability to engage in other relevant and valued occupations, their relationships with others and their contribution to society.

Leisure

In order to consider leisure it is first useful to ask what are leisure activities and what proportion are sedentary or physical. Current lifestyles are arguably tending towards limited physical activity with a decrease in levels of physical fitness and increased incidence of obesity and related cardiovascular disorders. Research has indicated that people with learning disabilities have limited opportunity to explore leisure options and can lead more sedentary lives (Messent et al 1999).

Suto (1998, p. 272) described leisure as '...an occupational performance area, a state of mind, time to be filled and a tangible activity through which therapeutic goals are met.' However, despite identification of the importance of leisure as an occupational domain within conceptual models such as The Model of Human Occupation (MOHO) (Keilhofner 2002) or The Canadian Model of Occupational Performance (CMOP) (Law et al 1997), for people with learning disabilities, the lack of leisure participation is often not fully explored or assessed.

As a result, leisure activities often get overlooked or are given low priority, the focus being limited to physical health needs rather than occupational health in its broadest spectrum. Occupational therapists can play an important role here, as demonstrated by Clark et al (1997) in their study of a 'well' elderly population. The study showed that people who received occupational therapy in what was known as 'the lifestyle redesign programme' showed significantly greater increases in health benefits over 9 months than those in the control groups receiving no intervention or participating only in increased social activities. Lessons from this study could usefully be applied to people with learning disabilities to enable them to improve their health and well-being through a lifestyle re-design approach to occupational therapy intervention. Such a programme could provide opportunity for participation in a range of leisure activity that people may not have previously experienced or to maintain new patterns and routines that have proved difficult in the past. Youngstrom et al (2002) suggest that leisure is about exploring opportunities and participating in those opportunities. People with learning disabilities often have little opportunity to explore new activities yet often have more time available with a lack of balance between this and other occupational areas. The occupational therapist may consider other factors that impact on limiting integration and access to leisure opportunities and these are discussed in Chapter 8 Leisure. An illustration of some of the factors that can limit leisure opportunity is given below in Box 3.2: Phillipa's situation.

Reader activity

- For Phillipa, what are the challenges to her leisure pursuits?
- What are the issues for Phillipa's parents?

Box 3.2

Case Illustration: Phillipa

Phillipa is 46 years old and has mild to moderate learning disabilities. She has limited vision and suffers from tinnitus in her left ear. Although she lives at home with her elderly parents, a support worker takes her out twice a week. She relies heavily on her support worker and they tend to go both days to the same shops and café as these are familiar to Phillipa. She has shown that once she has been somewhere a few times she can get around with minimal assistance and depends less on the support worker. Phillipa has expressed a wish to attend a local drama group but both her parents and carers are concerned that she will have difficulty coping with new people and places.

The occupational therapist can assess and intervene to address the lack of opportunity for autonomous choice and development of personal and social skills by broadening leisure opportunities at home and identifying community resources. As in Phillipa's situation, this can involve working not only with the clients or carers but with others from health and social services, voluntary agencies and self advocacy groups.

Another aspect to consider is the definition and outcome of leisure in terms of play and enjoyment. Kielhofner (2002) defines leisure as an occupational performance domain of 'adult play'. For people with learning disabilities, taking the opportunity to develop skills through leisure experiences can be described as activities that also provide enjoyment. These concepts are discussed further in Chapter 8. It is often through our 'play' and leisure activities that we are able to participate in social situations and build relationships with others outside our immediate circle, leading to development of social skills, opportunities for trying, succeeding and enjoying new activities, keeping fit and making informed choices, etc. (Clark et al 1997).

Productivity

Productivity includes the occupations aimed at economic preservation, home and family maintenance, service, or personal development (McColl et al 2003).

Productivity can include '…paid or unpaid work, household management, school or play' (Law et al 2005). For people with a learning disability there are considerable limitations on the range of options and potential for development in this area. Historically, work roles were linked to sheltered workshops (refer to Chapter 2, Historical perspectives) and roles in large institutions where there was limited acknowledgement of the importance of employment as a significant route toward personal development and self-esteem for people with learning disabilities. Employment opportunity, whether in supported employment, voluntary work, or work experience enables the individual to develop skills in daily habits and daily or weekly routines, valued roles, potential for social integration and financial gain (refer to Chapter 7, Occupational choices – choosing employment). However, although acknowledged through Government policy (Valuing people; DoH 2002) and the development of many local supported employment initiatives, occupational therapists do not always take a lead role in this area. This may be for reasons of lack of expertise, local tradition or simply that therapists have not considered this as part of core skills for working with people with learning disabilities. There is, however, potential for occupational therapists to be involved at different levels of productivity from introducing skills to enabling the individual to participate in chosen productive occupations, to supporting through the whole employment process. Further postgraduate training will be required to engage fully in the latter but occupational therapists should consider their role in a range of productive occupations alongside leisure and ADL.

For example, if education is viewed as a productive activity, occupational therapists have an important part to play in liaising with educational programmes, supporting people to find educational opportunities to meet their needs, reinforcing learning in everyday occupations and working in collaboration with educational colleagues. Educational activities can also play an important role in social participation, enabling the individual to be involved in their community, take on roles in the family environment or engage with friends and peers.

Work and educational opportunities often have spin-offs in other areas of people's lives and challenges in this area may enable or limit people from forming relationships, being able to contribute to the 'fabric of society' (Law et al 1997) or take on valued roles. Examples of how ADL issues can influence productivity can be seen in the case of Amy presented later in this chapter and in Chapter 7.

Reader activity

- How would you define a productive role?
- What factors impact on developing a productive role?
- Who else would influence carrying out a productive role?

The links between health and well-being and productivity and leisure are important considerations for occupational therapists in this field. Occupational therapists may also become involved with enabling people to manage their health through contributing to health action plans. The wider role of occupation and its influence on health is a key consideration alongside the access to ordinary health care services required to support physical and mental health.

Working within the occupational therapy process

At each stage of the occupational therapy process occupational therapists will consider relevant procedures, criteria, knowledge base, generic and core skills, documentation and other people involved. The next section takes you through each stage of an occupational therapy process considering some of the challenges to occupation for people with learning disabilities. We have used the term 'client' to refer to a person referred to the occupational therapy service.

Referral

Occupational therapists working in learning disability services provide a service for people whose primary reason for referral relates to the effect of their learning disability upon their occupational performance (COT 2003).

Occupational therapists will accept referrals based on their ability to meet the above principle and professional requirements. This involves adherence to service procedures, including obtaining relevant information to make decisions about the appropriateness of referrals and working '…to a documented system for prioritising referrals which recognises levels and degrees of need and optimises the use of resources' (COT 2005, p. 9).

The reasons for referrals may relate to the individual's needs in ADL, leisure or productivity or from carers' or service providers' concern of changes in ability, during a transition process or crisis in which increased risk has arisen. The individual may also visit the GP or be admitted to hospital for a physical ailment or changes in mental health. Occupational therapists can therefore receive a referral for an individual in either health or social care settings and will consider the challenges to occupations and occupational performance in the defined areas.

At the referral stage of the occupational therapy process occupational therapists will be involved, either directly or indirectly, in the inter-professional decision-making process about whether a referral is accepted by the team and then whether it is relevant for the occupational therapist. Each team will have different procedures and criteria for making these decisions. The occupational therapist may need to make further analysis to prioritize urgency of the referrals and to assess the level of risk that the referral may present. In most instances the community learning disabilities team act as gate-keepers to other statutory services.

Procedures

Procedures in place in learning disability services may include: service agreements, consent process, risk assessments, referral forms and criteria, literature about the service and links with other services such as general practitioners. Occupational therapists should familiarize themselves with these processes and clarify their role in implementing them within the inter-professional team.

Information gathering

Once a referral is accepted occupational therapists will draw on their relevant generic and professionmake a decision specific knowledge base to make a decision about a preferred course of action. At this stage wide-ranging information is sought to enable the therapist to consider the client in relation to their individual wishes, their occupations and the environment in which they take place. Environmental influences, including the views of significant others, may have strong emphasis to inform the occupational therapy intervention. As the client may be unable to communicate their own needs, the therapist may need to apply more than one strategy to obtain information including:

- talking to family and carers
- having an initial meeting with the client
- observing client reactions to occupations in ordinary environments
- referring to past records
- researching the evidence base.

Care must be taken, however, not to lose sight of the client as central to the process of information gathering and to check their awareness of the referral and the information that will be gathered. Considering the influence of family and carers is also important as the occupational therapist may have to work through them to resolve issues for the client, so thinking about 'who the client is becomes paramount' (Law et al 2005 p. 44).

In addition, the occupational therapist should establish consent with the individual before undertaking any assessments and interventions, to fully engage them in the process and ensure that they are aware of and happy with the plan of action. Occupational therapists working with people with learning disability will also need to consider the client's ability to give consent, ways of increasing understanding of what is being asked and using advocates where necessary. 'The important aspect of consent in learning disabilities is ensuring that someone is able to fully understand what is being suggested before they can give informed consent.' (Carnaby 2004 p. 239.) Consent to intervention may be by a formal record or agreement between therapist and client or may be an accepted part of the referral process.

It is possible that the individual will have a history of little or no skill in a given area due to limited opportunity in their lifestyle or environment. Occupational imbalance, especially for those with profound disability, is often long standing with minimal leisure or productivity development and a focus on managing physical health and care needs. An individual with a mild or moderate learning disability, who previously was independent, might lose or regress in behaviour, become withdrawn or forgetful or need prompting for familiar tasks for a number of reasons including health and social. Often the main reason for referral may be rather general and the first meeting with the client will establish the main focus for involvement with them and identify whether there are additional areas that also need addressing.

In some cases it may be difficult to work on the issue for which the client has been referred until other issues have been resolved.

Before considering specific health and social care needs it may be helpful to look at broad diagnostic categories of learning disability (refer to Appendix 3.1). This will give the therapist an overview of the type and level of need that may be associated with the referral and an awareness of what could be expected at the initial meeting with the client. It is important also to remember that just because a person has a label of learning disability their current challenges may not be directly attributable to their learning disability but may be to do with other physical health, mental health or social issues. Although these may still have an impact on occupational performance and be appropriate for intervention, occupational therapists should remember that the impact of the therapist learning disability in managing other challenges is central to the therapist role. Specialist learning disability occupational therapists may, therefore take on a liaison or advisory role if the client's needs are not directly related to their learning disability (See Chapter 12). During information gathering therapists should also consider the pace and level of understanding of the client. This may make the intervention process much longer than in other fields and for the new therapist can take quite an adjustment. The purpose of information gathering is to enable occupational therapists to start to:

- build an occupational history
- consider which areas of occupation present challenges
- consider the context for occupational performance
- get an initial idea of the client's priorities.

Occupational therapists will need to work closely with support workers and parents or carers in this field and may rely on their support to implement and maintain interventions as well as advocating for the clients' needs, as in the case of Amy Box 3.3.

The issues that arose involved not only Amy but also her employer and co-workers. The occupational therapist's role was initially to focus on the ADL aspects rather than productivity. Working interprofessionally with Amy, her case manager and support worker, the issues of ADL were overcome, leading to improvement in her productivity role.

Amy illustrates how issues may arise in terms of the occupational impact and social values of ADL

Box 3.3

Case Illustration: Amy

Amy was referred by her employment trainer for an occupational therapy assessment. The referral was in relation to her personal care routine, regarding her lack of personal hygiene and body odour that had recently become an issue. The employment trainer raised concerns as other staff were complaining and they are ostracizing Amy. The employer is threatening to refuse to continue with her employment training. Until recently, Amy has been independent in most aspects of personal care. She has a good relationship with her case manager who has spoken to her about personal hygiene but Amy does not see it as a problem. She does, however, agree to meet with the occupational therapist. Amy shares a flat with another woman and has input from a support worker twice a week to help her to carry out shopping and general household cleaning. During the occupational therapy assessment, it was raised by Amy that she now has a new support worker. A further discussion, with both Amy and her new support worker, on routines, identified that Amy had run out of deodorants and kept forgetting to buy shampoo. She was also finding it increasingly difficult to get in and out of the bath due to morning stiffness in her hip joints. Working with Amy and the support worker the occupational therapist prioritized the need to establish a new routine i.e. once a week Amy and her support worker checked and made a shopping list of any items needed for showering and washing her hair and together would shop for necessary replacements. A second routine was established in which the support worker ensured that Amy used a diary to remind her to shower and wash her hair. Amy also identified that she missed going to the hairdressers and this was something she would like to do again. Following an assessment of bath transfers and bathroom safety a referral was made to Social Services for provision of grab rails and bath seat. Amy re-established her self-esteem through her improved appearance and her employment status was reinstated.

and productivity. The myriad possible reasons for referral are seen here and the therapist will wish to ask some key questions to both the referrer and to Amy about the referral in order to make decisions about what to work on and in what order. These questions may be based on service criteria for referral to the occupational therapist as mentioned above or stem from the occupational therapist's knowledge base about the presenting factors when first meeting the client.

Relationship building

The entire process of service delivery begins with a collaborative relationship with the client (Youngstrom et al 2002, p. 615).

An important part of the success of an intervention in this field is establishing a relationship with the individual that can be effective throughout the intervention process. The initial meeting with the client will begin this process but for the individual with a learning disability it may take much longer to establish a relationship because of communication issues or degree of learning disability. Therefore, a significant part of the initial referral and ongoing assessment process may involve spending time getting to know the person or spending time in their environment to observe daily routines and influences. When building a relationship, the occupational therapist allows time to get to know the client's perspective in a familiar environment. It is worth considering what the therapist contributes to building this relationship (expertise and experience of diagnoses and intervention strategies) and what the client's contribution is (expertise and experience of own values, goals and priorities and the impact of learning disability on them) so that the focus is on shared understanding in a collaborative relationship (Fisher 2003).

Assessment

Following referral, the next phase is the exploration of issues through the assessment process. The aim of assessment is to gather information that will enable the therapist, in collaboration with the client, to develop and prioritize clinical goals for intervention (Duncan 2006,).

... the evaluation (assessment) process is focused on finding out what the client wants and needs to do and on identifying those factors that act as supports or barriers to performance. (Youngstrom et al 2002, p. 616)

Youngstrom et al (2002) suggest that two main purposes of assessment are to identify an occupational profile and to analyse occupational performance. An occupational profile involves drawing up a picture of the person from an occupational perspective by considering what is important to them, what experiences and history have contributed to their current situation and what their main concerns and priorities are now. An occupational profile will be based on information gathered from a range of assessment strategies and will provide a written record on which to base your intervention. The team may use a standard format to record, such as the framework of a model or standard report format, but will generally contain the following information:

- occupational history and experiences
- daily patterns and routines
- important values and interests
- occupational performance in aspects of ADL, leisure and productivity (from client, others, your observations)
- challenges to occupations within these areas (from client, others)
- environments for occupational performance
- demands of the occupations
- client priorities.

Reader activity

Referring back to Amy, consider the following questions to build up an occupational profile for her:

- What could she be asked about her history and occupational experiences?
- What are her daily patterns and routines?
- What are her interests?
- What does she value?
- What does she see as her needs? What do others say?
- What challenges, problems or concerns does she have? What do others say?
- What are the environmental influences on her occupational performance?
- What are the demands of the occupations?
- What are her priorities?

Both the range and choice of assessments in learning disability broadly cover all the occupational and performance domains. Making an analysis of occupational performance within the various areas for which the person has been referred includes assessing '…the quality of the person's occupational performance as he or she interacts with the physical and social environment …' (Fisher 2003, p. 2).

It is important that the assessments carried out by the occupational therapist fit with the principles and philosophies for assessing people with learning disabilities and they may form part of an overall individual care plan for the service user. Carnaby (2004) gives helpful criteria for good practice in interviewing people with learning disabilities as part of the assessment process and suggests explaining the purpose of the interview, avoiding use of jargon and long sentences and using additional materials to enhance communication where possible. Further reading is recommended in Chapter 7 and also Carnaby (2004), which provides a useful resource on assessment, planning and intervention in the field of learning disabilities. People with learning disabilities may have a wider range of activities that need assessment and planning than the general population and they will often need more support to help them to lead their lives in a satisfying way (Carnaby 2004). The role that the occupational therapist can play in the assessment process is therefore significant.

Fisher (2003) proposes a 'top-down approach to assessment' starting with the ability of the person to perform occupations that are meaningful to them and enable them to fulfil life roles competently and be satisfied with them. This is in contrast to an approach which focuses on 'impairments and capacity limitations' and the impact of these on ability to carry out daily living tasks and roles. A top-down approach to assessment is particularly relevant for people with learning disabilities if we are to ensure processes that consider individuals as 'people first'.

In order to approach assessment in this way occupational therapists also have to establish a relationship with the individual that can be effective throughout the intervention process. As mentioned earlier, this relationship can take much longer to develop than in other fields of practice, so allowing time for relationship building needs to become a significant part of the assessment process.

It is important at this stage to choose assessment tools that will gain the information that is required to evaluate the needs of the client and are within the range of experience of the therapist.

Both standardized and non-standardized assessment tools may be useful but their common purpose is to gather and make sense of objective information with and for the individual and involves applying the following criteria from Laver Fawcett (2002 p. 128):

- Evaluative – appropriate to and sensitive to degree of change in performance
- Descriptive – providing information that identifies functional status or circumstances at one moment in time and provides descriptive baseline data across all occupational domains and circumstances
- Predictive – establishes predefined categories and attempts to predict an event or functional status and the need for generalization into another situation or environment
- Discriminative – comparative between a normative group or another diagnostic group, for example level of dysfunction in relation to expectations of performance for health, age, developmental level, or against the individual's previous functional status.

Observing occupations is the preferred method for assessment in the field of learning disabilities and these observations can be recorded using standardized or non-standardized assessment tools. Before considering specific tools for assessment it is therefore important to consider what is meant by observation.

Observing occupations

One of the most common assessment methods used in the learning disabilities field is the observation of set tasks or occupations that have significance to the client. This is an opportunity to make observations about the person (how they manage the demands of the task), the occupation (occupational analysis and the demands it presents) and the context in which that occupation takes place. Observation of clients can be based on set tasks within familiar environments and it is recommended that the client is seen across a variety of contexts both individually and with others, depending on the desired outcome of assessment (Carnaby 2004).

The client is observed participating in a set task to assess function; for example in ADL – dressing, in leisure – playing bowls, or towards skills in productivity – handling money or filing in a correct sequence. The task may require practical or social skills or a combination of the two. Carnaby (2004) also suggests that observational assessments should be carefully planned and individual consent obtained wherever possible. Objective observation (Fisher 2003) and recording is recommended to capture both breadth and depth of information. Non-standardized checklists based on occupational analysis may be used to record observations of performance in order to promote accuracy and reduce subjectivity. Checklists enable the therapist to record the performance elements of the occupation and to grade level of independence to dependence. Having reviewed the range of checklists available, they generally encompass the following areas:

- Functional/physical skills (i.e. integrity and ability of sitting and standing, balance, walking, range of movement and strength in upper limbs, bilateral co-ordination, prehension (grips to hold objects)
- Behavioural/psychological skills (i.e. ability to read, write, count, remember names, memory)
- Communication/social skills (i.e. talk, turn-take, smile)
- Environment (i.e. difficulty with using tools/furniture, or interacting in home, shops, work or college environments)
- Physical appearance – physique, posture, facial expressions, mannerisms, gait, dress, etc.
- Form and content of speech – insight into client's mood, insight, cognitive functioning, thought disorder
- Performance patterns – client's energy levels, diurnal variation, e.g. worse in the evening, interaction with others, initiative and skills.

Occupational and environmental analysis

In order to develop checklists and assessment tools, one of the occupational therapist's core skills – occupational analysis – has an important purpose in addressing occupational challenges and using occupations within the intervention to enable optimum occupational performance (Duncan 2006). Occupational analysis enables therapists to evaluate the demands of an occupation in terms of the skills needed to achieve it, its level of complexity, its social or cultural value, its component parts, sequence, tools and equipment needed to complete it and any safety or risk factors involved (Duncan 2006). Occupations not only require certain skills in order to perform them, they are also part of a system of roles and habits to organize and make them manageable as part of a person's life. In addition, they are

based on an individual's self-conceptions, values and interests and the way he/she carries them out will change over time during a person's life.

All occupations are intricately bound up with the environment (people, objects and events) in which they take place. Occupational analysis provides a framework for observing how individuals carry daily living activities such as dressing self, road safety skills, taking part in a social outing or working in a supported employment situation (for further reading see Nelson & Jepson-Thomas 2003, Laver-Fawcett 2007). Occupational analysis can also be applied for an activity outside the individual's daily routine to assess or promote a specific skill/experience.

Environmental analysis also forms an important part of the assessment process, enabling the therapist to consider the benefits, constraints, challenges and supports afforded by the various environments in which the individual operates. This provides causal or explanatory information about the way that the individual functions.

Choosing assessment tools

Carnaby (2004) stresses the importance of choosing assessment tools that: (i) are directly linked to the individual, their context and the issues of concern; (ii) are reliable and valid; (iii) are efficient in that 'the outcome is worth the effort made' and; (iv) fulfil a useful purpose.

There has been a long history in the field of learning disabilities of the use of non-standardized assessments and using …home-grown evaluation tools without known validity and reliability' (Fisher 2001). It has been suggested that the use of norm referenced, standardized assessments not appropriate for clients with a learning disability as it is not viable to compare one client's performance with that of another. In addition, it is difficult to establish normative data in occupations such as self-care, productivity and leisure and constructing a reliable and valid test for this client group (Swee Hong et al 2000). However, it is important to acknowledge that standardized and well validated outcome measures can, and do, provide objective data to ensure a service is establishing results in line with clinical governance and evidence-based practice (Laver Fawcett 2007). For occupational therapists, there is a challenge to establish both good quality measures within the learning disability field, and to justify and evaluate the use of non-standardized assessment tools.

However, there are a wide range of assessment tools that have been specifically designed for use by occupational therapists that focus on occupational areas and performance within the from the perspectives of both client and occupational therapist. When choosing an assessment for use with people with learning disability the therapist should consider:

- appropriateness of referral request
- training needs
- appropriateness of assessment for people with learning disabilities
- how the assessment is implemented
- ensuring client-centred involvement
- outcome required.

Use of standardized assessments

Most standardized assessments, including those most frequently used by occupational therapists, assess performance components and specific areas such as balance, visual-motor skills and visual perceptual skills rather than actual performance in functional activities of self-care, leisure and productivity. They are generally, however, not standardized nor validated for people with a learning disability. The feasibility of using a standardized assessment tool can be limited with an individual who has poor verbal communication or who is profoundly disabled. Ability and skill of the individual can vary from one day to the next due to health status, medication or environmental stressors. Equally, the length of time to administer either interview or observation methods to complete a standardized instrument can impact on the individual's responses (refer to Chapter 4). Useful information can, however, be gained by ensuring a more informal approach to the assessment in a familiar environment. The occupational therapist needs to gauge the value of the information gained either from the client or carer and may well decide on a non standardized assessment to supplement the results of a standardized tool.

There are many other examples of standardized and self-report assessment tools that could be considered for their merits with people with learning disabilities. It is essential to choose tools that enable assessment of occupational performance and are adaptable for use with clients with specific communication or learning needs. Assessment tools that are embedded within the framework provided by a model of practice may also be a considered

choice as they are supported by a clear evidence base and provide technical tools for application to practice. Examples of this may be tools associated with the Model of Human Occupation (Kielhofner 2002) which '...are specifically built to support occupation-focused practice...' and include a range of assessments, case studies, published articles and manuals and record-keeping documentation (Forsyth & Kielhofner 2006).

Two examples of standardized tools available to occupational therapists are given below to demonstrate some of the considerations when choosing tools for use in the learning disabilities field.

The Assessment of Motor Process Skills (AMPS)

'[AMPS]...is a standardised method for implementing performance analyses' (Fisher 2006). It is designed to measure the quality of an individual's performance in domestic and self-care ADL by focusing on the motor and process skills required to successfully achieve them. ADL motor skills are described '...as observable goal directed actions....' used to move oneself and task objects, whilst ADL process skills are '...the observable actions of performance... .' that enable a person to sequence tasks, choose relevant tools and materials and make performance adjustments where necessary (Fisher 2003). A main benefit of using AMPS with people with learning disabilities is its focus on assessing the individual's ability in the occupations that are relevant and meaningful to them. The assessment has been validated with wide-ranging client groups, including people with learning disabilities, and is not diagnosis specific. As an outcome measure it enables the therapist to compare ability at initial assessment with re-evaluation and provides occupational therapists with a sensitive, validated and reliable tool for planning interventions and recording change. In administering the tool it is recognized that the assessor may need to rephrase questions and adapt the language used or involve a carer in order to involve the client in the process. Use of AMPS requires Raters to undergo training in its administration and scoring.

The Canadian Occupational Performance Measure (COPM)

The COPM (Law et al 2005), is a tool that focuses on a service users self-perception of their occupational performance in terms of rating of their priorities in ADL occupations, their perceived ability at their chosen tasks and their level of satisfaction with their performance. The COPM is described as '…an individualised measure designed for use by occupational therapists to detect change in a client's self-perception of occupational performance over time' (Law et al 2005, p. 1).

The COPM uses self-report as the main means of gathering data through interviewing the client and using self-rating scales. There can be difficulty in the use of self-rating scales with people with a learning disability. The concepts or language used for a rating scale (i.e. COPM – 'I do this extremely well') may cause lack of understanding or inability to acknowledge a difficulty. Willingness to comply with the therapist may also produce a positive rather than negative response to a question. There is limited literature on the use of the COPM with people with learning disabilities but the current manual (Law et al 2005, p. 41) does explore use of a proxy respondent or alternative respondent, both of which may be applicable to people with learning disability who are unable to respond fully themselves. In both these cases there are issues of who the respondent should be and how to implement client-centred practice, whilst also managing the views of different stakeholders in the assessment process. Law et al (2005 p. 41) state that '…the client is the one who is expected to make change as a result of therapy.' There may be a '…need to possibly modify the interviewing approach, the language of the assessment, or the scoring system…' (Law et al 2005) to enable the individual to acknowledge or communicate their own goals or needs. This is quite acceptable within the administration guidelines.

The COPM's intended use for client-centred practice makes it an appropriate framework for enabling occupation and placing the client at the centre of the assessment process from the start. This is a compelling reason for using it with this client group where historically they may have been marginalized during the assessment process.

Use of non-standardized assessments

Occupational therapists are faced with the task of establishing credible measures that record and respond to the interventions targeted, identify the elements to change for the individual with a learning disability and reflect occupational therapy ethos. For these reasons many assessments used in learning disabilities are non-standardized and this raises the question: Are assessments based on observation and interviews valid? Non-standardized assessment methods have attracted criticism, particularly in the development of assessment systems locally (Swee Hong et al 2000). The use of unreliable instruments to measure outcome is likely to seriously diminish the credibility of both the service and the professional (Chesson et al 1996). There is also the danger of subjective judgements by the occupational therapists on the effect of effort and time of intervention on a client. Ethical implications are paramount if intervention decisions are based on questionable assessment data (Laver Fawcett 2007). It is arguable, however, that non-standardized assessments are a legitimate tool for occupational therapy in learning disability as they can provide useful information when appropriate standardized assessments are not available. Also, people with learning disabilities may feel more comfortable with a less formal and systematic approach to assessment.

Occupational therapists use or develop specific non-standardized assessments based mainly on observational data of people with a learning disability, and more often a combination of observation of occupations, occupational analysis and inter-professional assessment tools.

Other non-standardized assessments

Occupational therapists working in an inter-professional team may also make use of assessment tools and checklists developed by others in the team or work in collaboration with others to jointly assess client needs. If the assessment contributes to health and social care assessment processes it is important to co-ordinate the information gathered through liaison with colleagues, carers and the client themselves.

Planning

… a plan that is developed based on the results of the evaluation (assessment) process and describes selected occupational therapy approaches and types of interventions to reach client's targeted outcomes (Youngstrom et al 2002).

Occupational therapists will be concerned at this stage with the options available to meet client goals, their own tools and processes for implementing these and most importantly how they can work in collaboration with the client to draw up an agreed plan of action that is client centred. For people with learning disability this last aspect is particularly important to ensure that they understand the purpose of the plan or the therapist may need to work through an advocate or carer.

The planning stage focuses on creating a plan that meets client goals, wishes and needs and considers what the therapist needs to do to put the plan into action.

Choosing models and frames of reference

The therapist and occupational therapy service may choose to work within a conceptual model of practice such as the person–environment model of occupational performance (PEOP) (Christiansen & Baum 1997), the Canadian Model of Occupational Performance (CMOP) (CAOT 1997) the Model of Human Occupation (MOHO) (Kielhofner 2002), or the Model of Competent Occupational Performance in the Environment (Hagedorn 2000). The application of a model to structure the occupational therapy process offers one way of naming, validating and prioritizing occupational performance problems and then to use relevant theoretical approaches, contextual conditions and strengths and resources to design an action plan that will meet goals. By using the framework of a model of occupational therapy the therapist can explore with the individual person (personality, needs, drives, desires and their capabilities) the components of their lifestyle and the context of the whole environment. In this way the concept of occupation and client-centeredness is ensured. For further reading on models, refer to Duncan (2006), Hagedorn (2000), Keilhofner (2002) and Law et al (1997).

Forsyth & McMillan (2001) propose the 'top-down' approach, discussed earlier, to demonstrate how the occupation paradigm influences the practice of occupational therapy and that knowledge from sources outside the occupational therapy domain needs to be 'filtered' by what they call the 'occupation filter' in order to use it in an occupational therapy specific way. The 'top-down' approach shows how occupational therapists use their profession-specific philosophies and knowledge base, including conceptual models of practice, to inform their practice and to inform the use of external bodies of knowledge such as frames of reference. For further reading on the top-down approach, refer to McMillan (2006).

Frames of reference

A frame of reference is the organization of theory, which may be from different disciplines (e.g. social or psychological theories). Within the learning disability field there are often complex needs of a physical, social and psychological nature which require intervention over a long period of time and the use of several complementary frames of reference to meet them. Occupational therapists working in the learning disabilities field can choose from the range of frames of reference available to guide their practice (Parker 2006) and act as 'a mechanism which links theory to practice' (Mosey 1981, cited in Duncan 2006). It is worth noting that the terms 'frame of reference', 'approach' or 'theoretical models' are often interchangeable or synonymous within current literature. Occupational therapists will therefore draw on complementary theories or bodies of knowledge to guide their practice depending on the reasons for referral. Those most commonly used by occupational therapists in the learning disabilities field include the developmental, rehabilitative and learning frame of references (Turner et al 2002). The developmental frame of reference refers to facilitating function through normal developmental stages. The rehabilitative frame of reference applies a variety of activities, techniques and methods to improve functional competence in everyday activities through enabling the client to develop or compensate. The theories within the learning frame of reference support the ethos that the individual's capacity to learn may promote positive change in occupational performance. This learning may be in acquisition of new knowledge and skills or insights into their behaviour. It is not the purpose of this chapter to discuss in detail frames of references as more detailed coverage of theory and current thinking on how they influence practice can be found in the recommended reading listed at the end of this chapter (Duncan 2006, Creek 2006, Turner et al 2002). However, these are briefly discussed below in choosing an approach to practice for people with learning disabilities.

Goal setting

Goals can be seen as '...targets that the client hopes to reach through involvement in occupational therapy' (Creek 2002 p. 129). When setting goals with people with learning disabilities it is particularly important to ensure that the goals are client centred.

There is a long history of service goals and carers' goals being met with the service users' needs coming low down on the priority list. 'It is important that care planning remains person centred in its approach and does not let organizational concerns and priorities make the individual's involvement in decision-making seem less important' (Carnaby 2004 p. 103). For this reason you may need to adapt terminology or grade the planning processes to help the client to actively participate in goal setting. Current service philosophies and principles encourage client-centred approaches and occupational therapy philosophy fits well with these values. Occupational therapists should also consider how goals for occupational therapy intervention fit with person-centred plans or health action plans if the client has them.

Goals should be both achievable and reviewable and practical measurements implemented so that both the therapist and the client know what will change or what new thing will be learnt to demonstrate that the goal has been achieved. People with learning disabilities may need support through this process and the therapist may need to work through others such as carers to implement goals and review progress. If this is the case it is important that the carer has been involved in negotiations with the therapist and client so that they also have ownership of the goals and are able to ensure that they are carried out when the therapist is not there. Deciding whose role it is to review progress on goals and at what point is also important. Occupational therapists need a flexible approach to acknowledge, understand and work with the individual or parent/carer to attain achievable, clearly defined, short-term and well-structured goals. In this way clear, tangible steps are developed leading to long-term goals of a more complex nature. It is important at this stage to hear what is being said, especially in relation to the long-term goals, and to consider how realistic and achievable they are and what resources should be employed to achieve them. Occupational therapists will focus on practical resources but also on client strengths that will enable them to work on the goals set.

By negotiating and adapting the activities within an occupation to the individual's pace, the client, carers and occupational therapist can agree methods of action towards short- and long-term goals. In some instances this may include the use of a written or verbal (i.e. on a tape) contract to enable the individual to understand and refer to the goals. At this point there may also be the need to involve other professionals or services such as a support worker for long-term maintenance of a programme.

Ultimately, the occupational aims for the intervention are towards achieving the goals and improving quality of life (Fresher-Samwaysk et al 2003). By applying the occupational therapy process to Amy's situation, some of these issues will be illustrated. At the start, the referral was for an assessment in relation to personal care and hygiene. The observational assessments identified that Amy's skill level had not diminished. However, Amy's change in support worker and environmental circumstances decreased her level of independence, which had implications for her social status, her productivity, her potential for appropriate choice and increased risk of injury in an activity of self-care. Through initial assessment and occupational self assessment (OSA) (Keilhofner 2002) Amy identified that 'I can't get into the bath'. For her case manager and work trainer the priority was concern about her lack of hygiene and the possibility of being withdrawn from the work training scheme appeared insurmountable. For Amy the main difficulty was the inaccessibility of the bath. To improve her quality of life her goals were identified in the following areas:

- *Personal growth accomplishments* – Amy wanted to re-establish her level of independent routines in the home and work especially her time keeping (e.g. getting up in the morning to have time to have a shower).

- *Physical independence improving self confidence and self esteem* – Amy wanted to improve her personal hygiene and go to the hairdressers. From the assessment, the occupational therapist identified that Amy had independent skills in self care, and making appropriate choices but lacked confidence. This was also because she did not have the opportunity to express these choices within the home and work routine. With the assistance of the support worker Amy established new daily and weekly routines. Purchase of a very loud alarm clock enabled Amy to get up in the morning on time. Amy wrote a shopping list each week for personal items and shopped for them with the assistance of the support worker. Amy practised telephone conversations to make an appointment with the local hairdresser.

- *Transportation/physical accessibility reducing risk factors* – Amy wanted to use the bath. The risk assessment identified that Amy had difficulty balancing to step into the bath to use the over-bath shower. Once grab rails and a bath seat had been provided the occupational therapist carried out a task analysis with Amy to enable her to learn to use the bath seat and grab rails to an independent level.
- *Personal and work relationships: i.e. awareness of issues of relationship, friendships* – Amy wanted to continue her work experience and make friends. Because of the issue of poor personal hygiene, Amy felt isolated and embarrassed. Improvement in her appearance and personal hygiene enabled Amy to integrate within the work place once more. A local women's group was identified and Amy agreed to attend with her support worker.

Outcome measures

Measuring success is often achieved using the same assessment measures used at the initial and ongoing assessment and looking for significant changes in the desired direction (Duncan 2006 p. 55).

As mentioned earlier under assessment, occupational therapists will want to consider measures that can demonstrate progress and achievement against goals set. Some assessment tools are designed to be used as outcome measures by being used to assess and then re-assess prior to discharge. However, at the planning stage the therapist may also consider other indicators of change in a client's performance such as repeat observational assessment. Choice of measure will depend on the client and therapist's discussion and identifying that which best or most easily reflects the goals that have been set and takes into account the client's needs.

Option appraisal

To make the most effective use of available resources and to choose actions that are relevant to meeting client goals occupational therapists should identify and appraise the range of available options. This will involve making decisions about resources, including time, expertise and practical resources, who will best carry out the goals set, where they will happen

and the level of intensity of the intervention. Some issues may be resolved quickly by provision of equipment or adaptation to physical environment whereas others may be more complex and time intensive. Option appraisal helps the therapist to ensure that the client is involved in both problem identification and problem solving. It also enables the therapist to negotiate a way forward with the individual that is best for them rather than relying on problem resolution based on past experience of working with similar clients. This is an opportunity for the therapist to share her clinical reasoning and consider practical ways of involving the client in decision making and brainstorming options for intervention.

Practical arrangements

The planning stage is also the place to decide on the practical arrangements for the intervention such as time, location, transport, frequency, who will be involved, equipment and materials and to set review dates. When working with people with learning disabilities or their advocates it may be particularly relevant to have written records or prompts to the client to remind them about the practical arrangements and to engage them in the process. It is also important at this stage to ensure that the roles of others that need to be carried out are agreed and made possible by establishing the importance and value of them in relation to meeting the client's needs.

Discharge

Setting goals also enables the therapist to establish with the client what is to be offered, why, and when it will end. Of course the same client may well be referred for additional issues or these may be spotted during intervention but they should be seen as distinct interventions rather than ongoing intervention for the same thing.

Intervention

Interventions are designed to foster engagement in occupations and activities to support participation in life...Intervention is the process of putting the plan into action (Youngstrom et al 2002 p. 618).

At this stage therapists will be implementing the action plan designed earlier by choosing approaches and occupations that can be used therapeutically or are already a part of the client's repertoire. For many people with learning disability the main aim will be to provide opportunities to try new occupations and experiences as their past may have been lacking in chances for real participation in valued, meaningful or age appropriate activities. This may be due to low expectations, residential constraints or carer's concerns of risk. Thus, enabling a person to become an active contributor and participator to their community can be central to occupational therapy practice in this field rather than the rehabilitation emphasis in other fields. Consequently, people with learning disabilities may not be aware of the choice of occupations available to help them meet their needs and the steps needed to achieve them realistically. Duncan (2006) states that choosing relevant occupations to be used in interventions requires a balance between the needs of the individual, the therapist's skills and resources and the conceptual model or frame of reference in which they are working. The important aspect is that occupations are chosen individually to enable people with learning disabilities to achieve their goals and quality of life.

Choosing approaches to practice

Occupational therapists working in the learning disabilities field can use different approaches to implement the knowledge base into practice. Creek (2002, p. 46) defines an 'approach' as '...ways and means of putting theory into practice'. The therapist will require an in-depth understanding of the relevant theory and body of knowledge (i.e. a frame of reference) to direct the approach towards achieving the desired outcome. Working with an individual with a learning disability may involve, for example, the therapist applying knowledge of development theories from the development frame of references. The occupational therapist may use a sensory integration approach based on a developmental frame of reference to encourage a more functional motor or sensory response for the client. The therapist 'requires a depth of knowledge about motor control and how the central nervous system works to produce controlled movement' in order to direct their approaches at '...recovery and improvement in motor performance.' (Feaver & Edmunds 2006 in Duncan 2006). Application of a developmental approach is presented in Chapter 6.

Biomechanical and compensatory approaches

For an individual with a learning disability changes to movement, musculoskeletal integrity and stamina issues can arise from birth or due to the ageing process, disease or injury that will have a direct bearing on changes to occupational performance rather than the learning disability. Duncan (2006) states the importance of the application of a biomechanical approach to involve interventions of meaningful occupation to '...restore, maintain or compensate for lost (temporary or permanent) occupational performance....'(p. 265). Working within the rehabilitation frame of reference the therapist uses biomechanical and compensatory principles to identify and address issues of occupational performance in ADL, productivity and leisure.

As in any field of work, occupations may need to be adapted with regard to environment, equipment, social, physical, cognitive, emotional, temporal or structural aspects in order to meet client needs. For people with learning disabilities it is most likely that the way the occupation is presented will have as much influence as the actual occupation chosen. Occupational therapists will put much thought into how they will introduce an occupation to the client, also whether grading will need to be considered to enable the client to develop occupational performance over time and with a positive experiences of success – something which many people with learning disability have not experienced due to others' low expectations or assuming failure before they have even tried.

The aim of compensation is not to change the individual's disability but to enable them to manage the impact of that disability through adaptation of the occupation or skill, use of equipment or support from others. Compensation thus involves the use of devices attached to the body (e.g. hand splint) or involves modifying or replacing objects to perform routine tasks. It may also involve the changing of procedures to accomplish a task including the use of others to assist with the activity. For an individual with a learning disability there is often a need for a graded, timed approach to the introduction of any compensatory mechanism to enable the individual to learn how to adapt or use the new method. This process may take months to achieve and require training of others as well as the individual. These considerations should be built into the intervention plan when using this approach.

Both the biomechanical and compensatory approaches have limitations. There is a danger of taking a reductionist view by focusing on fixing specific problem areas rather than using a holistic approach to overcome difficulties and enable occupation. Therapists should also consider the cognitive and/or psychological impact of introducing adaptations, new routines or new methods to the individual. Their willingness to accept compensatory approaches will be key to the success of the intervention.

In the case of Amy one of her major hurdles was getting in and out of the bath. Her inability to shower and wash her hair caused her to become flustered and embarrassed when faced with comments at work and at home. One way to overcome this was to compensate for her physical difficulties with the provision of a bath seat and grab rails. This also involved teaching Amy a new technique for getting in and out of the bath when using the new equipment. The learning frame of reference (see below) was also applied here to enable her to become independent in her personal care. Amy also needed help with identifying, making a choice and buying personal care items such as shampoo or deodorant. This was achieved by involving and informing Amy and the support worker in the use of prompts on a daily or weekly basis. In this way, Amy quickly, independently established daily routines of ADL and to make a shopping list for items needed once a week.

Learning frame of reference

A key element of change is some alteration in internal or external circumstances that results in the emergence of novel thoughts, feelings and behaviours (Keilhofner 2002, p. 41).

There are several learning approaches that can be used in the learning disabilities field that are based on the learning frame of reference. Understanding how people learn and what motivates learning in a particular setting is vital to ensure motivation for the individual to participate and learn. (Some of the theories underpinning learning are summarized in Box 3.4).

Educative approach

This approach is directed at providing specific information to enhance the knowledge base of the client, parent or carer (Foster 2002). The key word

Box 3.4

Examples of theories underpinning learning

- Humanistic – how the individual perceives and feels about themselves (self concept and striving for growth)
- Cognitive theory, e.g. attribution theory – self-perception. If success or failure is attributed to effort the individual will try again. If failure is attributed to task difficulty or lack of ability the individual will not put in effort or more time
- Social learning theory – importance of modelling behaviour to learning and emotions
- Behaviourism – importance of extrinsic and intrinsic motivation
- Experiential learning – use of discovery learning relates to the emotional connection of a learning experience.

---

is information and the importance of the appropriate method and level of communication to inform the person with a learning disability. By establishing clear outcomes, information is given to the individual or carer by visual (i.e. photographic) or verbal methods. For example the use of leaflets, symbolic or colour-coded cues, picture representation of a task sequence, information for carers on sensory integration, developing an individual audio tape or video for relaxation techniques or use of a diary (e.g. as used by Amy to remember hair appointments). Reinforcing aspects of the information can be made through discussion on a one to one or group basis.

Social learning approach

Poorly developed social skills are often prevalent in individuals with a learning disability. These can include poor conversational skills, inappropriate table manners, inappropriate or poorly groomed appearance, or impairment of work capacity such as lack of initiative or organizational skills. However, for individuals with a learning disability there is often a disparity in occupational knowledge and occupational action because of a lack of self-efficacy and opportunity to develop this belief or skill. This suggests that an individual may know how to do something but not perform. People with a high degree of self-efficacy believe that they can achieve and set personal goals, whilst people with a low degree of self-efficacy do not. Social skills training can be a key component of a client-centred approach if the individual has a lack of social or ADL skills and the assumption is that the individual can be independent. Social groups have a major impact on the development of positive roles and behaviours and can form the basis of both intervention and ongoing assessment of social skills development. Assertiveness training is an important area of social skills training. Amy's reliance on her previous support worker left her bereft of the self belief that she could ask for help both at home and at work. Attending the women's group gave her the opportunity to practise through role play and discussions assertive techniques to ask for help.

Experiential learning

We all learn by trial and error and in doing so we calculate the risks involved and the possibility of failure. It is likely that we rarely go into a situation without having some previous knowledge of that situation. Very often an individual with a learning disability has a long history of failure and rejection, or overprotection resulting in lack of opportunity to learn from new experiences. According to Gibbs (1988) learning from experience must involve links between the doing and the thinking. Gibbs suggests that using a four-stage model of learning as published by Kolb (1984) can help to explain how people learn from experience. The four-stage model of 'learning by doing' involves having an experience, reflecting on it, abstract conceptualization and then active experimentation based on reflections and learning (Kolb 1984). In this way individuals are encouraged to consider what they felt about the experience, what they might do differently, what information might support their experience and practising again based on new learning.

Occupational therapists working with people with learning disability can use this approach to learning as a non-specific way of offering a variety of life's opportunities to an individual. The aim would be that once an individual has experienced the opportunity, he or she is able to make an informed choice about doing it again. If offered in a safe environment with support from the occupational therapist to identify and address risks this can be a powerful way of providing guided learning opportunities. Risk assessment is therefore fundamental to planning and implementing any experiential learning opportunity. Risk of psychological, social or physical barriers to positive learning can be minimized by giving the individual the opportunity to identify and seek out information prior to undertaking new experiences and practising social skills on an individual or group basis with the occupational therapist. This can involve establishing what information is required such as times of opening, transport, or to produce prompt cards, or verbal instructions with appropriate cues (e.g. diagrams, leaflets, self-monitoring forms) to be incorporated later into ongoing homework for the individual's circumstances. Task-specific homework could include practising answering the telephone, asking for the price of an item when shopping or saying no in an appropriate way. Homework may also include self-evaluation of the outcome with feedback and discussion at the group's next meeting. For Amy her attendance at the group and homework enabled her to identify risks, practise assertiveness techniques of language, listening and initiating and ending conversations, and discuss issues of health in a safe environment.

Cognitive behavioural therapy (CBT)

CBT is the fusion of behavioural and cognitive theories. It is not the purpose of this chapter to discuss in detail these two theories as they are comprehensively discussed in other texts (refer to Stein & Cutler 2002, Creek 2002). However, it is useful to consider briefly the two components that underpin the CBT frame of reference. Cognitive therapy encourages the individual to verbalize thoughts and feelings to examine and interpret the emotional response such as fear or anxiety. By then using behavioural techniques, the individual is able to develop new ways of dealing with everyday situations. The concept of verbalizing thoughts and feelings has not historically been feasible for people with a learning disability. Historically, 'behavioural therapy' has been used with people with a learning disability seeking to address behavioural aspects rather than on an understanding of the internal schemas of the individual. Based on the principles of learning from Pavlov and Skinner the techniques include classical and operant conditioning through reward or punishment. Behavioural techniques used for people with learning disabilities include the following:

- Task analysis (*not* activity analysis) (forward, backward chaining by establishing criteria, steps, prompts)

- Systematic instruction has been used in relation to learning work tasks utilizing a prescribed task analysis with standardized conditions
- Gentle teaching for those with a profound learning disability; this is a method of communication, interaction with positive feedback.

Duncan (2006) states that CBT takes a '...problem-focused perspective of life difficulties' and focuses on them in relation to thoughts, behaviours, emotions physical responses and the environment (p. 220). The CBT approach uses techniques such as role play, reminiscence, reality orientation, or exploration of stress management techniques to enable the individual to gain insight into a particular situation and also others' perceptions of that situation. Exploration and practice of coping strategies can also be used for assertiveness, perception of risks or memory training (e.g. shopping route, bus training).

Specific occupational therapy interventions are discussed further in other chapters in more depth in relation to the individual needs of activities of daily living (Chapter 6), productivity (Chapter 7) and leisure (Chapter 8). Further reading on frames of reference is recommended in Duncan (2006) and underpinning theory of psychosocial approaches in Stein & Cutler (2002), Creek (2002).

Intervention review

Intervention review is defined as a continuous process for re-evaluating and reviewing the intervention plan, the effectiveness of its delivery and the progress towards targeted outcomes. (Youngstrom et al 2002).

This is an essential part of implementing the intervention plan and occupational therapists should continue to check progress against goals with the client as well as formal evaluation at an agreed time at the end of the intervention.

Evaluation

Evaluation is the process by which the client, the therapist and other relevant individuals (such as carers) or bodies (such as the multidisciplinary team) know if agreed goals have been met (Duncan 2006, p. 55).

As discussed previously, in the planning stage relevant outcome measures are chosen against which the success of the occupational therapy intervention can now be evaluated. For people with learning disabilities it is important to return to the earlier principles of considering ways that they and their supporters can be actively involved in the evaluation process so that they are aware of progress and achievements and can contribute to decisions that will be made as a result of the evaluation. The choice of assessments will influence the type of evaluation; for example, if COPM (Law et al 2005) is used then the client will be required to repeat the self-assessment questions to see if there have been changes in levels of satisfaction and ability for areas of occupation chosen as priorities. If AMPS (Fisher 2003) is used then a repeat of the assessment will be required to measure progress against agreed goals. For unstructured assessments the therapist may repeat the checklist or have put other measures into place to acknowledge when success will be noted, for instance observing the client carrying out an occupation independently on more than one occasion. Standardized and non-standardized assessments enable the occupational therapist to establish a base lines for evaluation of the client for the following reasons:

- Assessment and outcome information can provide important feedback to enable and improve occupational therapy clinical practice and decision making
- It can determine how and in what way interventions for clients can be improved or changed over a short or long period of time
- It can also allow benchmarking and comparison to provide effective and efficient services across this client group
- It can be used to monitor staff competency and identify training needs and staff continual professional development (CPD) – (e.g. postgraduate sensory integration training, AMPS training)
- Evidence of effectiveness for both clients and families is important in today's health and social service provision. Accountability is paramount to both clients and their families as well as commissioners of services.
- Feedback for families and clients to enable them to make appropriate choices as well as access

appropriate services through statutory or private means.

Developing good quality measures is something that takes several years and extensive research. If a standardized measure has been adapted or altered to fit a particular service or client group such as learning disability then '...once a measure has been altered or adapted, assessment results are no longer proven to be valid or reliable....' (Clarke et al 2001, p. 11).

Discharge and referral

Traditionally, in occupational therapy for people with learning disabilities there was often a blanket referral system and an unspoken expectation that occupational therapy would be ongoing across the person's lifespan. The move to community-based services has gradually seen a departure from this view; nevertheless, people with learning disabilities may be on the occupational therapist's case load for a long time due to the nature of the intervention. It is important to review each episode of care carefully and to demonstrate when one area has been resolved or handed back to the client/carer for continued work and which areas continue to need direct intervention.

Following evaluation a decision is made about aspects of the intervention that have been completed, for example by achieving goals set or the client deciding to end intervention. At this stage new needs may have been identified for further referral to the occupational therapist or to other members of the team. It is particularly important when working with clients with learning disabilities to inform them clearly about why the intervention has ended, what should happen if further needs occur and to share this information with relevant carers and other members of the team. It may be that the client is still involved with other members of the CLDT and therefore the occupational therapist can review progress and may choose to initiate a referral if ongoing occupational performance needs are identified.

From the referral phase of the occupational therapy process the occupational therapist should be able to demonstrate that the intervention implemented is evidence based. In learning disability services, there is a need to demonstrate an explicitly client-centred approach, to justify clinical judgement, and establish clinical expertise. Evidence-based practice can be demonstrated through a hierarchy of evidence either by systematic review, randomized controlled trials, non-randomized experimental studies, non-experimental studies, respected, expert opinion and client feedback. However, in the learning disabilities field the difficulty is that the occupational therapy evidence is not easily apparent. The challenge is to establish how this can be formulated (refer to Chapter 13) to demonstrate effective clinical practice for audit and evaluative purposes in line with clinical governance. As occupational therapists working in learning disabilities 'evidence' can be gained by searching and exploring the literature of both occupational therapy and other relevant texts on, for example, one or more of the following areas:

- sensory processing
- sensory integration
- adults – dual diagnosis
- learning disabilities
- developmental disabilities
- psychological theories
- occupational therapy
- occupations of ADL, leisure and productivity.

Evidence-based practice within a learning disability service can also be linked to the frame of reference as well as shared knowledge (e.g. with other professionals within a community learning disability team) to apply or change the type of interventions used with a client with a learning disability. Underpinning any occupational therapy intervention is the humanistic philosophy and client-centeredness of occupations. When working with a client with a learning disability the occupational therapist will identify that what can work with one client may not necessarily work with another.

Summary

This chapter has taken the reader through the stages of the occupational therapy process and highlighted some of the key considerations for the occupational therapist at each stage. Case illustrations have provided insights into the types of issues that therapists may encounter in their day-to-day practice and some ways of addressing them within the process. Further chapters in the book focus on specific issues and provide more detail.

Box 3.5

Case illustration: Freda

Freda is a 34-year-old woman with a moderate learning disability. She has recently recovered from a period of depression for which she was treated. However, she had withdrawn from college where she was attending a catering course and lost her confidence in going out on her own. Previously she was independent in going on her own to college and a friend's house. The referral for occupational therapy was received from her mother who was concerned about her withdrawn behaviour. Freda lives with her mother and stepfather. Through initial assessment Freda identified the following as her priority: '*To go on a bus on my own to go back to college and get a job*'. Following further assessments the occupational therapist identified that Freda had difficulty with remembering things and became anxious about going out. She has some basic ability in numeracy and literacy.

1. What assessments would you use for Freda?
2. What aims would be relevant for Freda?
3. What approach(es) would you implement to enable Freda to catch a bus? Indicate how you would record and monitor progression/improvement.
4. How would you evaluate the outcome?

Further reading

Creek J (ed.) 2006 Occupational therapy and mental health, 4th edn. Edinburgh, Churchill Livingstone

Duncan E (ed.) 2006 Foundations for practice in occupational therapy, 4th edn. Elsevier, Edinburgh

Gillman M 2004 Diagnosis and Assessment in the lives of disabled people: creating potential/limiting possibilities. In: Swain J, French S, Barnes C, Thomas C (eds) Disabling barriers – enabling environments, 2nd edn. London, Sage

Holt G, Hardy S, Bouras N (eds) 2005 Mental health in learning disabilities. Brighton, Pavilion Publishing

Stein F, Cutler SK 2002 Psychosocial occupational therapy. A holistic approach, 2nd edn. Albany, Delmar

Watson D 2003 Causes and manifestations of learning disabilities. In: Gates B (ed.) Learning disabilities towards inclusion, 4th edn. London, Elsevier

References

Canadian Association of Occupational Therapists 1997 Enabling occupation: An occupational therapy perspective. Ottawa ON, CAOT Publications ACE

Carnaby S (ed.) 2004 Learning disability today. Brighton, Pavilion Publishing Ltd

Chesson R, Macleod M, Massie S 1996 Outcome measures used in therapy departments in Scotland. Physiotherapy 82(12):673–679

Christiansen CH, Baum CM (eds) 1997 Occupational therapy: enabling function and well-being. New Jersey, Slack

Clarke C, Sealey-Lapes C, Kotsch L 2001 Outcome measures: information pack for occupational therapy. London, COT

Clark F, Azen SP, Zemke R et al 1997 Occupational therapy for independent-living older adults. JAMA 278:1321–1326

College of Occupational Therapists 2003 Principles for education and practice: occupational therapy services for adults with learning disability. London, COT

College of Occupational Therapists 2005 Code of Ethics and Professional Conduct. London, COT

Creek J 2002 Treatment planning and implementation. In: Creek J (ed.) Occupational therapy in mental health, 3rd edn. Edinburgh, Churchill Livingstone, pp 119–138

Creek J (ed.) 2006 Occupational therapy and mental health, 4th edn. Edinburgh, Churchill Livingstone

Department of Health 1995 The health of the nation: A strategy for people with learning disabilities. London, HMSO

Department of Health 2002 Valuing people a new strategy for the 21st century. London, HMSO

Duncan E (ed.) 2006 Foundations for practice in occupational therapy, 4th edn. Edinburgh, Elsevier

Fisher AG 2001 AMPS Assessment of motor and process skills

Volume 1: development, standardization, and administration manual, 4th edn. Colorado, USA, Three Star Press Inc

Fisher AG 2003 AMPS Assessment of motor and process skills Volume 1: development, standardization, and administration manual, 5th edn. Colorado, USA, Three Star Press Inc

Fisher AG 2006 AMPS Assessment of motor and process skills Volume 1: development, standardization, and administration manual, 6th edn. Colorado, USA, Three Star Press Inc

Forsyth K, Kielhofner G 2006 The model of human occupation: integrating theory into practice and practice into theory. In: Duncan E (ed.) Foundations for practice in occupational therapy, 4th edn. Edinburgh, Elsevier

Forsyth K, McMillan IR 2001 Introduction to theory. Unpublished material, Queen Margaret University College, Edinburgh. In: McMillan IR 2006 Assumptions underpinning a biomechanical frame of reference in occupational therapy. In: Duncan E. (ed) 2006 Foundations for practice in occupational therapy, 4th edn. Edinburgh, Elsevier pp 255–275

Foster M 2002 Theoretical frameworks. In: Turner A, Foster M, Johnson SE (eds) Occupational therapy and physical dysfunction; principles, skills and practice, 5th edn. London, Harcourt

Fresher-Samwaysk Roush SE, Choi K, Desrosiers Y, Steel G 2003 Perceived quality of life of adults with developmental and other significant disabilities. Disability and Rehabilitation 25(19):1097–1105

Gibbs G 1988 Learning by doing: a guide to teaching and learning methods. London, The Geography Discipline Network (GDN) Further Education Unit

Hagedorn R 2000 Tools for practice in occupational therapy: a structured approach to core skills and processes. Edinburgh, Churchill Livingstone

Holt G, Hardy S, Bouras N (eds) 2005 Mental health in learning disabilities. Brighton, Pavilion Publishing

Kielhofner G 2002 Model of human occupation – theory and application, 3rd edn. Baltimore, Lippincott, Williams & Wilkins

Kolb DA 1984 Experiential learning: experience as the source of learning & development. Upper Saddle River, NJ, Prentice-Hall

Laver Fawcett A 2002 Assessment. In: Turner A, Foster M, Johnson SE (eds) Occupational therapy and physical dysfunction: principles, skills and practice, 5th edn. London, Churchill Livingstone, pp 107–144

Laver Fawcett A 2007 Principles of assessment and outcome measurements for occupational therapists and physiotherapists: theory, skills and application. Chichester, Wiley

Law M, Baptiste S, Carswell A, McColl MA, Polatajko H, Pollock N 1997 The Canadian model of occupational performance. Toronto/Vancouver, CAOT Publications

Law M, Baptiste S, Carswell A, McColl MA, Polatajko H, Pollock N 2005 Canadian occupational performance measure, 4th edn. Ottawa, CAOT Publications ACE

McColl M, Law M, Stewert D, Doubt L, Pollock N, Krupa T 2003 Theoretical basis of occupational therapy, 2nd edn. Thorofare NJ, Slack Incorporated

McMillan IR 2006 Assumptions underpinning a biomechanical frame of reference in occupational therapy. In: Duncan EAS (ed.) Foundations for practice in occupational therapy, 4th edn. Edinburgh, Elsevier

Messent PR, Cooke CB, Long J 1999 Primary and secondary barriers to physically active healthy lifestyles for adults with learning disabilities. Disability and Rehabilitation 21(9):409–419

Mosey AC 1981 Legitimate tools of occupational therapy. In: Mosey A (ed.) Occupational therapy: configuration of a profession. New York, Raven, pp 89–118

Nelson DL, Jepson-Thomas 2003 Occupational form, occupational performance and a conceptual framework for therapeutic occupational. In: Kramer P, Hinojosa J, Brasic Royeen C (eds) Perspectives in Human occupation: participation in life. Philadelphia, Lippincott Williams & Wilkins

Parker D 2006 The client-centred frame of reference. In: Duncan E (ed.) Foundations for practice in occupational therapy, 4th edn. Edinburgh, Elsevier

Stein F, Cutler SK 2002 Psychosocial occupational therapy. A holistic approach, 2nd edn. Albany, Delmar

Strong S, Rigby P, Stewart D et al 1999 Application of the person–environment–occupation model: a practical tool. Canadian Journal of Occupational Therapy 66(3): 122–133

Suto M 1998 Leisure in occupational therapy. Canadian Journal of Occupational Therapy 65(5): 271–277

Swee Hong C, Smith Roper 2000 The development of an initial assessment for people with severe learning disabilities. British Journal of Occupational Therapy 63(2):83–86

Turner A, Foster M, Johnson SE (eds) 2002 Occupational therapy and physical dysfunction – principles, skills and practice, 5th edn. London, Churchill Livingstone

Watson D 2003 Causes and manifestations of learning disability. In: Gates B (ed.) Learning disabilities towards inclusion. London, Elsevier

Youngstrom MJ, Brayman SJ, Anthony P et al 2002 Occupational therapy practice framework: domain and process. American Journal of Occupational Therapy 56(6):609–639

Appendix 3.1 Defining learning disabilities

The term learning disability indicates the presence of reduced understanding of new or complex information or impaired skills of social functioning. It may also indicate that one or more of the following factors have occurred. Their presence may increase developmental and occupational challenges for an individual with a learning disability:

- Conditions which are syndrome-specific with related health affect
- Conditions with associated development disabilities arising from compromise of the central nervous system
- Conditions acquired from impact of maternal lifestyle/environment

Multifactoral causes of learning disability are comprehensively covered in a number of other texts and further useful reading is recommended in Watsons, in Gates (2004 Chapter 2) or Gillman (Chapter 38 in Swain et al 2004).

Broad diagnostic categories of learning disabilities are helpful to illustrate general principles that could indicate the possible outcome of occupational therapy interventions. However, the classification of learning disability alone will not clearly reflect either the individual's abilities or potentials. Definitions are based around the following:

- mild learning disabilities
- moderate/severe learning disabilities
- profound and multiple learning disabilities
- autism and learning disabilities
- dual diagnosis and learning disabilities.

Physical health considerations

When identifying physical health diagnosis for an individual with a learning disability it is useful to remember the impact of any condition on a person's feeling of well-being. The following systems approach illustrates the potential impact of physical health problems on occupation.

- Musculoskeletal system – conditions such as osteoarthritis, rheumatoid arthritis, dyskinesia, dystonia, e.g. causing limited range of moving, hindering dressing, or joint pain impacting on concentrating in leisure or work activities.

- Respiratory system – conditions such as infections, bronchitis or pneumonia, asthma leading to periods of ill health and immobility, e.g. resulting in loss or reduction of independent skill levels and social isolation.
- Endocrine system – such as hypo/ hyperthyroidism, obesity, e.g. reducing stamina and mobility levels to access community facilities and leading to development of a sedentary routine, lack of motivation to participate.
- Cardiovascular system – conditions including anaemia, cerebrovascular accident, myocardial infarction, hypotension, hypertension. Implications are tiredness, lack of energy, or paralysis, reduced fine and gross motor skills, e.g. can reduce or cause loss of skill levels for self care (such as washing and dressing routines or accessing leisure facilities).
- Digestive system – infections such as gastritis, appendicitis, hepatitis, mouth and duodenal ulcers, oral disorders caused by poor oral hygiene, gingival inflammation, teeth extractions 'acute abdomen', including pain and poor bowel function, e.g. resulting in poor diet, avoidance of certain foods and drink or difficulty with eating.
- Integumentary system – eczema, nutrition deficiencies resulting in xeroderma (dryness of skin), ulceration, pressure sores, e.g. avoidance of shaving, increase in self injury behaviour or increased levels of agitation reducing attention span.
- Nervous system – development of sensory disorders of vision and hearing related to congenital abnormalities and/or acquired through ageing such as cataracts, impacted ear wax, e.g. causing difficulty in perception either by sight or hearing and may lead to risk situations. Profound developmental impact on sensory integration and communication.
- Genitourinary system – implication of conditions such as menstruation, menopause, urinary tract infections, enlargement of prostate, e.g. causing change in routine and skill of toileting or managing washing, dressing.

Mental health considerations

Adults with learning disabilities are at increased risk of developing psychiatric disorders due to the complex interaction of often multiple biological, psychological, social and family factors (Holt et al 2005). It is important to note the difference between mental disorders classified in diagnostic terms from those behavioural disorders resulting from long-term patterns of maladaptive behaviours that interfere with typical life functioning. Behavioural disorders may be related to a mental health diagnosis and/or be a mismatch between expectations of the individual's capabilities and wishes, resources and level of support. Challenging behaviour is the most common reason for an individual with a learning disability to be referred to a psychiatrist and other professionals for assessment and accounts for a third of all admissions from the community to an assessment unit. A range of behaviours may present for a number of reasons and are summarized as follows:

- Self injurious behaviour e.g. self striking i.e. self injury to front of head, pica i.e. seeking out and eating cigarette ends, and biting i.e. self or others
- Severe challenging behaviours e.g. non-compliance, self or other injury (e.g. hair pulling) smearing faeces, stripping in public, temper tantrums, absconding, sexual disinhibition
- Moderately challenging behaviours e.g. over-activity, disturbing noises, stereotyped behaviour, stuffing fingers in body openings, sleep disorders.

Appendix 3.2 Case illustration: Freda, possible answers

1. What assessments would you use for Freda?

Following an initial visit Freda completed a MOHO Occupational Self Assessment form with the Occupational Therapist. Non-standardized assessments of interview and observation including numeracy, activity analysis, reading a bus timetable, and activity in the kitchen.

2. What aims would be relevant for Freda?

Possible aims of interventions for Freda were to improve her quality of life and establish her goals in relation to a number of areas:

- *Personal growth accomplishments* – Freda wanted to re-establish her level of independent activity in the home and college, especially her cooking ability.
- *Physical independence improving self confidence and self-esteem.* From the assessments the occupational therapist identified that Freda had independent skills in self care and making appropriate choices but lacked confidence. This was also due to the fact that she did not have the opportunity to express these within the home routine (e.g. cook a meal for her parents).
- *Transportation/physical accessibility reducing risk factors*, e.g. catching and travelling on the bus from home to college. Freda had good skills of communication and time keeping. She was able to read a bus timetable and knew the location of the bus stops from home and college. However, she was unable to handle money correctly on the bus.
- *Social and community involvement: i.e. identification of risk factors.* Freda had become very isolated and reliant on her mother. Equally, her mother was over-protective of her and

reluctant to allow her to go on the bus on her own as a risk situation had arisen the last time she was on the bus. Freda had kept up some contact with one friend from college by telephone.

- *Leisure activities: i.e. opportunity to identify and explore leisure interests.* Freda liked music and also was interested in swimming at the local leisure centre.
- *Personal and family relationships: i.e. awareness of issues of relationship, friendships, sexuality.* Due to her isolation, FREDA had few friends and her relationship with her mother was strained.

3. What approach(es) would you implement to enable Freda to catch a bus? Indicate how you would record and monitor progression/improvement?

For Freda one of the major hurdles for her to use the bus was her lack of numeracy skills which caused her to become flustered and embarrassed when faced with having to handle money on the bus. Using a compensatory approach one way to overcome this was to facilitate Freda to obtain a bus pass. Getting the bus pass was a major achievement for Freda and as she felt that she was like everyone else her anxiety before getting on the bus diminished. The intervention incorporated in a CBT programme using task analysis for road safety and getting on/off the bus, and was graded by supporting Freda to travel to the bus ticket office, complete the form, have her photo taken and pay for the bus pass.

4. How would you evaluate the outcome?

By revisiting the OSA to establish Freda's own evaluation of her progress and recording the progress of the task analysis and withdrawal of prompts and cues.

Chapter Four

The interface between communication and community living

4

Christine Griffiths

Overview

This chapter is intended to enable the reader to gain a greater insight into the communication difficulties that may be experienced and the impact this will have on the individual's ability to experience improved quality of life and to function appropriately in the community. The chapter will give an overview of communication with specific relevance to people with learning disabilities and is organized into four sections:

The first section provides an overview of the historical and current legislation and documents that have shaped our services and practice. The second encourages the reader to gain a wider perspective on the factors that can influence effective communication. In the third section the reader focuses on the crucial area of understanding and how this can easily be misinterpreted in adults with learning disabilities. Case scenarios are presented in the final section to enable the reader to identify some of the difficulties that may be encountered and examples of how effective communication can be supported by the occupational therapist in partnership with others.

Learning Objectives

By the end of the chapter, you will be able:
- Identify individual potential effects of significant others and the environment on the ability of people with learning disabilities to communicate effectively
- Explore the range and variability of communication strategies that may be required to support the rights, expectations and needs of people with learning disabilities
- Recognize three different levels of understanding and their significance in developing appropriate communication skills to support community living
- Consider the role of occupational therapy and the importance of multidisciplinary working.

Historical and current background

There are a number of Government, Trust and Professional policies and guidelines that shape the services we provide for people with learning disabilities, which will be referred to throughout this book. Valuing People (Government White Paper, DoH 2001) and Fulfilling the Promises (Welsh Assembly Government 2001) lay out clearly the rights of people with learning disabilities and highlight the following principles:

1. The right to be treated as an equal citizen to other citizens of the same age.

2. The right to expect an ordinary pattern of life within the community.

3. The right to make their own decisions, with support if necessary.

4. The right to additional help and support from their families and their communities to improve their chosen quality of life.

In order to respond to these rights we, as therapists, need to embrace a much wider, holistic overview of an individual's needs, embedding this within a social model of intervention and support. This will mean moving away from a medical model that focuses on 'deficits' and difficulties and instead taking account of the whole person and the way they want to live their life. We of course need to identify these difficulties but then to determine the impact they will have on the person's life, building on skills within functional environments. Although it is crucial that the occupational therapist contributes their specific professional skills, this will frequently be most effective within a multidisciplinary approach that supports close working relationships with a variety of statutory, voluntary and private organizations.

In addition to this, more recent national documents such as Our Health, Our Care, Our Say (DoH 2006), Independence, Well-being and Choice (DoH 2005) and the Welsh Assembly's Service Principles and Service Responses (WAG 2004) identify more explicitly the health and social care service aims for people with learning disability and how we might achieve them. In particular, in these documents and more specifically in occupational therapy services for adults with learning disabilities (OTPLD) (National Association of Occupational Therapists 2003), a person-centered approach is stressed as essential to enable individuals to drive what happens to them during their lifetimes. A more detailed description of this approach, stressing the importance of the community, is included in a book entitled *Friendship and Community* (Kennedy et al 2002). At a higher level, this may involve participation in policy-making decisions about whether to access direct payments to pay for daily activities. At a more basic level, this could involve making choices about the kind of activities they want to participate in, deciding which CD to play, but also indicating when and how they need help and support or who they want to sit next to.

Communication is an essential element in achieving the aims and principles set out in these documents. Meaningful involvement is impossible in any activity if we are unable to understand what is going on and are unable to contribute by expressing ourselves in a way that is understandable by others and valued by them. It is therefore important to remember that, as a human being, communication is a basic human right (DoH 2001) and that we all have a responsibility to ensure that individuals achieve this. It is also essential to pitch communication at the right level and that the methods give appropriate support. Communication cannot be separated off into a 'skill area' to be taught in isolation events or activities happening in the person's life. It overarches everything that we do and therefore support should provide meaningful opportunities in the individual's environment to enable successful and effective communication to occur. The Means, Reasons and Opportunities Model described by Money & Thurman (2002) demonstrates this further.

This chapter will aim to identify some key factors that may inhibit this interaction and to suggest strategies to enable the occupational therapist to develop more effective communication skills when working with individuals with learning disabilities and when supporting them to access their community.

Barriers to communication

In order to determine where barriers may occur, it may first be helpful to think about where communication has an impact on the life of a person with a learning disability. First, it is helpful to look at how communication influences service provision, applying this to the five accomplishments (O'Brien 1987):

- to be part of your community
- to be respected by those around you
- to form relationships
- to build skills and learn new things
- to make meaningful choices.

Reader activity

- What do you need to effectively communicate with others to achieve the five accomplishments?
- What are factors that could hinder effective communication to achieve the five accomplishments?

Broadly we can divide the factors that can act as a barrier to communication into three areas:

- the individual
- significant others
- the environment.

The individual

Communication is a higher cognitive function and therefore the level of learning disability undoubtedly plays a part in the ability and capacity to understand and express oneself. It is also of significance that the individual is able to integrate sensory information appropriately, as this will directly influence the 'building blocks' of their development and ultimately, effective communication in their environment. This point is discussed in more detail in Chapter 6, Sensory integration and self-care. However, there are other factors that need to be considered which are highlighted in the following reader activity:

Reader activity

Reflect on:

- How well do you communicate with your colleagues when you have had a late night, are feeling unwell or are taking medication?
- How effective is your communication when you are feeling very emotional?

People with learning disabilities, especially those who have epilepsy, may be taking medication that will affect their level of concentration, motivation and level of alertness. They may have difficulty sleeping, be emotionally labile and generally take longer to digest what you are saying to them or what is going on around them. This can be further influenced by physical difficulties, sensory loss (particularly hearing or visual), genetic disorders that specifically affect communication or conditions such as autistic spectrum disorder. In all these situations it is likely that the individual will be unable to respond in ways that we might expect, e.g. reduced eye contact, standing too close or not answering when we expect them to.

The individual can also experience difficulties in expressing themselves as they may be unable to choose an appropriate method of communication as they are reliant on others, or the chosen method

is not available e.g. symbol book left at home, objects of reference lost (refer to Table 4.1 for definitions of strategies). People with more severe learning disabilities often develop their own specific ways of communicating, which may or may not be understood by others. The work of Hewitt & Nind (1998) on the subject of 'intensive interaction' and of Caldwell (2005) explores ways of responding to behaviours of individuals that value their unique way of communicating, allowing the individual choice and greater control in the interaction.

Unclear speech can be difficult to understand if we are not 'tuned' in to it. The individual may be unable to improve intelligibility significantly due to conditions such as cleft palate or dyspraxia, the latter also affecting the ability to sign effectively. In addition to this, if attempts at communication in the past have been unsuccessful, ridiculed or ignored, then this will ultimately affect their confidence, self-esteem and motivation to try again in the future.

Significant others

Communication can only occur between two or more people and so the communication skills of others significantly affect the likelihood and quality of any interaction. Now think about the questions in the following reader activity:

Reader activity

- How well do you listen to what is going on if you are not interested in the subject area or do not understand the words being used?
- How easy is it to communicate if other people do not seem to be listening to you, patronize you or try to 'help' too much?
- Do you find it easier or more difficult to communicate with people whose personality may be different from yours, e.g. loud/shy, impatient/methodical and does this depend on what mood *you* are in?
- Does it take more effort to listen to someone with a foreign accent or who has had an aesthetic at the dentist?

Language is frequently complex, often assumes prior knowledge and can be delivered quickly. Verbal communication alone can be extremely difficult to follow.

Table 4.1 Strategies to support understanding

Aim	Think about	Try out
Plan your own communicative approach to support therapeutic interventions	The amount of key words that can be understood effectively (supported from comprehensive speech and language therapy assessment)	Do not overload, keep sentences short
Support the individual to understand what is happening and what is required of them	How to decrease the reliance on verbal skills	Use extra cues, e.g. appropriate facial expressions, tone of voice, eye/finger pointing, gestures, non-verbal communication
Help to sequence a task and follow an explanation	How to increase participation	Split important information into smaller, manageable parts, e.g. instead of 'We're going to make beans on toast for dinner, so you open the beans first with the tin opener and we'll put them in the pan', you might say, 'Let's make beans on toast' (while you get the items together); 'open the beans with this' (while you offer the tin opener) and 'Now put them in the pan' (when you offer or point to the saucepan)
Offering choices	We often tend to remember the beginnings or endings of sentences, look towards one corner of a symbol board or remember the last place you pointed	Change the order occasionally to check that the person is making an informed choice e.g. 'Do you want coffee or tea?' and then the next time changing the choices around
Avoid confusion	Your choice of vocabulary	Use vocabulary that the individual is familiar with and be consistent
Maintain concentration	Distractions in the environment	Reduce distractions
Retain or process information appropriately when given commands	Is the person doing something else at the same time, e.g. walking from one room to another, particularly if they have poor mobility?	Wait until the individual has stopped whatever else they are doing so that you have their full attention
Support people who have difficulty in retaining information	People may appear to understand much of what you say, but become anxious or constantly ask repetitive questions	Use visual reminders so that the individual can keep checking back on information given to them (this could be in a clock format for somebody who is anxious about time)

We normally, therefore, also rely on additional cues, which we gain from body language, the situation and the environment. Staff or carers (including ourselves), however, can often be inconsistent in responses and may send out confusing mixed messages leading to verbal and non-verbal communication that does not match, e.g. saying 'Yes, I'm listening' when turning around putting something away in a cupboard. These complexities and mixed messages can frequently be misinterpreted, leading to breakdown in communication.

The listener may also experience difficulties of their own in responding to the chosen method of communication, e.g. a hearing/visual loss (which is not always obvious) or little knowledge of the symbols or signs being used. It is therefore our responsibility to ensure that we, as therapists, develop a basic knowledge of the chosen system and use it appropriately. The communication of others can be influential if we have preconceived ideas about how people with a range of learning disabilities communicate, or we are prejudiced about particular cultures or social backgrounds. Do we see behaviours that challenge our services purely as acts of aggression or as a means of communicating feelings and choices in a way that is different from the norm? Are vocalizations and facial expressions viewed as valid? Is a symbol board a 'lesser' form of communication with speech being the ultimate aim? How we value the communication skills and choices of others will easily influence our interpretation of the situation and how we positively respond to them.

Environment

The environment itself has a profound influence on the effectiveness of communication. It is clear that if the setting is not conducive for the individual or if the opportunities are not available then it is unlikely that meaningful communication will occur at all. To consider the influence of the environment think about the following and what they mean in practical terms.

Reader activity

- What kind of environments do you work in, e.g. day centres, homes, clinics, hospitals?
- How 'busy' are they, in terms of people, activity and furnishings?
- How noisy, comfortable, hot/cold are they?
- How familiar are they to the individual?
- How easy is it for the individual to get their message across, e.g. are objects of reference readily available, are choices offered in an appropriate way and at the appropriate time or do routines mean that he/she does not need to communicate?

A great deal of concentration and motivation is required in order to interact with others and therefore distractions in the environment will impede this process. Noise and visual stimulation from televisions, radios and cluttered environments may cause sensory overload for some, leading to withdrawal or challenging behaviours, whereas for others an environment that is too sterile with too little to interest

them will further reduce motivation and the ability to initiate any activity. We also tend to communicate much more freely in familiar environments where we feel relaxed and know what is going on.

Coping with distractions will place more demands on the individual so that they will experience difficulties in listening or processing information given to them, thereby reducing their level of understanding (this will be discussed later in this chapter). People with communication difficulties are often reliant on staff, carers and others to organize the environment so that opportunities are available for meaningful communication to occur. Colleagues may inform or write in clinical notes that a service user, having learnt a particular method of communication such as signing, does not use it. However, if we observe the behaviour of others around the individual, including ourselves, we may notice that in fact nobody else is signing either! This is unlikely to encourage the individual and is not conducive to effective interactions occurring. Activities introduced through active support, discussed in more detail later in this chapter and in Chapter 13, provide the opportunity for encouraging shared communication through demonstration and modelling as well as through verbal means, as communication strategies can easily be included in this structured approach. Signs, symbols or other methods used can then be reinforced in other situations as this will help to generalize the vocabulary learned, enabling more meaningful participation in the activities. For example, if an individual has learnt signs/symbols for a particular activity such as dressing, they should be encouraged to use them, perhaps in a structured way in a variety of situations – choosing clothes in the morning, when out shopping, washing clothes, etc. This facilitates communication that is valued and effective. If choices are not offered in an appropriate way or the most effective methods of communication are not readily available and reinforced by others, then attempts to communicate may either not occur or be unsuccessful.

Levels of understanding

It is crucial that at an early stage the appropriate level of understanding is identified as, without it, it is impossible to engage meaningfully with an individual or to work in a person-centered way. It is also questionable how well informed the individual is about our involvement and therefore raises issues of consent. It is an area that can be easily misjudged as people frequently tend to nod their head or smile in the right place or respond to the situation rather than the words we are saying. All too often we hear the expression 'he can understand everything I say but can't tell me what he wants'. We need to question why this is in order to provide the right kind of support to enable the person to be properly engaged in what we are doing.

This section will identify the various levels of understanding and how they develop. It will specifically cover:

- Situational understanding and routines
- Symbolic understanding
- Verbal understanding.

Situational understanding and routines

Situational understanding describes how we gain information from the situation or events around us i.e. how we pick up on cues. In order to understand, for example, that it is teatime, we do not have to know what these words mean because we can smell the food, hear the pans clanking around in the kitchen and food being served onto the plates and it is probably about the same time that we always have tea. Another example might be that if the window is open on a cold day and I point to the window asking you to close it, you do not need to understand any language to know what I want. You can gain this information from the situation, the draught, my actions and my tone of voice. How often have you been on a railway platform but followed the crowd to another platform because you could not really hear the announcement? Acknowledging that the individual may not be gaining a great deal of information from the actual words we have used will help us to understand why they may respond to something we have said or done in one setting but appear totally confused or non-cooperative on another occasion.

Situational understanding, however, can be a very useful means of enhancing and developing the understanding of a person with a learning disability as it will help them interpret what is going on and what might be happening next. It is also imperative that this information is clear and that there are no mixed messages being given, as this can cause great

anxiety and distress. Some examples of situations that provide information are:

- Environmental cues, e.g. smells, noises, the activity itself and the materials involved, the time, the room used (does it have multiple uses or is it normally used for lunch-time?), where furniture, etc. is situated
- Non-verbal cues, e.g. tone of voice, body language, gestures
- Familiarity with the situation, e.g. do they enjoy the activity, have they done it before and how often?
- People's roles, e.g. is it always the same person who would do a particular activity with them?
- Routines, e.g. is there a framework to what usually happens and when?

If we fail to recognize that an individual is relying on these cues we are likely to place far too many verbal demands on them and experience greater difficulty in engaging them in specific activities. This may also lead us to make the wrong assumptions about people's preferences, level of concentration or motivation. However, situational understanding can be gradually built up over time so that the individual can learn, through repetition, what usually happens during an activity and what this means. This can be developed into a useful routine to further enhance effective communication. Strategies to develop routines during therapeutic interventions are discussed later in this chapter. Routines offer a framework on which to build future learning and provide a feeling of stability, helping to reduce levels of anxiety as well as enabling us to look forward to regular events. When we are able to understand what is going on around us we generally feel more in control of our lives and more motivated to participate and interact with others. Routines enable us to build on this process by providing appropriate levels of support to encourage effective communication to occur.

Finally, it should be recognized that this is a very important part of understanding and interpreting our world. We all need this information but a non-verbal person or an individual who has difficulty following verbal communication may be entirely dependent on the situation in order to feel safe in their environment and make decisions that affect their lives.

Symbolic understanding

The way in which we learn to represent our world develops from understanding a range of methods from the real object to the written word. People with learning disabilities may be functioning at any point on this continuum and for this reason it will not always be helpful to provide a picture or photo for somebody who does not understand or cannot communicate verbally. It is therefore essential that we determine the appropriate level and form of understanding in order to communicate in the most appropriate way with the individual. Advice should be sought from a speech and language therapist to ascertain information from a detailed assessment, particularly when working with individuals with more complex communication difficulties. However, for many individuals careful observation would provide basic information as to the method found to be most easily understood in a particular setting.

Figure 4.1 gives some simple examples of types of symbolic understanding (i.e. down) and the sensory information that is gained from them (i.e. across). Try this out with different objects, e.g. a piece of fruit, a block of wood, a flower and tick the sections that give you information. It is clear that the real thing provides a lot of sensory information whereas the spoken (or written) words are only a series of representative noises or marks and provide no sensory information at all. For this reason, real objects are by far the easiest means of understanding and often hold some universal messages e.g. jangling your keys means you are ready to go, holding your money out in a shop means you want to pay.

There are, however, some points that should be considered:

- We rely on previous knowledge and experiences to interpret new information. We need to link this information, old and new, in order to understand what we are experiencing. People with learning disabilities will therefore need time to process new information and become accustomed to new vocabulary/signs/pictures or objects (and have the opportunity to use them appropriately).
- There is a significant developmental leap when moving from objects (three-dimensional) to pictures and photographs (two-dimensional).
- There is generally a considerable amount of developmental learning between each stage. For this reason, it is not advisable to use miniature objects when developing programmes for people with more profound learning disabilities as the real thing is much easier to understand.

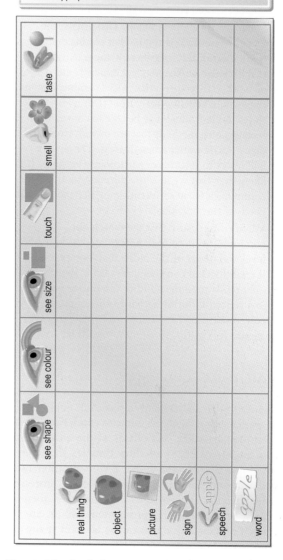

Consider how much sensory information is available for each representation of "apple" (left hand column). Tick the appropriate boxes

Figure 4.1 • Symbolic understanding. Copyright Bro Morgannwg Inclusive Communication Initiative 2005.

- Development in adults with learning disabilities can be patchy for a variety of reasons. Individuals may show some understanding of photographs of family members, but not respond consistently to photographs of objects. Alternatively, some photos or symbols may be meaningful while others are not. It is therefore important that this is carefully assessed before assumptions are made and, in many situations, a combination of methods may prove more effective.

- Under times of stress, we all resort to easier or more familiar ways of doing things. This may be the case when we are making requests or placing demands on an individual during therapeutic activities so that although he/she may not appear to need signs or symbols during everyday social communication they would benefit greatly from their use at these times. An individual may be able to convey their feelings using methods that are more formal on many occasions but when distressed or anxious will resort to gestures or particular behaviours. It is likely then that we may use different methods of communication at different times, depending on the needs of the individual.

- We need to ensure that we match our communication to the appropriate method, level and needs of the individual. For example, if an individual communicates using signs but only tends to understand or use one or two in a sentence during activities then our own communication (including our verbal language) should reflect this to be most effective.

Verbal understanding

The ability to understand verbal communication is dependent on many things, some of which have already been mentioned e.g. the effects of the environment, how quickly people speak, how complex the topic or vocabulary is, the non-verbal communication used. Verbal information must be fully listened to, processed, remembered and then acted on. Therefore, memory plays a large part in this process and will dictate the amount of information that can be taken in at any one time. We also tend to concentrate on key words within a sentence, which carry the main message. Therefore, for example, if somebody hands us a biscuit and asks if we want one, we do not have to understand any words (remember situational understanding?). However, if there is a choice of a biscuit and a drink and somebody asks if we want a biscuit, then 'biscuit' is a key word.

The ability to develop verbal understanding is a higher cognitive function (as shown in Figure 4.1). However, there are ways that we can support the effectiveness of verbal understanding, which are summarized in Table 4.1.

It is important to remember that although our interactions may not seem very long or complicated to us, they probably are! We very often use jargon, complex sentence structures and include lots of information. When staff/carers are learning to sign, they are often amazed by the amount they are trying to put into one sentence. We should also recognize that we all rely on using a range of other methods to support our understanding in different situations in everyday life e.g. responding to road signs when driving, reading maps, reading diagrams to put furniture together.

We therefore need to be aware of the general level of understanding of the individuals we are working with and additionally take account of any other demands that are placed on them. This will help to ensure that we do not overestimate the level of understanding of those who function with apparently mild to moderate learning disabilities. Our interactions can then be adapted accordingly to suit the needs of the individual at that time, by either simplifying our own language or providing more cues, using other methods of communication as required or adapting the environment or structure of our therapy. Even working with clients with a mild learning disability it is advisable that all verbal communication uses non-complex vocabulary, avoids using too many 'unnecessary' words and is not overtly rapid (in a manner which values the individual).

Methods of communication/ communication strategies

There are many texts available that explain in detail the origins and development of different strategies. Table 4.2 provides some key information on the strategies identified in this section.

For the purposes of this chapter the author has concentrated on the practical application of these strategies by providing examples of their use.

When faced with the possibility of meeting somebody with a learning disability for the first time many people initially begin to panic about how they will interact with them, how they will be able to carry out an assessment properly and how they will be able to ensure a person-centred approach. What they forget, however, is that there are many forms of communication available to all of us and we rarely use one form in isolation. Speech or verbal communication is

Table 4.2 Methods of communication/communication strategies

Strategy	Summary of use	Reference
Visual strategies	These can take various forms, e.g. objects, photos, symbols, pictures, drawings. It is a concrete reminder of an activity, person or event and is extremely useful for portraying concepts such as time, feelings, abstract ideas and sequencing of events	Hodgdon 2003
Symbols	Symbols are a visual means of portraying an idea or concept and range from those that are transparent (guessable), those that are learnable as the link can be understood when explained, and those that are abstract	Detheridge et al 2004 Abbott 2000
Signs	British Sign Language (BSL) is a manual system developed by the deaf community and is a language in its own right. Systems such as Makaton and SignAlong have been based on BSL and support key words to assist communication, i.e. Sign Supported English	Kennard 1997
Talking Mats	This is a visual framework that helps people with communication difficulties to think about topics while providing them with a means of expressing themselves	Murphy & Cameron 2002
Objects of reference	An object that is specifically chosen to represent an activity, person, place or event	Ockelford 1994
Personal Passport	Personal Passports are a positive means by which individuals who cannot speak for themselves can describe themselves and their personality, their communication, how others can best support them and other useful information to share with others. Their style and content are very personal to the individual	Millar 2003

therefore only one method and becomes less of an issue as we get to know the individual over time and so learn which are the most effective methods to use at any given time to support them, and also begin to understand what the various behaviours they use may mean.

Below are some examples of various situations where difficulties may arise and some suggestions for communication strategies that we can use.

Scenario 1

Sarah has a short attention span, seems to get confused when doing her laundry and constantly asks staff/carers for help.

Needs

In this example, even though Sarah normally seems to understand simple verbal communication she has difficulty retaining the information required when completing a task and becomes overloaded and anxious. The task needs to be broken down and sequenced into measurable chunks, providing the information required at each stage. In this way, the instructions will be short and more easily remembered. Sarah also needs a more concrete reminder of what she has to do so that she can check back herself at any time and does not need to ask questions constantly.

Strategy

Visual strategies are extremely helpful in providing concrete reminders of the task in hand. They allow the task to be broken down into smaller elements, the information being as limited or as detailed as required. An example of each is given in Figures 4.2 and 4.3 using Widgit symbols (Widgit Software Ltd 2004). Additionally, when first introducing the

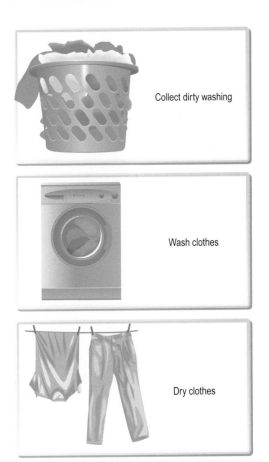

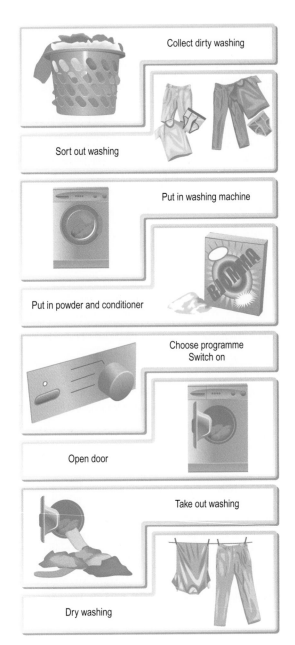

Figure 4.2 • An example of a chart identifying key aspects of the task. Pictures and symbols copyright Widgit Software 2004.

activity, sections can be demonstrated by the carer or occupational therapist but Sarah would be encouraged to open the door of the washing machine herself or help with sorting. The amount of involvement can be increased as the routine becomes more established. Obviously, instructions are given verbally but the table (which could be laminated and put next to the washing machine) is a concrete reminder of what needs to happen and when. If at any stage Sarah becomes confused and does not want to consent it is easier to see where the breakdown has occurred. The use of appropriate signs such as Signalong (Kennard 1994) or Makaton (Makaton Vocabulary Development Project 2007) may also help to maintain Sarah's attention and reinforce key vocabulary.

Figure 4.3 • An example of a chart visualizing more detailed information. Pictures and symbols copyright Widgit Software 2004.

Scenario 2

Michael wants to be involved in choosing the food for the week. He doesn't seem to recognize formal symbols but can identify labels from familiar foods.

Needs

Michael requires a method that enables him to choose the foods he would like and then make up a meaningful shopping list before going shopping.

Strategy

Initially staff/carers need to establish that Michael knows what the labels are. They could be asked to collect the labels from familiar foods during the week and then check out on the weekend whether Michael knows what they are by asking him to find the matching food in the cupboard or fridge. A 'Talking Mats©' (Murphy & Cameron 2002) activity could then be set up to encourage Michael to make up a shopping list.

To do this stick, the labels on to card and fix small pieces of Velcro© on to the back (by including Michael in this activity other areas could be assessed or worked on, for example, eye/hand co-ordination, hand function, pincer grip, etc.). Take a large carpet tile or similar and chalk a line down the middle. At the top half of one put a symbol of a happy face and at the top of the other put a symbol of a sad face (or a tick and a cross but make sure Michael understands). Present the labels in groups of about three to Michael asking him which side he wants to put them. Gradually work through the labels. If he seems a bit unsure at any time show him the actual food. At the end collect all the labels from the 'happy' side and arrange them in a plastic wallet – this is the shopping list.

Many activities can be developed from involving the individual in this kind of activity which will include them meaningfully in community living, i.e. learning about money and transport when shopping, buying the items needed to prepare a meal, developing physical skills by actually making up a visual or tactile list. The vocabulary, in whatever format, can be reinforced when first buying the food, when unpacking it and when collecting it together to cook a meal and so on.

Scenario 3

Gillian is not keen to join in with the group cookery sessions and seems distressed when she first comes into the kitchen. She is partially sighted with a profound hearing loss, does not appear to understand any formal methods of communication and tends to use behaviours that are interpreted by staff/carers to indicate what she wants.

Needs

Gillian needs information to let her know where she is, what she is going to be doing and with whom, so that she is prepared. This will encourage her to participate meaningfully in the chosen activity. The others involved also need to understand what Gillian's behaviours mean, particularly how she communicates whether she wants to do something or not and whether she is happy, or to recognize the signs that she is becoming distressed. They then need to establish a shared method of communication with her.

Strategy

The problem may not actually be with the cookery session but perhaps Gillian is confused because she is in the kitchen expecting to have a cup of tea or something to eat. She also may not know who she is with and what is expected of her. Objects of reference can be developed by staff, carers and others to represent themselves; for example, a distinctive key ring, badge or bracelet (items should be safe and easily replaceable so avoid expensive jewellery or characteristics such as beards or length of hair that might change). Gillian would first need to have some indication of your presence so that her personal space is not invaded too quickly. The item could be shown to Gillian when you first meet her as you say her name and get down to eye level. An object of reference would also be useful here to represent the activity, such as a wooden spoon, which should again be shown to Gillian immediately before starting every cookery session. A wooden spoon can also be placed on the kitchen door for Gillian to see/feel on her way in so that she knows what the room will be used for.

This may be a group activity where others have a structured visual plan of what they need to do. However, Gillian will be able to participate by helping the others to collect together the materials and foods needed and she will undoubtedly gain a great deal of social and sensory learning from the experiences of preparation and cooking. From a communication point of view it would be helpful to remember some of the earlier points raised:

- Ensure that the environment is not too cluttered or distracting
- Ensure that you have Gillian's full attention when including her, e.g. call her name or touch her arm first

- Ensure you use appropriate body language and tone of voice
- Where possible offer real objects and encourage Gillian to make choices
- Observe closely for ways that she communicates likes/dislikes. This information may also be available from a Personal Passport (Millar 2003). Ask the staff or the speech and language therapist if one has been developed.

Scenario 4

Jean is able to live on her own with a few hours daily support from a care worker. She has a list of phone numbers of her friends and relatives, including some emergency numbers. Many of the numbers she knows by heart but she sometimes gets them mixed up and might panic in an emergency.

Needs

Jean needs a system that will help her to identify who the numbers belong to that is clear and easily accessible.

Strategy

Photographs could be taken with a digital camera of friends, relatives, doctor, police, ambulance, etc. A chart or clearly laid out phone book of corresponding numbers and photos could then be made up and kept by the phone.

The examples above give an indication of how a variety of communication methods can be adapted to support individuals with learning disabilities to engage meaningfully in a range of community activities. This will ultimately provide them with greater independence and the means to make choices that are understood and valued by others.

Summary

A great deal of information can be gained from taking the time to get to know the people we support and also in working closely with carers, staff and other professional colleagues to ensure that we share information and provide integrated care. As therapists, we have a unique opportunity to enable appropriate opportunities within the home and wider community to occur and to adapt our own communication to meet the needs of those with communication difficulties, particularly where additional physical and/or sensory impairments are evident. This chapter has identified some of the barriers to this occurring and has highlighted the importance of establishing the appropriate level of communicative support. Adjustments to the environment and our own communication can have a major impact on the success of our interactions. If we can add to this the establishment of a shared method of communication, whether this is through interpreting individual behaviours or gestures used or by utilizing a range of more formal methods, then this will further enhance the process. Speech and language therapists will also help to provide more detailed information and support when working with individuals with more complex communication difficulties or when developing multidisciplinary approaches.

Effective communication is an essential element of community living if this is to be a meaningful experience. Enabling effective communication allows an individual a degree of control over their lives and a means of conveying their own thoughts and feelings. This will then enable us to shape our services accordingly to support the appropriate skill development and opportunities required to foster those aspects of community living that are important to the individual.

Box 4.1

Case illustration: Alan

Alan will soon be moving out of the family home to a staffed house, sharing with two other residents, one of whom he already knows from attending the day centre. Alan is a 21-year-old, and has a moderate learning disability. Although normally happy and relaxed in very familiar circumstances, he does become easily upset in unfamiliar environments and if confused. On these occasions, he frequently hits his head and paces around in an agitated manner. He understands small amounts of information but his parents are apprehensive that the move will be confusing for him. They are also worried that any preparation will confuse him into thinking that he is moving immediately. The staff at the house are also concerned that he will be unsure of his surroundings and the layout of the rooms in the new house and will not be able to remember the plans leading up to the move.

Reader activity

1. How would the occupational therapist identify the issues for Alan bearing in mind the concerns of both his parents and staff?

2. What strategies are required to support the above? How could the occupational therapist and speech and language therapist work together to achieve joint aims?

Further reading

Abbott C 2000 Symbols now. Cambridge, Widgit Software pp 63–76

Abudarham S, Hurd A 2002 Management of communication needs in people with learning disability. London and Philadelphia, Whurr Publishers

Bogdashina O 2005 Communication issues in autism and Asperger syndrome. London, Jessica Kingsley Publishers

Child C 2004 Choices, changes and challenges. South Devon Healthcare NHS Trust

Edwards L 1999 Epilepsy – a speech and language therapist's guide. Speech and Language Therapy in Practice Spring:4–8

Gates B (ed.) 2007 Learning disabilities toward inclusion, 5th edn. Edinburgh, Churchill Livingstone

Hodgdon L 2003 Visual strategies for improving communication. Troy, Michigan, Quirk Roberts Publishing

Kelly A 2002 Working with adults with a learning disability. Bicester, Speechmark

McGill J 1998 Listening to users. Talking Sense Winter:16–17

Millar S 2003 Communication – by the book. Speech and Language Therapy in Practice Winter: 25–27

Munro S 2004 Jabadao – Making a song and dance about communication. Speech and Language Therapy in Practice Autumn:4–6

Murphy J, Cameron L 2002 Let your mats do the talking. Speech and Language Therapy in Practice Spring:18–20

Ockelford A 1994 Objects of reference. London, RNIB

Park K 1999 Whose needs come first? Speech and Language Therapy in Practice Summer:4–6

Powell G 1999 Current research findings to support the use of signs with adults and children who have intellectual and communication difficulties. Makaton Vocabulary Development Project. www.makaton.org (accessed 29 February 2008)

Roberts J 1997 The scent system. Talking Sense Autumn:20–21

Scott J 2003 Get out there and use it. Speech and Language Therapy in Practice Winter: 24–25

Sense South East 1996 Communication – good practice. Talking Sense Spring:16–18

Useful resources

Caldwell P 2005 Person to person. Brighton, Pavilion Publishers

www.signalong.org.uk (accessed 29 February 2008)

www.makaton.org (accessed 29 February 2008)

www.widgit.com (accessed 29 February 2008)

References

Abbott C 2000 Symbols now. Cambridge, Widgit Software

Caldwell P 2005 Person to person. Brighton, Pavilion Publishers

Department of Health 2001 Valuing people: a new strategy for learning disability for the 21st century. London, HSMO

Department of Health 2005 Independence, well-being and choice. Our vision for the future of social care for adults in England. London, HSMO

Department of Health 2006 Our health, our care, our say. A new direction for community services. London, HSMO

Detheridge T, Whittle H, Detheridge C 2004 The Widgit Rebus Symbol Collection. Cambridge, Widgit Software Ltd

Hewitt D, Nind M Widgit Software Ltd 1998 Interaction in action. London, David Fulton Publishers

Hodgdon 2003 Visual strategies for improving communication. Troy, Michigan, Quirk Roberts Publishing

Kennard G 1997 SignAlong Phase 1 (Basic Vocabulary). Rochester, The SignAlong Group

Kennedy J, Sanderson H, Wilson H 2002 Friendship and community. Manchester, Northwest Training and Development Team

Makaton Vocabulary Development Project 2001–2007. 31 Firwood Drive, Camberley, Surrey GU15 3QD UK. Tel: 01276 61390. www. makaton.org

Millar S 2003 Personal communication passports. Edinburgh, Call Centre

Money D, Thurman S 2002 Inclusive communication. Speech and Language Therapy in Practice Autumn:4–6

Murphy J, Cameron L 2002 Talking mats and learning disability. Derbyshire, Winslow Press

National Association of Occupational Therapists 2003 Working with people with learning disabilities. Lingfield, OTPLD Prisma Press

Ockelford A 1994 Objects of reference. London, RNIB

O'Brien 1987 A guide to lifestyle planning. In: Wilcox B, Bellamy T (eds) A comprehensive guide to activities catalogue. Baltimore, Paul H Brookes Publishing

Sign Along Group 2001 Stratford House, Waterside Court, Neptune Close, Rochester, Kent ME2 4NZ, UK Tel: 0870 7743752. www. signalong.org.uk

Welsh Assembly Government 2001 Fulfilling the promises. A report to the National Assembly for Wales, Cardiff

Welsh Assembly Government 2004 Learning disability strategy: Section 7 Guidance on service principles and service responses. Cardiff, Welsh Assembly Government

Welsh Assembly Government 2005 Designed for life: creating world class health and social care for Wales in the 21st century. Cardiff, Welsh Assembly Government

Widgit Software Ltd 2004 The Widgit Rebus Symbol Collection. Cambridge, Widgit Software Ltd

Appendix 4.1 Case Illustration: Alan, possible answers

1. How would the occupational therapist identify the issues for Alan bearing in mind the concerns of both his parents and staff?

2. What strategies are required to support the above? How could the occupational therapist and speech and language therapist work together to achieve joint aims?

Identifying needs

Completing an initial assessment, the occupational therapist can explore the issues for Alan and his parents and also separately with the house manager, issues for staff. At this stage, it is important to be introduced to Alan in a familiar environment and in a way that is appropriate for him to understand (refer to Table 4.1). Using a model framework such as the Model of Human Occupation, several assessments can be carried out including observations of Alan's occupation and routines in a number of settings at home and the day centre, a familiar car journey, volitional questionnaire and a sensory inventory. Frequent contact would also enable Alan to feel comfortable with the occupational therapist and establish a relationship. Talking with his parents and staff at the day centre could identify key communication strategies. The assessments could identify specific environmental triggers that cause Alan to become anxious and exacerbate his self-injuries behaviour. These may include unexpected noises, large open spaces and manoeuvering around furniture. Alan might keep to strict daily routines at home and during the day, therefore it is important to identify any preferences in relation to his occupations (e.g. cues for brushing his teeth, how he indicates when he wants to have a drink).

Through meeting with the house manager, staff and the two other tenants, the occupational therapist could identify both physical and social factors that have a potential positive or negative effect. By considering the ergonomic aspects of the house layout including the size and location of his bedroom, the garden and location, the occupational therapist could match possible stresses such as noise levels, enclosed spaces, with his needs in this unfamiliar environment.

Identifying strategies

Strategies to support understanding: the problem may not be that Alan will not be able to manage the actual move to his new home but that others' expectations are not clearly communicated to him. By identifying Alan's occupational strengths, including the communication strategies he uses with his family, familiar routines, and objects that could be transferred to his new home, the physical environment can be designed to his preferences. This may include a routine based on sensory aspects. The speech and language therapist and occupational therapist from their joint assessments can also introduce a stepped strategy to enable him to firstly be introduced to the staff and other tenants and then encouraged and supported to make known his preferences (refer to Table 4.1).

Methods of communication/ communication strategies

The staff will need to be informed of both the importance of using consistent methods of communication (e.g. may include cues, prompts and gestures) and Alan's methods of communication (refer to Table 4.2). This may involve identifying how he communicates when he wants to do something or not and if he is happy or to recognize the signs that he is becoming distressed. Routines and participation can be phased in to familiar routines from home (i.e. time of going to bed or time of meals). The amount of participation can then be increased once the routine becomes more established in his new home.

5

Occupation and health promotion

Jenni Hurst

Overview

Health and wellness are of major importance to the current United Kingdom (UK) government and this is reflected in their expectation of the service you will deliver as a health professional. This means that the National Health Service (NHS) is no longer viewed as primarily a service for people who are ill (Department of Health 2000). The move towards a patient-led NHS reflecting a client-centred approach to medical interventions demonstrates the changes required within the context of the medical model (DoH 2000). This approach is also reflected in the policies for people with a learning disability in the White Paper Valuing People: a new strategy for learning disability for the 21st century (DoH 2001a). In particular, Chapter 6: Improving health for people with learning disabilities, provides clear guidance on future service provision. People with a learning disability should be able to access their primary care team and receive the level of service detailed in any relevant National Service Framework (NSF); for example, NSF for Diabetes or Mental Health. The National Cancer Plan also makes specific reference to people with a learning disability,

with the expectation that there will be equality of health screening available from mainstream services.

Occupational therapists view the health and wellness of the individual from an occupational perspective so that promoting the importance of a healthy lifestyle to the individual is seen as essential to a meaningful intervention within a cultural context (Wilcock 1998, Watson 2006). Reynolds (2001) also proposed that occupational therapists should facilitate physical activity as a means of promoting well-being. This is in line with the current recommendations of the Medical Officer for Health, who recommends five sessions of 30 minutes excercise five times a week. Current recommendations also acknowledge that specific tasks such as gardening and housework provide useful exercise and give additional meaning to the contribution of these daily or weekly tasks to a healthy lifestyle. Occupational therapists are increasingly developing their role in a variety of settings that will give them an opportunity to promote the role of a healthy lifestyle as part of the intervention that they plan with their clients. This chapter will explore the role of the occupational therapist working

with people with learning disability in the wider community. It will also consider the occupational deprivation and health implications for the population of people with a learning disability and mental health problems who are currently detained in prisons (Couldrick & Alred 2003).

Learning Outcomes

By the end of the chapter you will be able to:

- Discuss the occupational factors that can influence a healthy lifestyle for a person with a learning disability
- Understand how an occupation filter can be applied by an occupational therapist when assisting a person with a learning disability to enjoy a healthy lifestyle
- Discuss how working as a member of a multi-disciplinary team you can help raise awareness of the issues.

Factors that influence a healthy lifestyle

To understand what a healthy lifestyle is one firstly has to have a concept of health and this should be viewed from the broadest perspective. A well-used definition comes from the Ottawa Charter:

Health promotion is the process of enabling people to increase control over, and to improve their health. To reach a state of complete physical, mental and social well being, an individual or group must be able to identify and to realize aspirations, to satisfy needs, and to change or cope with the environment (WHO 1986 p. 1).

One of the difficulties with this definition is that it aspires to a state of health that is difficult to achieve, let alone maintain. Whilst you can, as an individual and as a health professional, try to work towards enabling health, reflect for a minute how often you can describe yourself as in a state of complete physical, mental and social well-being. To begin to understand the proposed changes you need to start by consulting Chapter 6 of Valuing People for an overview of what

is required of a health professional working with people with a learning disability. The White Paper highlights the problems and challenges that changing the service for people with a learning disability will entail and records the poor provision of some services. This places the focus on improving primary and secondary health services to address some of the main health problems and the implications of the changes to these services. The chronic health difficulties of people with severe and profound disabilities are also highlighted; this is of major importance because of the above average death rate of young people with learning disabilities. Research has demonstrated that people with learning disabilities do not use current screening services and specific symptoms that would benefit from early treatment are not always diagnosed (DoH 2001a).

One of the main recommendations in Chapter 6 is the need to improve the consistency of service provision across the NHS for people with a learning disability. This involves changes in the role of the specialist community learning disability team in helping to overcome barriers that people with a learning disability may encounter when accessing their primary care team. The role of health facilitator is identified as influential in overcoming barriers and providing educational opportunities for the primary care team. Hames & Carlson (2006) studied how these recommendations have been applied and found that change is still needed. Their research found that members of the primary care team did not always appreciate the implications of the White Paper and specialist teams still had difficulties in communicating their role. They also found that some general practitioners still did not fully understand the health needs of their patients who have a learning disability. To ensure awareness of these issues and as part of their good practice, occupational therapists should always consider the range of conditions relevant to their client when completing an initial assessment. Links with the primary care team are essential for health checks and should be established as part of good practice.

Additionally, when working with individuals from different ethnic backgrounds, you need to be aware that cultural differences may affect the way a person with a learning disability is perceived. Changing the perceptions and attitudes of the general population so that the individual takes on more responsibility for managing their own health is currently a concern of public health legislators internationally. Factors such as lack of income, ability to communicate their needs clearly and, until recently, a lack of advocates on their behalf have all contributed to the social exclusion and lack of access to mainstream health services experienced by people with a learning disability. Occupational therapists are currently exploring the profession's view that health and wellness is inextricably linked to occupation. Occupational science also explores the current view on psychological and sociological concepts of the individual's adherence to and understanding of a healthy lifestyle. Hurst (2004) found that occupational therapists believed that they did influence the health and wellness of the people they worked with, especially in providing health education in tertiary and secondary settings. Occupational therapists, through the use of a client-centred approach, already have the skills to engage in a health promoting encounter with service users and that is demonstrated in Table 5.1.

Whilst service users should not be defined by a clinical diagnosis such as Down's syndrome or Fragile X syndrome, as part of your intervention you do need to take into consideration how these may influence their health needs. For occupational therapists the main focus of any client-centred intervention will be how they can assist the service user to improve their occupational performance.

It can be difficult to differentiate between health, wellness and illness so that people with learning disability may have difficulty in highlighting their health needs (Seedhouse 2004). In recent years the emphasis has changed from the predominance of the medical model to that of a social model of health. It can be argued that neither of these models can adequately cover the needs of an individual with a learning disability. In particular, people with a profound and multiple learning disability may have physical health needs linked directly to their medical diagnosis. Sometimes health inequalities are compounded by the poor communication skills of mainstream health professionals or the lack of awareness of the staff working with people with a learning disability (Sheeby & Nind 2005). Young & Chesson (2006) found that through using a variety of resources it was possible to include some people with learning disabilities and severe mental health problems in discussions regarding their health. They highlighted the gap between the inclusion required by government policy and the need for further training and support for staff. However, the

Table 5.1 Comparison of skills needed for a health promotion encounter with the occupational therapy process

	Health promotion intervention	Occupational therapy process
Communication	Establish rapport	Establish rapport with client and relevant others
	Note non-verbal messages	Aware of all aspects of communication
	Check for understanding	Check for understanding
Motivation	Explore existing beliefs, attitudes and skills	Assess existing beliefs, attitudes and skills
	Provide information and skills	Explore locus of control
	Negotiate and agree contract	Collaboration and negotiation with client
	Check learning	Check understanding of the planned intervention
Support	Provide opportunity for acquiring knowledge	Provide opportunity to relearn/learn skills
	Act as advocate for social and environmental change	Act as an advocate for client with relevant others
	Evaluate progress	Evaluate progress

Hurst (2004) adapted from Tones & Tilford (2001) and Creek (2003).

importance of good communication between health and social care professionals and the service users does need to be highlighted. It is essential that service users are given appropriate and timely information about their health needs in a way that they will understand (Hart 2003, Thurman et al 2005).

It is important to remember that health promotion and health education are therefore no longer the domain of a specific band of health professionals but the responsibility of the whole specialist team. People with a learning disability have a higher incidence of additional health needs and the ethical debate continues as to how much health screening should be offered to those individuals who are at increased risk (Heason et al 2001). This is linked to the difficulty all health professionals face, which is being able to communicate clearly to ensure that you really have obtained informed consent (DoH 2001b). The challenge is to further develop the links between the specialist teams and general health provision. One of the methods devised to improve communication on all levels is the implementation of a health action plan.

The health action plan

The role of a health action plan (HAP) is to support the person-centred plan and, whilst it should be regularly and clearly updated, it is envisaged that it will be useful to ensure that support is offered to individuals at times of transition (DoH 2001b). Transitions are of considerable importance in the lifespan of a person with learning disability and they may have more than an average number of these events to cope with. Transitions are therefore discussed in more depth in Chapter 9. People with mild learning disability may wish to use health action plans as an approach that would enable them to be actively involved in managing their own health needs. As discussed earlier in the chapter, this should be a way of ensuring access to primary health care, for a group of people whose health needs have traditionally not been met by mainstream health services.

Health action plans should include not just health needs such as having regular hearing and/or eyesight tests, but also aspirations for a healthy lifestyle, e.g. joining an exercise session at the gym. With the permission of the service user, a copy of the HAP can also be kept with their notes in their GP's surgery. This can be an aid to communication if they see someone who does not know them well, as well as providing valuable insight for the primary care worker. A useful paper 'Treat me right!' (MENCAP 2004) can be found on their website. It relates experiences of using health services and identifies the main health difficulties with illustrative stories of what can go wrong when health professionals fail to understand the current UK government expectations of their role with people with a learning disability. Whilst the focus of client-centred care is important, there is a danger of ignoring the role of the family and formal or informal carers in the services used.

As an example, Thurman et al (2005) suggest the knowledge and skills that carers acquire can sometimes not be appreciated when health professionals struggle to communicate with their patients. Further reading is recommended on defining health and wellness in Chapter 6 of Valuing People (DoH 2001a), before attempting the following reader activity.

Reader activity

Read Chapter 6 of Valuing People – improving health for people with learning disabilities and:

- Make a summary of the key action points.
- How much do you know about keeping yourself healthy? Make a list of five things that you have done this week to keep yourself healthy, for example: eating a minimum of five portions of fruit and vegetables or taking a thirty minute walk.
- Now write your own health action plan.

Whilst health action plans can be used to promote an awareness of health when working with people with a mild learning disability, they can also be used as performance indicators. They can also be audited to provide evidence of the awareness of the health needs for people with profound and multiple disability. Access to the same range of health and social care services as the rest of the population allows service users to demonstrate community presence and for the community to promote choice for them to manage their health needs (O'Brien 1989). Promoting health by careful assessment and intervention planning when encouraging the development of knowledge and skills is an essential part of the occupational therapist's role. In striving to achieve the inclusion of health promotion, therapists should also be aware of not imposing their own standards on a person with a learning disability. It can be argued that, ethically, it is essential to explain the consequences of health behaviour, as with most health behaviours, this can usually be argued from different perspectives by anyone determined to continue with the behaviour, especially when it is eating, drinking or smoking (Seedhouse 2004). When working with someone who has a learning disability it is important to ensure good practice when obtaining consent and to note that consent does not have to be verbal (Gates 2003). A decision to act in 'best interest' could be made in exceptional circumstances but would always be based on a multidisciplinary decision. This has implications for the specialist team and is one occasion when the medical and social models may conflict. Effective communication between the team at this time means that those working with the service user understand the implications and consequences of any condition and the actions needed.

Promoting health through occupation

Sumsion (2005) suggests that client-centred practice, although difficult to achieve, is important for an effective intervention. Working within the framework of the Canadian Model of Occupational Performance (Law et al 1997) will help promote client-centred practice. Although not all service users will be able to use the Canadian Occupational Performance Measure (COPM; Law et al 2005), it can be useful for assessment and evaluation purposes for people with a mild learning disability. One of the difficulties that people with learning disability face is that they are often unaware that they have choices. Using the COPM to promote autonomy and empowerment allows the service user to become actively engaged in the intervention. Insight into what is important for the service user will also give the occupational therapist a way of presenting healthy options that they may not have had an opportunity to consider. For people with a learning disability their occupational form can be very complex. Whilst health and social care professionals are concerned that a unified approach is used, it is important to remember that people will exhibit different behaviours depending on the context of their occupational performance. Temporal aspects of the occupation are therefore of equal importance when considering the individual occupational balance. Having your life organized for you means that you are often not offered choices. People with learning disabilities often have a weekly programme and always mix with the same people during the day and evening. Lack of safe and reliable transport, especially in rural areas, limits choice for anyone who does not have a car.

Reader activity

Think about the choices that you make about your occupational performance and your behaviour:

- If you have had a stressful time what do you do about cooking a healthy meal or taking some exercise?
- Do you have some time when you just want to be alone and relax and not have to be polite to anyone? How do you let others know this?

This chapter will now look in more depth at the occupational domains of self-care, productivity and leisure and discuss how occupation links to the health needs of a person with a learning disability (Sumsion 2005).

Occupation and activities of daily living/self care (ADL)

Promoting self-care occupations as part of a healthy lifestyle is important and relevant health education provided at the same time as skills acquisition means that there is some occupational significance to carrying out a task such as cleaning teeth. For example, when you learnt to clean your teeth you may have acquired the skill through imitation or some more structured learning, but it remains a complex occupational performance. Service users who live with their parents or in supported accommodation may have support for their ADL tasks, but those who live alone may lack physical dexterity and/or motivation to clean their teeth. Overall general health can be affected by problems in the mouth; an individual with tooth decay and gum disease may find difficulties in chewing food and may avoid food because of pain from sensitive teeth. If someone with limited communication skills changes their reaction to food at meal times any dental problems should be the first thing eliminated. People with a learning disability can be less aware of non-verbal signals from others and so bad breath may not be acknowledged.

Inclusion in the health action plan of a regular dental check and advice from a dental hygienist will all contribute to a healthy mouth. The occupational therapist can provide support by advising on aspects of self-care, providing equipment and appropriate graded opportunity to learn new skills. Cleaning teeth properly requires a range of complex skills to complete the occupational performance and mastery is often ignored until dental decay is advanced. Dentists as well as other mainstream health professionals may need support to understand how to communicate with someone who has a learning disability. A wide range of resources on dental care is now available and liaison with the speech and language therapist will ensure that a suitable text or tape is selected. There is a range of suitable resources available; for example, both MENCAP and the British Institute of Learning Disabilities (BILD) publish resources to assist health professionals when talking to service users about specific health issues and healthy lifestyles.

Reader activity

- How important is communication in a health care encounter – consider the last time you went to see your GP or dentist, how effectively did they communicate with you?
- Next time you clean your teeth, consider the complexity of the task and reflect on the following questions:

  (i) Cognitive: do you know what the recommended time is to clean your teeth properly? If you do, how do you measure this time?

  (ii) Physical performance: how difficult is it to brush the molars at the back of your mouth?

  (iii) Sensory: how would it feel if someone else brushed your teeth? Do you have a favourite brand of toothpaste?

Sight and hearing are also essential to good health and problems with these can result in the individual having difficulties with daily self-care routines. Difficulties with foot care can also lead to problems with balance and gait and a referral to a podiatrist may be required. Although some of these problems appear minor, collectively they can affect an individual's occupational performance and ability to engage with and communicate effectively within their environment and so are essential parts of a healthy lifestyle.

Programmes to encourage people with profound and multiple disability to increase their range of self-care skills should be carefully discussed with all those involved with the service user. Choice and control are difficult to ascertain in these situations and it is important to try and balance the probability of learning the skill with the value placed on that occupation by the service user. To illustrate this further, Ruben provides an example of conflicting approaches.

Staff in the day centre had been following a feeding programme with Ruben for over a year with no signs of him being able to eat independently. This programme had been initiated by his keyworker and although a heated plate and a spoon with a padded handle were used Ruben still needed hand over hand assistance. This meant that lunch was prolonged and the food was cold and inedible. Staff in his residential setting fed Ruben and felt that this was a more pleasant experience for him. The occupational therapist queried the programme as Ruben had sensory and physical difficulties with partial sight and cerebral palsy that resulted in a weak grip. All the staff working with Ruben were asked to discuss how eating a meal became a valued and meaningful occupation and how they identified Ruben's preferences. All involved agreed that the occupation of eating food should be a pleasurable experience. As a result, the feeding programme was abandoned; Ruben then really enjoyed his food in both settings and the next problem was weight gain. It is important to remember that, whilst occupational therapists in conjunction with other members of the specialist team do use both backward and forward chaining as a way of teaching skills, such programmes should be reviewed regularly. It may take people with a learning disability longer to learn a new skill but unless some progress is made then it may be that particular aspects of self-care will always need assistance. Valued and meaningful occupations are more likely to be adopted and it can be more difficult to identify what the service user values if communication is difficult.

Many people with learning disability live in staffed homes and therefore budget and staff time, knowledge and skills in food purchase and preparation can limit the choice of food. Scriven & Atwal (2004) suggest that occupational therapists should consider looking for upstream roles relating to prevention. One method of engaging in a wider upstream, preventative role could be to encourage training sessions on nutrition from a dietitian for staff working with people with learning disabilities. Occupational therapists can then work with individual service users who need to learn new skills for nutrition, food purchase and preparation prior to a move to more independent living. This will ensure that the service user gets support on a daily basis from a more informed staff group who will understand and support the programme agreed between service user and therapist. This idea relates well to O'Brien (1989) who suggested a basis for evaluation of community participation and produced five service accomplishments to measure how effectively a person with a learning disability engages in their community. These are listed as community presence, participation, respect, choice and competence. The five accomplishments can be used to inform the approaches used by occupational therapists viewing health promotion from an occupational perspective.

Occupation and productivity

People with a learning disability need to perceive themselves as a productive part of society to ensure mental and physical health. A person with a mild learning disability living independently in the community will have a more complex range of tasks to perform to ensure that they remain healthy than someone who lives in a residential setting. When considering productivity occupational therapists usually receive referrals to assist someone in budgeting, cooking and other domestic skills and through careful assessment and working in a client-centred way can assist independence. Using occupation to assist them to identify what they believe are productive roles will contribute to self-esteem and promote health and wellness. Occupational performance analysis with the use of AMPS, if required, can highlight the occupational strengths and needs of the individual. This will provide insight for the person with a mild learning disability and additionally, as part of a specialist assessment from the team, assist support workers to provide appropriate levels of assistance. Additionally, stress levels can be reduced and contribute to the health of those service users faced with unrealistic expectations from support staff.

Increasingly, people with a learning disability are finding employment and will need to understand how to provide a healthy balanced meal within the time and budget available. At the end of a busy day cooking a meal may not be possible, and like other people, they may find that they do not enjoy eating alone. Even if they have a carer's role, confidence in ability may be lacking simply because the task appears to be too complicated. This occurred when working with Ruth.

Ruth was referred to the specialist team because her children were in care and she wanted to be able to provide meals with her own cooking during her access visits to them. Ruth wanted to work with the occupational therapist to learn to cook lasagne for her children. She had decided that only being able feed them from tins was not good enough and wanted to be able to give them what she describes as a 'proper meal'. The occupational therapist found that Ruth had very basic reading skills, lacked understanding of basic nutrition and confidence in choosing fresh ingredients. An occupational performance analysis of her cooking skills resulted in a method of acquiring these skills being devised. Ruth learnt to cook several simple dishes that had components of the lasagne, which could be combined to produce the main dish. She started with a white sauce for cauliflower cheese and then cooked pasta and a meat sauce. These recipes were photographed and provided with useful text so that in the end Ruth had her own recipe book. She also learnt to shop for the ingredients and ultimately could cook them independently for her children. Ruth's children enjoyed the dishes and provided such positive feedback that she then went on to take a cookery course at her local college. Introducing choice and the power to make her own decisions gave Ruth the opportunity to contribute both to her own and her children's health (Hollins & Flynn 2003, Sumsion 2005).

Other factors that may prevent people with a learning disability from leading productive lives need to be set in the context of the expectations of others, the physical environment and, if appropriate, the support of employers. Occupational therapists may be involved in assisting service users to prepare for work. The use of occupational performance analysis to provide structured opportunities for individuals to use public transport and develop interpersonal skills needed in the workplace all underpin successful employment. Communication is again an issue and for a potential employer to able to ask, in a way that can be comprehended by their employee, for tasks to be completed usually leads to a successful working relationship. However, these factors do not just apply to people with a learning disability, which you will be able to reflect on as you complete the next reader activity.

Reader activity

Think about a work situation that you have experienced.

- Did you have the knowledge and skills required for the job?

- Did your employer support you if you were having difficulties?
- How did you get to work; how complicated were the travel arrangements?
- What interpersonal skills did the job require?

Reflect on your answers and think about how difficult these factors could make finding employment if you were a person with a learning disability.

Occupation and leisure

Leisure is a concept that is open to interpretation and exists because people in the developed world can earn enough money through work to spend time choosing what they do for some of the time while not in paid employment. Recently, the enjoyment of exercise as a productive use of leisure time has been linked to health and wellness. Walking in particular has been identified as an inexpensive means of keeping fit and occupational therapists are encouraging exercise by using walking groups to support people as part of their occupational balance. People with learning disability are very dependent on others for opportunities to enjoy their leisure time. They are less likely to walk or go to a gym on a regular basis, which means that they are unable to meet the recommended requirements of 30 minutes of exercise five times a week (DoH, 2006). As part of the health action plan, health and social care professionals need to support service users in accessing community resources. People with a learning disability find it difficult not to lead a sedentary lifestyle, as they are often dependent on others for transport. In particular, service users with profound and multiple disability are particularly vulnerable as they can be dependent on families or support workers for their leisure opportunities. Hawkins & Look (2006) found that the barriers usually identified applied to the group of 19 adults included in their study. These are: lack of understanding of the health benefits of physical activity, lack of awareness of options and issues relating to risk and finance.

When completing an assessment with a service user it is important that occupational therapists include leisure, even if the referral is for another aspect of occupation. People with learning disabilities need to have access to a range of resources, and occupational therapists, by awareness of the importance of occupational balance to health and wellness, can become involved in primary health promotion. Through visiting the local library, links to community associations can be found and explored further. By talking to service users you can also find out about other leisure resources that exist locally and are linked specifically to learning disability. These may include voluntary groups, adult leisure libraries and fitness groups.

Consider the following questions about how you use leisure to contribute to your own occupational balance.

Reader activity

- How do you define a leisure activity?
- How do you keep fit?
- How would you feel if someone organized your leisure time for you?

Reflect on the importance of leisure for yourself. This will help you consider the leisure needs of Susan in the case study at the end of the chapter.

Occupational disruption

Self-care can also relate to health-damaging behaviours and, whilst a limited budget may reduce the number of people with a learning disability who smoke or abuse other substances, this still can be an issue in some settings. In particular, those people who have a learning disability and additional mental health or behavioural difficulties may be encountered in mental health or forensic settings (Roy 2000). Occupational deprivation through the lack of control and choice that occurs in these settings may require a different approach to that used by staff working in community settings. Occupational therapists working in these settings may need to look at behavioural issues as well as providing opportunities to develop and improve occupational performance skills. Prentice & Wilson (2003) suggest that the occupational therapist will need to help a service user by improving their occupational performance, which may include the opportunity to:

- improve coping skills by learning techniques for anger or anxiety management
- improve memory and concentration
- increase self confidence

- develop independent living skills
- improve social networks and increase leisure interests
- develop employment skills, especially communication and self expression.

Building relationships between forensic settings and specialist teams are important to maintain continuity for a person with a learning disability before they return to their own community.

Occupation, health and wellness in context

For the general population, health and wellness are not only affected by medical conditions that influence lifestyle choices but by other environmental elements such as housing and employment. The influence of the environment on the lifestyle of a person with a learning disability is not confined to where they live or the day services they use. The influence of the family and their expectations has and always will be important in shaping the health of the person with a learning disability. The status of family in the community and the culture that they are part of will have implications that can influence how they use health and social care services. With the rise in public awareness of the health implications of social exclusion, this is now recognized as influential in health and wellness. For example, obesity places a responsibility on health professionals to support the individual to gain knowledge and skills by appropriate interventions, including basic dietary information alongside budgeting or cooking skills. This may be an issue for parents with a learning disability, as discussed in the example of Ruth, who may also be subjected to more detailed scrutiny (for further reading refer to Chapter 10: Working with parents with a learning disability). How a family or individual copes with a loss or bereavement will also need to be explored. The health implications of bereavement and how to promote the health of the service user while they are experiencing the grieving process is discussed in Chapter 11. The transition from childhood and adolescence to adulthood and how this is viewed in terms of promoting independence and the future has implications especially for the mental health of the service user and these issues are discussed in Chapter 9.

Changing behaviours that risk health

At a service level the occupational therapist may be asked to participate in the specialist team's contribution to any health needs assessment for people with a learning disability within the Primary Care Trust. This should provide a sound multidisciplinary basis for identifying specific health needs and ensuring that the service user has access to the health professional qualified to assess and meet these needs. Providing information and support to enable a person with a learning disability to identify and change behaviours detrimental to their health also needs a framework so that the therapist can explain the approach to the service user, their family and other carers. As mentioned previously there are always ethical implications to consider when explaining health and wellness and professionals have to be careful not to impose their view of health and wellness on others.

When working with any individual who is currently identified as putting their health at risk, the occupational therapist should select an appropriate occupational therapy model and frame of reference. Consider the use of a health empowerment frame of reference/model as this could help both the therapist and service user understand how they could change. The Trans-theoretical (stages of change) Model (Prochaska & DiClemente 1982) describes the individual who does not acknowledge the need to change as 'precontemplative'. This means that if an individual smokes or drinks to excess they have yet to acknowledge that this will damage their health. Only when they are prepared to contemplate ceasing smoking will they be ready for the next stage and be able to prepare and plan, and they should be encouraged to seek support from the primary health team. Having succeeded in ceasing smoking they then have to maintain the new role of a non-smoker. One of the positive aspects of this model for occupational therapists is that lack of success in the behavioural change is viewed as an opportunity to try again rather than failure. The specialist nurse in the multidisciplinary team will usually be able to advise on the range of resources that are available to help support service users. The opportunity to promote health can be integrated in the occupational therapy intervention and it is important that the occupational therapist is able to communicate this aspect of their role to both the specialist team and other health and social care professionals (Hurst 2004).

Summary

This chapter has examined how the selection of meaningful occupations can enhance the health and wellness of people with a learning disability. A range of opportunities for promoting health have been discussed in relation to the occupational therapist's role in this area. Occupational therapist working in specialist teams that relate to primary care services need to be able to ensure that equity exists in relation to health for this sector of the population. It is therefore important that they are able to explain that occupation has a direct influence on health an wellness. The following Case Illustration gives an opportunity to reflect on the contents of this chapter.

Box 5.1

Case illustration: Susan

Susan Jones (aged 35) has Down's syndrome and a mild learning disability. She is able to communicate effectively but has a limited vocabulary and cannot always express herself clearly. Susan has a problem with her weight but is supported and encouraged by her mother to eat a healthy diet. Susan enjoys her food and is proud of the fact that she can make simple snacks and her own drinks at the day centre, although she is not allowed to do this at home. Her mother has always run the home and sees herself as caring for Susan completely.

Susan lives with her mother (aged 70), in a two-bedroomed flat; but since her father died two years ago her life has changed. She no longer goes out at weekends because her mother sold the car and they have not been on holiday since his death. Susan asks to go out to social events but her mother says that she likes her company

at home. She has attended the local day centre since her family moved to the town 20 years ago. Currently, changes are happening at the day centre such that she is worried that it may be closing down. She enjoys spending her time there and has lots of friends, who she only sees at the centre.

Her keyworker has noticed a change in her behaviour recently. Susan now gets angry when one of her best friends, Denise, tells her about what she has done at the weekend. Denise lives in supported sheltered housing and helps to cook her own meals and goes out to the shops, cinema and pub and always talks about what she has done at the weekend on a Monday morning. When Susan is asked why she is angry she says that she is 'fed up and unhappy and does not know what to do'. Denise is very concerned as she found Susan sitting and crying in the toilets the other day. Her keyworker has tried to talk to Mrs Jones but she insists that Susan is happy at home.

At a recent person-centred planning meeting Susan said she wanted make her own snacks and a cup of tea at home and her mother insisted that she could not be allowed to this. To prevent the argument developing her keyworker suggested a referral to the occupational therapist working in the specialist learning disability team. Susan and her keyworker were very keen for this to happen and Mrs Jones has reluctantly agreed.

Reader activity

1. In what way is Susan's health and wellness affected by her current situation?

2. How would an occupational therapist assist Susan to identify the meaningful occupations of ADL, productivity and leisure to promote her health and wellness?

3. Which other members of the specialist learning disability team or primary care team would the occupational therapist liaise with?

Further reading

Prentice R, Wilson K 2003 Forensic occupational therapy within learning disability services. In: Couldrick L, Alred D (eds) Forensic occupational therapy. London, Whurr

Scriven A, Atwal A 2004 Occupational therapists as primary health promoters: opportunities and barriers. British Journal of Occupational Therapy 67(10):424–429

Watson RM 2006 Being before doing: the cultural identity (essence) of occupational therapy. Australian Occupational Therapy Journal 53:151–158

Useful resources

The Valuing People support team has produced a useful site with health information and resources you can download: http://valuingpeople. gov.uk/index.jsp (accessed 3 March 2008)

You can also find information that is constantly being updated if you check on the Department of Health website and search for information on diet and exercise.

References

Adams L, Beadle-Brown J, Mansell J 2006 Individual planning: an exploration of the link between quality of plan and quality of life. British Journal of Learning Disability 34:68–76

Couldrick L, Alred D 2003 Forensic occupational therapy. London, Whurr

Creek J 2003 Occupational therapy defined as a complex intervention. London, College of Occupational Therapists

Department of Health 2000 The NHS Plan: a plan for investment, a plan for reform. London, The Stationery Office

Department of Health 2001a Valuing People: a new strategy for learning disability for the 21st century. London, The Stationery Office

Department of Health 2001b Seeking consent working with people with learning disabilities. London, The Stationery Office

Department of Health 2006 At least five a week: evidence on the impact of physical activity and its relationship to health – a report from the Chief Medical Officer. London, DoH

Gates B (ed.) 2003 Learning disabilities: towards inclusion, 4th edn. Edinburgh, Churchill Livingstone

Hames A, Carlson T 2006 Are primary health care staff aware of the role of community learning disability teams in relation to health promotion and health facilitation? British Journal of Learning Disabilities 34:6–10

Hart S 2003 Health and health promotion. In: Gates B (ed.) Learning disabilities: towards inclusion, 4th edn. Edinburgh, Churchill Livingstone

Hawkins A, Look R 2006 Levels of engagement and barriers to physical activity in a population of adults with learning disabilities. British Journal of Learning Disabilities 34:220–226

Heason C, Stracey L, Rey D 2001 Valued occupation for people who have a learning disability. In: Thomson J, Pickering S (eds) Meeting the health needs of people who have a learning disability. Edinburgh, Baillière Tindall

Hollins S, Flynn M 2003 Food, fun, healthy and safe. London, Royal College of Psychiatrists

Hurst J 2004 Health promotion in student practice placements: occupational therapists' use of related activities. Unpublished Masters Thesis, London, College of Occupational Therapists Library

Law M, Baptiste S, Carswell A, McColl MA, Polatajko H, Pollock N 1997 The Canadian model of occupational performance. Toronto, CAOT Publications

Law M, Baptiste S, Carswell A, McColl MA, Polatajko H, Pollock N 2005 Canadian occupational performance measure, 4th edn. Ottawa, CAOT publications ACE

MENCAP 2004 Treat me right! – better health care for people with a learning disability. MENCAP website http://www.mencap.org. uk (accessed 3 March 2008)

O'Brien J 1989 What's worth working for? Leadership for better quality human services. Georgia, Responsive Systems Associates

Prentice R, Wilson K 2003 Forensic occupational therapy within learning disability services. In: Couldrick L, Alred D (eds) Forensic occupational therapy. London, Whurr

Prochaska J, DiClemente C 1982 Transtheoretical therapy: Toward a more integrative model of change. Psychotherapy Theory, Research and Practice 19:276–288

Reynolds F 2001 Strategies for facilitating physical activity and wellbeing: a health promotion perspective. British Journal of Occupational Therapy 64(7): 330–336

Roy A 2000 The care programme approach in learning disability psychiatry. Advances in Psychiatric Treatment 6:380–387

Scriven A, Atwal A 2004 Occupational therapists as primary health promoters: opportunities and barriers. British Journal of Occupational Therapy 67(10):424–429

Seedhouse D 2004 Health Promotion: philosophy, prejudice and practice, 2nd edn. Chichester, John Wiley

Sheeby K, Nind M 2005 Emotional well-being for all: mental health and people with profound and multiple learning disabilities. British Journal of Learning Disability 33:34–38

Sumsion T 2005 Promoting health through client centred occupational therapy practice. In: Scriven A (ed.) Health promoting practice: the contribution of nurses and allied health professionals. Basingstoke, Palgrave Macmillan

Thompson J, Pickering S (eds) 2001 Meeting the health needs of people who have a learning disability. Edinburgh, Baillière Tindall

Thurman S, Jones J, Tarleton B 2005 Without words: meaningful information for people with high individual communication needs. British Journal of Learning Disabilities 33(2):83–89

Tones K, Tilford S 2001 Health promotion: effectiveness, efficiency and equity. Cheltenham, Nelson Thornes

Watson RM 2006 Being before doing: the cultural identity (essence) of occupational therapy. Australian Occupational Therapy Journal 53:151–158

Wilcock A 1998 Occupation for health. British Journal of Occupational Therapy 61(8): 340–345

World Health Organization 1986 Ottawa Charter for Health Promotion. Geneva, WHO

Young A, Chesson RA 2006 Obtaining views on health care from people with learning disabilities and severe mental health problems. British Journal of Learning Disabilities 34:11–19

Appendix 5.1 Case illustration: Susan, possible answers

1. In what way is Susan's health and wellness affected by her current situation?

Susan may have mental health problems as she has exhibited behavioural changes and is clearly confused and angry. If these are not resolved it could lead to further disruption to her life and she needs to be listened to and have the opportunity to express her needs. Although Susan's mother is helping her by watching her diet for her, this is not her choice and her physical exercise is also limited in as she has no real chance to do this apart from at her day centre activities.

2. How would an occupational therapist assist Susan to identify the meaningful occupations of ADL, productivity and leisure to promote her health and wellness?

The occupational therapist initially listened to Susan's narrative and heard she was still upset at her father's death and not being able to go to his funeral. She was also angry that her mother had sold the car. She wanted to be able to do more at home and was bored at the weekends because all they did was go to the shops and then she watched television or she played her CD player. She also felt that her mother would not let her choose her own clothes or have a television in her room. She said that she was upset because she had asked her mother if she could go out with Denise and the friends she shared her house with and her mother had said no. At the moment she has no money of her own as her mother takes all her benefits and she has to ask her mother if she wants something. She says that the usual reply is that they cannot afford it. Susan obviously cares for her mother but as she listens to the others talking about all that they have done at the weekends she feels very angry and wants them to 'shut up'. She also wants her mother to let her have some money and to make a cup of hot chocolate when she wants it. She knows from making her drinks at the day centre that you can get a 'special type of hot chocolate' so her mother telling her that it is too fattening is not necessarily true.

Client-centred work with Susan highlighted the following priorities:

- having some money of her own is very important
- being able to go out with Denise
- making her own chocolate drink
- making her own breakfast.

Staff at the day centre and support workers at Denise's house cannot understand what all the fuss is about as they have assured Mrs Jones that Susan is very safe making hot drinks and that they would be supporting Denise, Susan and other friends on social outings. Mrs Jones remains adamant that she will not let Susan do these things because she is not capable.

Mrs Jones is rather annoyed that someone else is now involved but she does agree to have a chat with the therapist. Given the opportunity she starts to talk about the distress that Susan's birth caused and the social isolation that ensued for her and her husband. Having been told that they could never have children they were both overjoyed when she became pregnant. Her husband was very upset by the attitudes of his family and she believes that he never 'got over' having a daughter with Down's syndrome. In fact she had to fight to bring up Susan at home rather than letting her go into care. She cannot grasp that attitudes about and expectations to people with a learning disability have changed and is very worried about what will happen to Susan when she dies. In fact she rather expects Susan to die before her because that would solve her problem although she feels very guilty about this. She also talks about her husband's death and how lonely she has been since, especially as she also has money problems.

The occupational therapist now has a clear picture of the current situation and can begin to plan an intervention. If this is to remain client centred, it has to focus on Susan's wants and needs but it also has to take into account Mrs Jones's concerns for the future and how the loss of her husband and subsequent financial difficulties could be affecting the situation. Clearly some support for Mrs Jones at this stage will allow the therapist to focus on Susan and her occupational performance and form.

3. Which other members of the specialist learning disability team or primary care team would the occupational therapist liaise with?

Mrs Jones agrees to meet with the social worker from the multidisciplinary team to talk about the future opportunities for Susan. She will also be advised how to get information on benefits so she can check that she and Susan are receiving the correct benefits. She also agrees to have the telephone number of CRUSE bereavement counselling services (as it is still causing her distress).

With support Mrs Jones began to realize that it was in Susan's best interests to look to the future and Susan and the occupational therapist began to focus on the occupations she had identified. Susan's long-term goal was to move out and live in the house with Denise when a space became available. Adams et al (2006) highlight the way that the quality of the person-centred plan influences the quality of life and Susan's example illustrates this.

Section **Two**

The chapters in this section explore the barriers and opportunities for people with learning disabilities to develop and maintain occupational integrity in activities of daily living, employment and leisure.

Activities of daily living broadly cover the spectrum of the skills and routines for self maintenance or self-care, safety aspects in the home and home management. Very often an individual will present with an inability to be independent in relation to one or many self-care occupations. Activities such as washing, combing hair or brushing teeth can provoke maladaptive or emotional responses, such as avoidance or atypical seeking out of stimuli, that prove difficult and confusing for the individual and their carers. In Chapter 6, Vanessa Townsend focuses on the relevance of sensory integration to personal activities of daily living. The chapter explores the theory, process and application of sensory integration approaches for people with learning disabilities.

In Chapter 7, Angela Kelsall discusses the issues of developing and supporting employment opportunities for people with a learning disability. Employment perspectives are explored in relation to transition into the work place and development of individual self efficacy. The chapter identifies some of the barriers and opportunities for employment, the implications of policy changes and models of employment. These are presented as a challenge for occupational therapists to take a role in developing opportunities for people with learning disability into employment.

The last chapter in this section discusses the meaning and complexity of leisure as an occupational performance area. Chapter 8 explores the barriers and opportunities of leisure for people with a learning disability. Although leisure is an important occupational domain, it is often considered a low priority from a service provision perspective. Leisure is acknowledged as having intrinsic attributes and benefits to improve self-esteem, personal growth and just having fun. The occupational therapy role is discussed in relation to maintaining client-centred approaches, ensuring choice and participation in leisure pursuits.

The reader activities in all the chapters give you the opportunity to reflect on your understanding of the meaning of self-care, work and leisure for people with a learning disability.

Chapter Six

Activities of daily living for individuals with a learning disability: using a sensory integrative approach

6

Vanessa Townsend

Overview

Activities of daily living (ADL) involve routines of self-care necessary to maintain health and well-being. In our daily lives we also develop our own preferred routines, and express ourselves through, for example, choice of clothing or food tastes. To enable people to become independent in these activities, occupational therapists need to understand how from childhood we develop the necessary skills to dress, wash, feed, and groom ourselves. In doing this we acknowledge both the impact of our bodies and the environment on our ability to carry out these activities. The process of integrating both sensory and motor stimuli to override physiological and emotional reflex responses is a development that underpins how we acquire skills. This complex developmental process is termed sensory integration (SI).

Although SI is not exclusive to the learning disabilities field there are particular reasons why occupational therapists need to consider SI dysfunction in individuals with a learning disability. To do this, occupational therapists should have a clear understanding of neuroanatomy, physiology and development. Postgraduate training in SI techniques is vital before involvement in implementing SI interventions and as a therapist new to the learning disability field and SI it is likely that initial involvement will involve 'shadowing' a senior therapist.

This chapter therefore aims to introduce you to the context for using SI for people with learning disabilities and its application to some of the problems of self-care. It starts with a brief overview of the foundations of SI, acknowledges, recent evidence and makes links with the occupational therapy role. The chapter does not provide a comprehensive text on SI theory but identifies key sources of evidence for further reading. By integrating a case illustration, the chapter explores the types of issues that may present in self-care with an individual with SI dysfunction.

Learning Outcomes

By the end of the chapter you will be able to:
- Identify how a sensory processing dysfunction may present during self-care activities
- Define SI, the sensory systems involved in sensory processing and the most recent classifications of sensory processing dysfunction

- Appreciate how the SI approach is applicable to individuals with a learning disability
- Define the role of the occupational therapist from assessment through to the provision of direct therapy and consultative advice.

ADL and development of SI

ADL broadly cover the spectrum of self-maintenance tasks including grooming, personal hygiene, routines for health maintenance, socialization for communication, functional mobility, safety and home management, i.e. clothing care, cleaning, etc. This chapter focuses on the relevance of SI to aspects of personal hygiene rather than home management aspects. People with a learning disability very often present with complex problems and inability to be independent in relation to one or many ADL occupations. Difficulty with ADL often presents itself in people with learning disabilities as avoidance, seeking out high levels of stimuli or atypical maladaptive emotional behaviour towards activities such as bathing, washing, combing hair, brushing teeth or eating certain types of food.

Ordinarily, we interpret sensory information from our bodies and environment as demonstrated in the following example showing the processes that occur for an individual to do this.

Consider what happens if you accidentally sip a very hot drink. Immediately there is a 'protective' reaction and withdrawal from the source of the hot drink. Second, you take actions to reduce the heat in your mouth by opening your mouth wide and possibly fanning your mouth with your hand. Finally, there is an emotional reaction to the pain by possibly showing annoyance and avoidance of further risk by either putting the cup aside or waiting until it cools. All three processes demonstrate involvement of a SI process (Ayres 1972a) as follows:

- Sensory registration – the tea is hot
- Sensory modulation – responding to the heat by a physical response (withdrawing), and emotional response (heightened level of arousal)
- Sensory discrimination – make a critical immediate adjustment or future change by adjusting behaviour to avoid sipping the tea when it is still hot.

From her observations when working with children Ayres (1972b) identified that a subgroup of children with learning disabilities had difficulty interpreting sensory information from their bodies and environment, whereas in most situations we can 'control' our reactions to sensory stimuli and demands from our own bodies and the environment. Consider the following reader activity to identify the type of stimuli we experience from everyday self-care activities.

Reader activity

- What sensations can you experience when combing your hair?
- How do you feel when you smell bread baking?
- Does listening to your favourite music relax or excite you?
- What is your response to rocking back and forward rapidly?
- What happens when water gets in your eyes when showering?

Some of your responses to the above will be momentary, manageable, positive reactions such as relaxing to music or negative such as discomfort when getting water in your eyes. However, for people with a learning disability adverse responses can result in reactions that are maladaptive and pose significant problems of occupational performance.

Classifications of SI systems

Sensory systems

Sensory information is received through sensory systems involving seven senses, which are detailed in the Glossary:

- tactile (touch)
- vestibular (movement)
- proprioception (body position)
- auditory (sound)
- vision
- olfactory (smell)
- gustatory (taste).

All of the above individual senses do not operate in isolation but are integrated to enable us to carry out everyday activities. Sensory processing occurs both at a conscious and unconscious level by which an activity, such as running a tap, will involve registering a number of stimuli simultaneously. For example, identifying by seeing (visually) and hearing (auditory) if the water is running too fast or too slowly, or feeling (touch) whether the water is hot or cold and its wetness on the skin. The processes of registration, orientation and response are illustrated in Figure 6.1. Together, the senses contribute to adaptive responses involving:

- Reflex integration – e.g. removing hand if water is too hot
- Movement skills – e.g. whilst standing and using arms to turn taps, involving lateral dominance, midline crossing, left–right orientation, maintenance of tonic muscle tone, slow, graded, rhythmical and reciprocal movements, gross and fine motor coordination and balance
- Auditory, language and visual spatial processing functions – perceiving and adjusting to the sounds and objects whilst adjusting taps to moderate water flow.

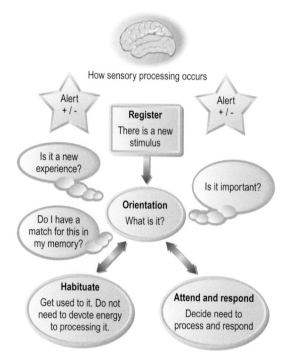

Figure 6.1 • How sensory processing occurs. Adapted from Green D 2003 Applied clinical reasoning using a sensory integrative approach in the treatment of individuals with pervasive developmental disorders and learning disabilities. Revision from the 7th edition.

Proprioceptive and visual information enables us to lift or turn objects with the appropriate amount of force. Simultaneously, integration of tactile, vestibular, proprioceptive and visual senses creates a stable frame of reference against which other sensations are interpreted. The auditory cortex also receives information from the visual and somatosensory systems to register and make sense of environmental stimuli. Further reading can be found in Cohen (1999) and refer to the Glossary for the above terms.

The developmental theory underlying SI

It is important to be aware of the developmental theories and terminology used to classify SI dysfunctions. There are five assumptions underpinning SI theory.

Neural plasticity – Ayres (1972a) believed that the brain, especially the young brain, is naturally malleable and capable of change, given the correct input. By providing enhanced sensory experiences within the context of meaningful activities that involve the planning and execution of an adaptive response, we can increase SI and improve learning

Developmental sequence – SI in a normal child occurs in a developmental sequence. SI theory reasons that by systematically providing sensory motor experiences to facilitate normal neuromotor development, we can assist the brain to function more normally and establish normal developmental sequences

Nervous system hierarchy – Ayres (1972a) recognized that the brain functions as a whole, but that higher level, 'executive functions' such as abstract thinking, reasoning, perception and language, evolve from and are dependent on the integrity of lower level, subcortical structures of the brain. These subcortical structures develop and mature through sensorimotor experiences. Further reading is recommended in Tyldesley & Grieve (2002)

Adaptive interaction – when an individual learns through interaction with the environment something new or meets a new challenge, is indicative of effective SI and continues to develop effective SI further

Inner drive – people have an inner drive to participate in activities with sensory motor components.

Most recent classifications of sensory processing dysfunction

Initially, the five syndromes attributed by Ayres (1972b) as deficits in SI obtained from the senses included: tactile defensiveness, disorders of postural and bilateral integration, apraxia, deficits in form and space perception, and auditory/language disorders. Dyspraxia is a developmentally based difficulty in motor planning of unfamiliar motor tasks. Ayres (1985) stated that dyspraxia is a problem of organizing the motor plan and hypothesized four major expressions of dysfunction in praxis: somatodyspraxia, bilateral integration and sequencing (BIS) deficits, visuodyspraxia, and dyspraxia on verbal command (refer to the Glossary). For further reading, a comprehensive coverage of the foundations for SI can be found in Ayres (2005). The development of SI within paediatrics is clearly linked to developmental theory and is also described fully in *Sensory Integration Theory and Practice* (Bundy et al 2002). The recent classifications of SI dysfunctions found in the occupational therapy literature and briefly introduced below are:

1. Dysfunctions in sensory modulation (Lane et al 2000) include dyspraxia (dysfunction in movement responses), and sensory discrimination (dysfunction in responses to sensory input). The sensory discrimination dysfunction can present with three response patterns: over-responsivity (over-arousal to sensory input), under-responsivity, and fluctuating responsivity.

2. Sensory modulation disorders are defined by Murray-Slutsky & Paris (2000) as difficulties with registration, orientation or arousal (ROA) such as:

   - Predictable sensory ROA disorders – discrete under- or over-responsiveness in ROA, or a specific sensory system, (e.g. avoidance or dislike of certain clothes' textures, light touch, motion sickness)
   - Fluctuating or defensive ROA disorders – hypersensitive or fluctuating responses in ROA or a specific sensory system, including tactile defensiveness (e.g. withdraws from hair combing), gravitational insecurity (e.g. avoids walking on different carpets or grass, clumsy, stumbles, falls), aversive response to movement and sensory under-responsiveness to touch, movement, sight or sound
   - Tactile discrimination difficulties (the somatosensory system) (e.g. decreased awareness or has difficulty feeling clothes are not on straight)
   - Somatodyspraxia (e.g. difficulty with gross and fine motor tasks and is often accompanied by deficits in tactile discrimination – may avoid putting hands into water or using hands to touch).

3. Sensory modulation dysfunctions: Bundy et al (2002) further categorize SI dysfunctions as 'sensory modulation dysfunctions' (SMD) including sensory defensiveness in tactile, auditory and visual systems, gravitational insecurity, aversive response to movement and sensory under-responsivity, and practic dysfunctions including bilateral integration and sequencing deficits (BIS) and somatodyspraxia. For a summary of these terms, refer to Box 6.1.

To summarize, sensory modulation is the ability to regulate and organize the degree, intensity and nature of responses to sensory input in a graded and adaptive manner. This enables the individual to maintain optimal performance. Where the individual reacts in a disproportionate way to a non-noxious sensation (e.g. when drying, to the touch of towel on the skin) it may suggest that they have a sensory modulation dysfunction. The behaviour may result in avoidance or seeking out high levels of stimuli. Sensory modulation is not a linear process, so an individual can jump from defensiveness to under-responsiveness in a matter of seconds.

How the SI approach is applicable to individuals with a learning disability

Historically, the development of SI within paediatrics is clearly linked to developmental theory (Ayres 1972, Bundy et al 2002). More recently, Urwin & Ballinger (2005) have established the relevance of SI as an

Box 6.1

Summarized classifications of SI dysfunctions

Sensory modulation dysfunctions (SMD)

Sensory defensiveness in the tactile, auditory and visual systems

Presents disproportionate over-responsivity response to non-noxious touch, which may result in extreme anxiety, hitting out, or avoidance and causes:

- Disrupted milestone, social, emotional and academic achievement,
- Disrupted personal care routines,
- Distractibility,
- Irregular emotional tone,
- Often the need for extreme personal space.

Sensory under-responsivity (under-responsiveness)

Presents as a failure to respond to sensory stimuli in an expected way and the individual may appear:

- Passive, lethargic and unengaged,
- Require an excessive amount of stimulation to achieve engagement,
- May demonstrate extreme behaviours to obtain or avoid sensation – strange postures, rocking, etc., fluctuating responsivity.

Gravitational insecurity

- Individual shows an extreme reluctance to move,
- Experience autonomic system reactions: sweating, clamminess, pallor, hyperventilation.

Aversive response to movement

Is characterized by the individual experiencing physical responses to movement including vertigo, nausea, dizziness. The individual may present by:

- Avoiding movement,
- Exhibiting an increase in arousal or restlessness following movement,
- Experiencing motion sickness,
- Exhibiting self-injurious behaviour.

Practic dysfunctions – dyspraxia

Bilateral integration and somatodyspraxia (BIS) is a type of SI dyspraxia in which there is evidence of impaired vestibular and proprioceptive processing. The individual may present with difficulties of

Bilateral integration:

- Ability to perform unfamiliar motor tasks is impaired,
- Dyspraxia deficits such as left–right confusion and avoidance of crossing midline and often postural deficits.

Somatodyspraxia

Evidence of poor processing of at least somatosensory information is characterized by difficulty across the whole spectrum of gross and fine motor tasks and is often accompanied by deficits in tactile discrimination.

Sequencing deficits

Poor motor planning, not simply poor execution, and their motor planning is significantly poorer than their performance in other areas of cognition.

intervention for people with learning disabilities in the UK. Research (Smith-Roley et al 2001) has identified the main learning disability diagnostic groups linked with SI difficulties as:

- Pervasive developmental disorder (including autism and Asperger's syndrome)
- Attention deficit hyperactivity disorder (ADHD/ADD)
- Learning disorders (specific learning difficulties)
- Fragile X syndrome
- Developmental coordination delay (DCD) (including dementia).

However, the sensory modulation model generally is considered more relevant for persons with mild to moderate problems in learning and behaviour and excludes those with overt neurological damage such as stroke, cerebral palsy and spina bifida (Kielhofner 2002). This section will highlight how the occupational therapist might intervene in relation to possible sensory modulation dysfunction. In Box 6.2 a case illustration (Sarah) will be used to integrate the issues that can arise from a SI dysfunction in ADL and to demonstrate the role of the occupational therapist.

Rationale for accepting referral

The first step taken by the occupational therapist was to obtain a clearer rationale for accepting the referral.

Box 6.2

Case illustration: Sarah

A referral made to occupational therapy by Sarah's case manager requested assessment and advice about how best to support Sarah's transition into adult services. Sarah is an 18-year-old with severe learning disability, who lives at home with her parents, older sister and nephew of 2 years. Sarah's transition into adult services is causing some concern as the school have described her as difficult to engage, nervous and distractible, often demonstrating self-injurious behaviours, and on some occasions hitting out or throwing items within her vicinity. Sarah is wheelchair dependent, and communicates via gesture, body language and differing non-vocal sounds. She receives total support during personal ADL, which she finds distressing.

The referral was initiated by reports from staff carrying out personal care for Sarah. There had been an escalation of self-injurious behaviour evident during changing of incontinence aids and at meal times when others, especially unpredictable peers, came too close. Secondary to this was Sarah's lack of engagement in 'table-top' activities, as she would not hold items. The case manager reported that all these behaviours had been present throughout her schooling. Sarah's mother and father were finding it increasingly difficult to cope with Sarah, and their older daughter and grandson who had recently moved back into the parental home. They were insisting on a 5-day service out of the home environment for Sarah. However, within the existing service provision the case manager could not envisage how to maintain support for Sarah to meet her needs, especially in relation to risk to herself and others.

How sensory processing dysfunction may present during ADL

SI assessments

It is important to carefully consider the elements impacting on an individual suspected of having a SI dysfunction. When an occupational therapist suspects a SI dysfunction a holistic assessment resembling that undertaken for any other condition is made: obtain a full history, utilize a range of standardized and non-standardized assessments, including clinical observations.

Specific standardized SI assessments for adults with learning disabilities include the Sensory Integration Inventory – Revised for Individuals with Developmental Disabilities (SII-R) (Reisman & Hanschu 1992). This is the most commonly used assessment for adults with a learning disability and limited verbal skills. It has a criterion-referenced checklist of 111 tactile, proprioceptive, and vestibular behaviours and general reactions that may have a relationship with poor sensory processing. The assessment is completed by carer interview and/or observation.

Alternatively, there is a self-questionnaire, The Adolescent/Adult Sensory Profile (Brown & Dunn 2002). Based on self-rating responses to specific sensations it produces a sensory processing profile of the individual across four quadrants: low registration, sensation seeking, sensory sensitivity and sensation avoiding. It also results in an intervention matrix based on taste, smell, movement, visual, touch, activity level and activity processing.

As this tool depends on individuals being able to verbalize about their sensory experiences it was not ideal for Sarah. Therefore, the Sensory Integration Inventory – Revised for Individuals with Developmental Disabilities (SII-R) was chosen and completed with Sarah's mother and father on an additional home visit. The inventory was also completed with Sarah's teacher to establish consistency checking. Observation of Sarah during the school day verified the descriptions provided by her teacher and family.

Sarah: initial assessment (obtaining a full history)

A home visit to interview Sarah's parents was carried out to gain as full a history as possible and a clear picture of current life circumstances and any wider issues affecting the family. Sarah's mother and father described Sarah as a difficult baby who had always cried at every occasion of self-care, particularly nail trimming, combing and cutting hair, and teeth cleaning. Any physical contact, except for being hugged, tightly wrapped in a blanket, resulted in distress behaviours. Sarah's acquisition of basic skills such as reaching, grasping and manual exploration had never been realized, as she would immediately discard toys. At 'primary' school she disliked children coming near her and reacted with self-injurious behaviour when offered messy tasks such as finger painting – a pattern repeated in 'junior' school when offered collage, pottery, etc. Sarah did, however, love to be pushed on a swing, and to be cuddled tightly, and historically showed pleasure when travelling in the car. The other current variables in Sarah's life included her sister and nephew returning to the family home, which according to her parents appeared to have increased Sarah's anxiety levels. There had been increased difficulty caring for her because of her reactions to self-care tasks and physical contact. Her parents were very concerned about her provision on leaving school. In all other respects Sarah's routines remained stable.

From the information gathered, the occupational therapist identified a possible 'cluster' of factors, which may be indicative of a SI dysfunction:

- Sarah could not tolerate self-care activities, or light touch
- She discarded items and did not develop manual exploration
- She avoided 'messy' activities
- She disliked 'unpredictable' peers in her vicinity and yet she liked tight cuddling and motion in a vehicle.

The 'wider issue' voiced by Sarah's parents was assisting her physically during self-care. Historically, Sarah's father had lifted her in and out of the bath, and her mother had washed, dried and dressed her. This posed a significant manual handling risk and gender-specific issues. Referral to the physical disabilities occupational therapist was made to assess for the provision of appropriate manual handling equipment for use in the home, and also an assessment of manual handling practices within the school environment where Sarah was also hoisted.

The resulting 'clusters' from the SII-R assessment supported the hypothesis that Sarah was hypersensitive to tactile sensation. Sarah's behaviours illustrate one way in which an individual with a learning disability may over-respond, (e.g. hyper-sensitivity) to sensory input. Individuals can also under-respond (e.g. hypo-sensitivity) or demonstrate a fluctuating response to a sensory input (seeks out or avoids sensation) in an atypical or disproportionate manner to what would normally be expected, and this is called a sensory modulation disorder (SMD).

However, as illustrated by Sarah, the difficulty in determining SI dysfunction is that many people with learning disabilities will present with behaviours that are long standing. The occupational therapist may need to consider a number of alternative explanations of long-established behaviours or habits. Self-injurious behaviour could function as demand avoidance, a communicative function, a means to control a situation or others for non-sensory based reasons. There may be gain for the individual in positive or negative attention or behaviour stemming from lack of occupational opportunities, control or choice. The behaviours might serve as a retaliatory function, either reactive to a novel circumstance, or a historical response from one to another. Behaviours can be established and carried over from other environments or previous routines. Behaviours should also be considered in relation to the possibility or indication of abuse, response to life changes or inconsistency in interactions.

Anxiety and level of arousal during activities

Stress-related anxiety can amplify and exaggerate the behavioural response to the sensory input as indicated with Sarah when new or unpredictable situations arise. Sensory defensiveness may generate unfounded apprehension or fear, concentration difficulties and restlessness. An individual's generalized responses with tactile defensiveness may include an aversive response to non-harmful touch ranging from pulling away from, or hitting out to deflect the touch – The fight or flight mechanism illustrated in Figure 6.2. For example, if a friendly touch feels painful (a mismatch to expectation), the behavioural inhibition system is activated, taking control of behaviour, leading to increased arousal, anxiety and attention to the stimulus. The individual may exhibit extreme avoidance of touch through social activity or care activities. Sarah illustrates the difficulties presented within personal care tasks with high levels of touch, especially to the face, hands, feet; hair washing or nail trimming for example, may be extremely anxiety provoking. Observable anxiety at anticipated touch is often interpreted as emotional lability. The individual may be visually alert in an attempt to foresee (and avoid) potential touch, making the individual appear distractible.

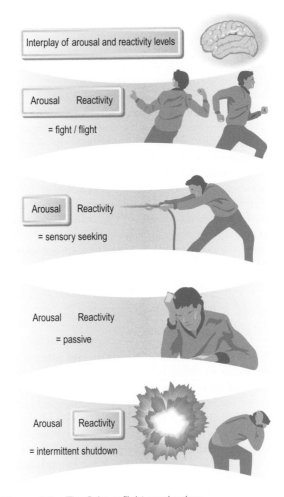

Figure 6.2 • The fight or flight mechanism.

Impaired sensory processing on occupational performance during ADL

Blanche & Schaaf (2001) depict the relationship between SI and engagement in daily occupations as a 'rolling wheel'. The 'rolling wheel' model demonstrates the inter-dependence of effective sensory processing and participation in ADL. Research has confirmed the relationship of SI to functioning in daily occupations (Spitzer & Roley 2001). All ADL impose a high demand on sensory modulation. Observation during ADL must, therefore, be explored fully before possible SI dysfunction is established. When observing the client engaged in ADL, remember that establishment of SI dysfunction must be based on a pervasive 'cluster' of presentations across wide-ranging activities, contexts and environments, and throughout the individual's historical presentation. The following gives a basic outline of how SI impacts and manifests during ADL.

Bathing or showering

Presented in Box 6.3 is an illustration of how SI dysfunctions may present during washing, bathing, showering and grooming. Consider the amount of sensory processing necessary to make bearable washing your face in cold water with foaming facial wash and then drying it with a coarse towel. Also, teeth cleaning, nail trimming, hair brushing, face washing are all commonly disrupted by SI dysfunction.

Box 6.3

How SI dysfunctions may present during washing, bathing, showering

Occupational behaviour	Sensory system/dysfunction
Difficulty adjusting to reasonable water temperature	Tactile processing
Seeming distress at non-noxious touch such as wiping forearm Aversion to fluffy texture of towel Intolerance of light jets of water from the shower/withdraws from splashes	Tactile processing
Difficulty locating and wiping soap off self	Tactile processing
Difficulty stepping in/out of bath in absence of any physical condition or visual impairment Fear response/inability to tip head back/forward for hair washing Reluctance to move freely during the activity	Vestibular proprioceptive processing
Collapses down into the bath in an uncontrolled manner, in the absence of a physical disability Difficulty maintaining dynamic standing balance in the shower, in the absence of a physical disability Requires assistance to move from lying to sitting to standing in the bath, in the absence of a physical disability	Vestibular proprioceptive processing
Overly attentive to/distracted by the smell of toiletries	Olfactory processing
Overly attentive to/distracted by an auditory aspect of the task, such as the sound of running water Overly upset at common noises such as water running, toilet flushing	Auditory processing
Overly attentive to/distracted by a visual aspect of the task such as pattern on a towel/tiles in the bathroom, the bristles on the hairbrush Knows which items are required for task: soap, flannel, etc., but unable to locate them although within visual field	Visual processing
Difficulty initiating washing or sequencing during the activity	Practic dysfunction
During personal care posture is floppy, with the individual having to lean on surfaces, or 'prop' themselves whilst washing at the basin Does not position self squarely on the shower seat, in the absence of physical cause Is overly rough with wash items/can not grade the force of actions	Proprioceptive processing hypo-responsivity
Emotional tone throughout washing/bathing/grooming anything from anxiety, distress, avoidance by removal of self or hitting out	General modulation difficulties
Inability to habituate to unimportant background noises such as the tap running	Modulation difficulties

SI dysfunctions may present as follows:

- Impaired balance and distress at stepping into the bath due to poor vestibular–proprioceptive processing
- Difficulties adjusting to changes in water temperature arising from tactile modulation problems
- Aversive response to components of bathing or showering, such as the feel of being showered, having water poured over the head, being wiped with a flannel/towel, arising from tactile hypersensitivity. This could manifest as avoidance, fear, or hitting out
- Aversive responses to tipping the head back or forward for hair washing due to gravitational insecurity, often resulting in complaining, crying or hitting out.

Dressing

Dressing requires basic motor planning, sensory processing of visual, tactile and vestibular–proprioceptive input and organization of behaviour (Inamura 1998). Sensory processing dysfunction manifests itself in many ways as the individual attempts to dress:

- Impaired balance and execution of dynamic postures due to poor vestibular-proprioceptive processing
- Difficulty pushing extremities through clothing due to poor proprioceptive ability with vision occluded, and poor body scheme
- Difficulties with sequencing the activity arising from practic and organizational difficulties
- An aversive response to tactile qualities of clothing, particularly light, tickly fabrics, or garments that brush/move against the body. In extreme cases the individual may find clothes intolerable and seek to remove them
- An aversive response to bending down to put on lower garments, or lift feet off the floor to do so, due to gravitational insecurity.

Eating and drinking

In order to eat and drink independently the individual must have basic practic skills, oral and upper extremity motor skills and cognitive ability. Indeed, the ability to process tactile and proprioceptive input in the oral area is key to the development of adequate eating and drinking skills. Sensory processing dysfunction may manifest itself in many ways as the individual attempts to eat and drink:

- Immature eating patterns can present as inability to close lips around a spoon and suck food from it, inadequate oral motor manipulation of food and drooling
- Impaired ability to scoop food with utensils due to poor proprioceptive feedback
- Difficulty holding and taking utensils to the mouth. These actions require tactile and proprioceptive discrimination, basic motor coordination and overall differentiation (Coley 1978)
- An aversive response to food textures.

An individual can also present with a visual, auditory and motor SI dysfunction. Visual hypersensitivity may entail visual acuteness to such a degree that the individual describes seeing things invisible to others, such as the air's particles, or separate strands of hair as if magnified, and may cause a retreat into stereotypes such as rocking, hand flapping to calm, or covering the eyes as defence.

Grandin (1996) describes audio hypersensitivity as having her hearing set on maximum loudness. Others describe hearing sounds that are inaudible to others or of a frequency that only animals can hear. Common defensive reactions include withdrawing from sources of sound, or trying to destroy them or covering the ears.

An aversive response to movement is a hyper-responsivity hypothesized to occur as a result of poor modulation of vestibular-proprioceptive input. An individual such as Sarah may experience physical responses to movement including vertigo, nausea, sweating, pallor and dizziness. They may also react to this sensation with self-injurious behaviour and/or demonstrate increased arousal levels following movement.

Sensory under-responsiveness presents as a failure to respond to a sensory stimulus in an expected way – an under-reaction, or less intense reaction than typical. The individual with sensory under-responsivity may require a higher than average amount of stimulus to alert them, and without this they may seem passive, and unengaged. Alternatively, the individual may present as being driven to participate in particular activities/actions in an attempt to seek a level of sensation that they actually appreciate and feel.

Intervention for an individual suspected of having a SI dysfunction

There are three elements of intervention for SI – direct intervention, indirect intervention and consultation (Bundy et al 2002). Direct intervention is the creation and graded presentation of sensory input by the occupational therapist to assess and ameliorate sensory dysfunction. Indirect intervention or monitoring is the 'skilling up' of a third party to undertake particular activities with the individual, monitored by the occupational therapist. Consultation is the provision of education, advice and strategies to carers enabling them to 'reframe' their understanding of the individual, and modify their approach and the environment to better suit the sensory needs of the individual.

Principles of direct intervention

Intervention is aimed at maximizing client motivation and participation by providing a controlled amount of sensory challenge through activities that 'stretch' the individual's skills and abilities, but not so far as to be unobtainable and therefore de-motivating. The individual is offered controlled sensory input to develop effective sensory processing which in turn enables an 'adaptive response' to the environment and occupations. Sessions for Sarah were provided three times per week, lasting half an hour each, for 12 weeks. Direct intervention traditionally occurs in a large room containing a range of suspended items – hammock swings, linear swings, rubber tyres, trapeze swing, rocker boards, mini trampolines, soft matting, ramps, large balls.

Intervention for tactile defensiveness

As is common in adult learning disability services, no specialized SI room existed in which to provide direct intervention for Sarah. Therefore, direct intervention by the occupational therapist was limited to a quiet private room and adapted to what could be easily be provided. Small, confined, warm spaces with cushions and weighted blankets are often comforting and calming and offer the features of the womb environment, as is stated by Oetter & Richter (1990), cited in Williams & Shellenberger, (1996).

Low lighting, a quiet environment and a soft interaction style are also calming. Calming or inhibitory activities are those that involve deep touch pressure, proprioception, slow, sustained, rhythmical, or linear movements. In this way the environment is organized and presented to offer whole body containment and minimal stimulation.

The occupational therapist provided Sarah with deep tactile pressure by hugging, interspersed with slow linear rocking, whilst seated together on soft matting. Ayres (1972b) found that clients with tactile defensiveness responded best to deep pressure and proprioception. She believed that the provision of specific tactile and proprioceptive stimuli would activate the dorsal column medial lemniscal system to close a 'gating mechanism' controlling the passage of defence-eliciting stimuli and thereby diminish the defensive response. Deep tactile contact by wrapping Sarah in a blanket and applying firm massage was also provided and Sarah visibly calmed. Small items were gradually offered, such as a low frequency vibrating 'snake' which she began briefly to touch. This level of interaction, which had not been previously observed in Sarah, was monitored, recorded and evaluated using Goal Attainment Scale scoring (Tobbell & Burns 1997).

Similar findings have been noted by Green et al (2003) working with a client with tactile defensiveness. The rationale for the 'Sensory Integration Therapy' was to combine tactile input with more calming proprioceptive and vestibular stimuli in order to promote the ability to engage appropriately with her environment. The importance of the creation of a safe environment and graded introduction of calming inhibitory techniques such as brushing, deep pressure, low frequency vibration, and slow linear movement on a swing is also described by Urwin & Ballinger (2005).

Principles of indirect intervention and consultancy advice

Occupational therapists traditionally work through a third person (i.e. parent or carer) and this occurs even more so when working with people with a learning disability. This role is fully discussed in Chapter 14: Working with people with learning disabilities and their networks. When considering the role of the occupational therapist in indirect SI intervention, the aspect of training and information giving is paramount. For Sarah's carers and parents the issue was how could they interact safely with her in activities of personal care and not increase her stress and anxiety. The staff were trained in SI techniques and Sarah's specific dysfunction. Her SI profile was utilized to identify and adapt interactions – avoiding unnecessary physical contact, and using deep touch pressure before assisting Sarah with personal care activities. The occupational therapist was therefore both a trainer and role model in these techniques. During showering staff used firm movements to wash and dry Sarah, coupled with wrapping in a towel. Similarly, hair brushing utilized firm strokes and teeth cleaning was carried out using a vibrating tooth-brush. 'Messy' activities were not included in Sarah's daytime plan – but instead those that capitalized on the other senses such as wheelchair movement to music, olfactory and auditory 'quizzes', music, vehicle outings and quiet time in a 'womb' environment of soft matting, cushions, weighted blanket, low lighting and sounds.

Sarah's parents were also educated about tactile defensiveness, enabling them to reframe their understanding of her behaviours, and modify their approach and methods of assisting her in ADL. The physical disability occupational therapist provided a mobile hoist, which Sarah clearly enjoyed being lifted in and which coincidently calmed her prior to personal care.

Lastly, advice was provided to the case manager about the types of day service environment that would best meet Sarah's needs, and this was utilized to modify an existing environment, including redecoration in neutral colours, removal of visual clutter and adjustable lighting. The social elements of the environment were also tailored, by choice of peers with needs compatible with Sarah's, and the possibility of quiet time, dependent on Sarah's arousal levels.

Other specific SI dysfunctions and intervention

Intervention for decreased tactile discrimination

For those individuals that present with decreased tactile discrimination Jaarsveld (2005) suggests that stimulation of the tactile, vibratory, deep touch pressure, proprioceptive and linear vestibular senses should be incorporated into intervention. Activities that are fast, erratic, include movement with speed, and/or direction changes are arousing and excitatory. Intervention includes brushing the skin with various textures, vibratory equipment, deep pressure to large areas of the body and the hands. As tactile processing improves, discriminatory skills are furthered challenged by asking the individual to find objects hidden amongst other textures such as dried beans or pasta.

Intervention for gravitational insecurity

Bundy et al (2002) advocate that intervention for gravitational insecurity centre on activities that provide enhanced proprioceptive and linear vestibular sensation, initially with feet remaining on the ground in order to maximize the individual's ability to control the movement. Intervention may utilize bouncing on a large ball, or trampet, commencing with a tolerable degree of movement. Progress to a linear swing may be made and then onto equipment which moves less predictably. Activating the swing by pulling on a rope also serves to enhance proprioception. Fun and meaningful activities with the naturally occurring components of bending, change of head position or stepping can be gradually incorporated into the session.

Intervention for aversive response to movement

Again, intervention utilizes activities that provide linear vestibular and proprioceptive input, progressing from controllable, predictable movement as the individual's progress allows. Naturally occurring ADL requiring movement should be introduced into intervention.

Intervention for practic dysfunction

Intervention is based on the principles of conceptualizing a plan – ideation, planning, sequencing and organizing sensory information, and carrying out the plan. The first step in intervention is to facilitate an optimum state of arousal – calm, yet alert. With this achieved the individual can be supported to develop ideation. To do this the therapist may have to model activities for the individual to imitate, give physical and verbal prompts and instructions and employ objects that are familiar to the individual. Prompts, cues and instructions are faded out as the individual begins to show signs of spontaneity. Slowly, more novel objects and activities are introduced. The activities chosen should promote bilateral coordination, crossing the midline, and executing sequences of movement in both feed-forward and feedback dependent tasks. Examples include: catching a ball with two hands, propelling self on a swing, 'games' involving picking up objects placed to one side, kicking and throwing objects at a target whilst moving, riding a bike around obstacles, physically negotiating an 'obstacle course' of soft items, etc. The vestibular and proprioceptive systems receive information about the body's movement through space, muscle tone, balance, coordination of the two sides of the body and the timing and sequencing of movements through these activities. Successful processing of this information contributes to the development of body scheme, neuronal 'memory' models of movement and the planning and programming of projected (feed-forward) action sequences, supporting execution of actions.

Summary

This chapter has given a brief overview of how SI dysfunction can present in an individual with a profound learning disability. As Sarah demonstrates, SI theory can provide a useful framework for describing an individual's presentation in ADL. By critical assessment, planned interventions can be based on tactile, vestibular and proprioceptive sensation. It is crucial to grade sensory stimuli to elicit an adaptive response, whilst challenging the individual by just the right amount. The success of any direct intervention should be determined by the impact on the individual's ability to improve in purposeful

occupations such as bathing, dressing and feeding. SI therapy is not a 'stand-alone' approach; it must be coupled with improving occupational function. The role of the occupational therapist can also involve indirect intervention and consultation with parents and others to inform them of effective strategies and approaches during ADL. By using a combination of training opportunities, advice and acting as a role model, carers can be informed on how to implement SI to minimize SI dysfunction and promote function. However, it should be considered amongst all other theories and approaches and requires the practitioner to have undertaken postgraduate training.

Box 6.4

Case illustration: Simon

A referral has been made to occupational therapy for advice on how to support Simon in learning dressing skills. On initial questioning about Simon's performance he is described as reluctant to move, especially bending to put on lower garments, or lift his feet off the floor to do so. Support staff are questioning if this is just laziness on Simon's part, as he is far more participative in activities presented to him whilst he is sitting at the table.

Reader activity

1. By referring to the 'sensory modulation dysfunction model' explain why might Simon be reluctant to dress his lower half?

2. How would you further assess Simon?

3. What format does intervention normally take?

Further reading

Arkwright N 1998 An introduction to sensory integration. Arizona, Therapy Skill Builders

Ayres AJ 2005 Sensory integration and the child: 25th anniversary edition. Los Angeles, Cresport Press

Bear MF, Connors BW, Paradiso MA 2007 Neuroscience – exploring the brain, 3rd edn. Philadelphia, Lippincott Williams & Wilkins

Cribbin V 2003 Sensory integration information booklet – a resource for parents and therapists. Ireland, Sensory Integration Network

Spitzer S, Roley SS, Clark F, Parham D 1996 Sensory integration – current trends in the United States. Scandinavian Journal of Occupational Therapy 3:123–138

Tyldesley B, Grieve JI 2002 Muscles, nerves and movement in human occupation, 3rd edn. Oxford, Blackwell Science

References

Ayres AJ 1972a Sensory integration and learning disorders. Los Angeles, Western Psychological Services

Ayres AJ 1972b Types of sensory integrative dysfunction among disabled learners. American Journal of Occupational Therapy 26:13–18

Ayres AJ 1985 Developmental dyspraxia and adult-onset apraxia. Torrance CA, Sensory Integration International

Ayres AJ 2005 Sensory integration and the child: 25th anniversary edition. Los Angeles, Cresport Press

Blanche EI, Schaaf RC 2001 Proprioception: a cornerstone of sensory integrative intervention Chap 6. In: Smith-Roley S, Blanche EL, Schaaf R (eds) Understanding the nature of sensory integration with diverse populations. Arizona, Therapy Skill Builders, pp 109–124

Brown C, Dunn W 2002 Adolescent/adult sensory profile. Oxford, Harcourt

Bundy AC, Lane SJ, Murray EA 2002 Sensory integration theory and practice, 2nd edn. Philadelphia, FA Davis Company

Cohen H (ed.) 1999 Neuroscience for rehabilitation, 2nd edn. Philadelphia, Lippincott Williams & Wilkins

Coley I 1978 Paediatric self-assessment of self-care activities. St Louis, Mosby

Grandin T 1996 Thinking in pictures and other reports from my life with autism. New York, Vintage Books.

Green D, Beaton L, Moore D et al 2003 Clinical incidence of sensory difficulties in adults with learning disabilities and illustration of management. British Journal of Occupational Therapy 66(10):454–463

Inamura KN (ed.) 1998 SI for early intervention: a team approach. Arizona, Therapy Skill Builders

Jaarsveld AV 2005 Sensory integration in mental retardation and pervasive developmental disorders. In: Crouch R, Alers V (eds) Occupational therapy in psychiatry and mental health, 4th edn. London, Whurr, pp 369–392

Kielhofner G 2002 Model of human occupation, 3rd edn. Baltimore, Lippincott Williams & Wilkins

Lane SJ, Miller LJ, Hanft BE 2000 Towards a consensus in terminology in sensory integration theory and practice, Part 2: Sensory integration patterns of function and dysfunction. Sensory Integration Special Interest Section Quarterly 23(2):1–3

Murray-Slutsky C, Paris BA 2000 Exploring the spectrum of autism and pervasive developmental disorder – intervention strategies. San Antonio, The Psychological Corporation USA, Elsevier Health Sciences

Reisman LE, Hanschu B 1992 Sensory integration inventory – revised for individuals with developmental disabilities. Minnesota, PDP Press

Smith-Roley S, Blanche EL, Schaaf R (eds) 2001 Understanding the nature of sensory integration with diverse populations. Arizona, Therapy Skill Builders

Spitzer S, Roley SS 2001 Sensory integration revisited: a philosophy of practice. In: Smith-Roley S, Blanche EL, Schaaf R (eds) Understanding the nature of sensory integration with diverse populations. Arizona, Therapy Skill Builders, pp 3–27

Tobbell J, Burns J 1997 Goal attainment scaling for people with learning disabilities. Oxford, Winslow

Tyldesley B, Grieve JI 2002 Muscles, nerves and movement in human occupation, 3rd edn. Oxford, Blackwell Science

Urwin R, Ballinger C 2005 The effectiveness of sensory integration therapy to improve functional behaviour in adults with learning disabilities: five single-case experimental designs. British Journal of Occupational Therapy 68(2):56–66

Williams MS, Shellenberger S 1996 How does your engine run? – a leader's guide to the alert program for self regulation. Albuquerque, Therapy Works Inc

Appendix 6.1 Case illustration: Simon, possible answers

1. Simon's behaviour may be a result of gravitational insecurity causing dizziness. This may also be apparent when having to bend down for anything in a cupboard or/he may be reluctant to step up into a bus or climb stairs.

2. How would you further assess Simon?

Assessment would involve initial assessment, observation and interview to complete SI inventory and carers' assessment. This may be carried out over a period of several weeks to gain a full picture of Simon's abilities.

3. What format does intervention normally take?

Direct intervention means working with Simon probably on proprioceptive and tactile input. Indirect intervention with staff is to establish that he is not lazy and that he would require some tactile stimulation before having to bend down. Consultation with the staff team for training on SI approach, including methods of tactile stimulation and routines to be used prior to ADL and possibly advice regarding environmental changes to bedroom/bathroom.

Chapter Seven

7

Occupational choices – choosing employment

Angela Kelsall

Overview

Throughout the period of adolescence, choices and performance capacity refine towards occupational identities and competencies associated with early adulthood. The pattern related to achieving the one important day of getting a first job and thereby becoming a worker is an example of the process Keilhofner (2002) refers to as evolving 'a sense of who one is and wanting to become' and 'putting that identity into action in an ongoing way'.

This chapter will explore understanding of the occupational meaning of work and the huge diversity between human accomplishments in adaptation to adult occupations and roles within employment. Accomplishments are dependent, first on whether an individual has past and present experiences of appropriate opportunities in employment settings, and second on whether they perceive themselves as capable and are enabled to respond to employment opportunities. People with learning disabilities, as part of normal life, do not often have exposure to these adaptive conditions. This limits how they advance their learning and expectancy of future adult working lives. They are unlikely to share with peer groups entering mainstream work-related training, employment programmes and job opportunities. Their closest worker role models may be parents, siblings and family friends. The relevance of employment as an occupational choice for people with a learning disability is discussed in this chapter in relation to these points.

The chapter will also explore the implications of policy changes and opportunities for employment in the current climate within the UK. The Government's present strategic programme to increase employment for disabled adults, mainly via the route of vocational rehabilitation practice, may not help individuals with a learning disability. However, legislation (such as the Disability Discrimination Act 2005 and the Human Rights Act 1998) combined with a number of working groups actively reporting to ministers, is urging change. There are many Supported Employment Agencies in the United Kingdom supporting people with learning disabilities. Their emphasis is on real jobs with recruitment by a real employer; wages at the going rate; fully integrated workplaces and full conditions of employment. Within the present day context two employment models, the Work Readiness Model and the Supported Employment Model, will be discussed in relation to supported employment theory. The occupational therapist's role parallels the theory of supported employment by application of the assessment, support and to develop employment opportunities for people with a learning disability. This role will be outlined in the chapter.

Learning Outcomes

By the end of this chapter you will be able to:

- Describe how people explore and obtain employment and compare this process with that for an individual with a learning disability
- Identify the choice-making process of employment for an individual with a learning disability
- Define employment models to support people with learning disabilities
- Describe the role of occupational therapy in establishing employment opportunities.

Getting a Job

It may be helpful to begin at this point by reflecting on how you have explored and identified work-based opportunities and choices ultimately leading towards a career in occupational therapy. The types of activities that ordinarily exist for people to progress towards employment may include visiting career fairs, work site visits from school and subsequent work experience. Generally, a significant portion of time is allocated to recognizing and developing basic interests and abilities, prior to adolescents finishing schooling or young adults leaving college, with aspirations of a future career that may lead to employment in the area of choice. For example, through having a Saturday job or paper round, enhanced freedom is created from a small income and also the young person builds a belief within themselves and from those around (i.e. families, peers and workplace colleagues) as behaviours, skills and responsibilities of work emerge. This development towards employment as productive occupation engenders:

- competent performance of actual job tasks

- interaction with colleagues and people in charge in the workplace
- associated organizational tasks such as applying for a job, time management, orienting and getting to work, dressing accordingly, etc.

These are all factors that contribute to changes in occupational behaviour which are epitomized through the years of adolescence to careers in adulthood. This typical pursuit of work and careers in adolescence and early adult life is the essence of the process of occupational adaptation. That is, a continuous process of participation in work-related experiences is highly desirable to generate an identity and competence towards a future working life and a valued life role. Adaptation is a central part of occupational therapy philosophy. Hagedorn (2002) refers to adaptation promoting survival and self-actualization throughout the life cycle and suggests that purposeful activity (occupation), including its interpersonal and environment components, facilitates the adaptive process. Identifying employment opportunities typically involves prioritizing and organizing appropriate activities towards their pursuit, including exploration of employment roles and types to develop personal preferences. Guidance to help the individual make work-related choices and identify constraints to their chosen goals, in the first instance, may be obtained by discussing and seeking help from family and school.

The outcome elicited by all these opportunities, is that, in most instances, young people go on to have expectations that they will, in early adulthood, end up on the first step to employment with real money and social status. This, in turn, triggers more trial and effort leading to further performance development and strengthened understanding of themselves in an adult worker role. The process of developing personal perspectives of meaningful occupation also arises from relationships between factors originating in the past and present.

This is summarized as follows:

- Feelings and thoughts that influence growth of an interest and ultimately grow into worthwhile occupational pursuits
- Self and others' belief in one's capabilities to perform the skills of chosen occupations
- The influence of the personal perception and others' view of productivity roles as socially valuable.

To summarize, by the time of reaching adulthood, some aspects of life's aspirations are already about to become satisfied. A foundation is achieved of adult aspirations based on accumulated life experiences and knowledge. The individual has established inclination towards choices of related work and career activity, looking forward to prospects of new meaningful occupations and activities. Others, however, through different circumstances, may shape their life in other types of productive and leisure occupations at this stage. To put the above into context, ask yourself the following questions in relation to your own experience.

Reader activity

1. What was your first experience of employment?

    - Visits to careers fairs, voluntary work, a weekend job and work site visits?
    - Discussion with family and school peers about choices of career pursuit and sharing the experiences of mainstream training programmes and career pursuit activities.

2. How and when did you identify your first job?

    - During adolescent years, there was an expectancy of employment in adulthood and a significant portion of time allotted to developing interests, abilities and attributes towards this
    - Identification and exploration of work-based opportunities was sought via job agencies, media, direct employer contact, college sources, local friend and family networks
    - This activity of securing a job typically occurred leading up to and following leaving school or college.

3. What did you gain from your first job?

    - Manifestation of choices towards certain career decisions
    - Adaptation to the (adult) responsibilities and benefits of having a job
    - Insight to suited and unsuited job tasks and environments
    - Enhanced degree of independence, self-understanding and sense of status
    - Increased direct job skills and associated organizational skills such as applying and interviewing for jobs.

'I want to work' – an occupational choice?

Individuals with learning disabilities are not exposed to the ordinary situations described above and the majority simply move from education to day centres. The approach to person-centred planning described in Valuing People (DoH 2001) as a '...mechanism reflecting the needs and preferences of a person with a learning disability and covers such issues as housing, education, employment and leisure (4.17)'. This expresses the importance of including people with learning disabilities and supporting them to take part in all forms of empowerment. The government's commitment to moving people with learning disabilities into employment is demonstrated in Objective 8 of Valuing People (2.9).

However, specialist services are currently generally failing to provide support to people with learning disabilities to overcome the barriers to employment both in terms of physical, social and psychological factors. The complex service networks and systems that should facilitate opportunities for young people with a learning disability to develop career pathways after school life in fact can inhibit their progress. On leaving school or college there is little opportunity to participate in pursuing work, even if expressed as something they would like to do. The special education system has tended not to hold paid work as a central objective for adult life. For many adults with learning disabilities who are already recipients of adult services systems, there is exclusive provision in segregated day care centres. Streamlining into adult day care becomes a lifetime destiny that often realistically:

- separates people from community opportunities
- offers only a narrow range of occupations
- provides few opportunities to progress from day care
- limits development towards a productive and valued role.

Other factors include financial disincentives within the benefits system for people with a learning disability: 'benefits rules and regulations continue to be regarded as a major barrier, perceived or real, and deter both carers and day services from encouraging people with learning disabilities to find work' as outlined in the Improving Work Opportunities

Report: Working Group (Department for Work and Pensions 2006a). The focus of the benefits system is on capacity rather than being able to assist individuals to seek employment whilst also able to provide their security and flexibility. Many are debating the case for reform of the benefits system. The aforementioned report to Ministers and the Learning Disability Task Force (Department for Work and Pensions 2006b) also integrated several recommendations from an earlier study by Beyer et al (2004), including a review of the current Income Support benefit disregard level, to allow people to work more hours. A large number of people with learning disabilities depend on this benefit, particularly people in residential care. Currently, an individual may earn £20 per week, which represents less than 4 hours at the national minimum wage. Earning more than this means an individual is no better off (each pound earned from working reduces income support by a pound) and worse, may risk their passport to other critical benefits.

At the present time an individual may receive benefits that:

- permit a limited number of hours of work whilst remaining on benefits
- allow returning to benefits after a while if the job does not work out
- allow remaining on benefits when undertaking voluntary work with no limit to hours or expenses that can be reclaimed.

For further reading and information on benefits, refer to the Useful Resources at the end of this chapter.

Ultimately, people with a learning disability are separated from normal opportunities of jobs in real work settings, which if offered are only in a narrow range of occupations. The socially common view of young people with learning disabilities leaving school or college is that they are incapable of performing and holding down a job. Equally, a consequence of this is that an individual with a learning disability may not develop earnest aspirations of having a job. There is also a continual failure to provide people with learning disabilities with information to underpin their decision of whether employment might be an occupational choice. Nor is subsequent support offered to seek employment and master their potential as an employee.

Evidence supporting this has been accumulating in the United Kingdom over the past decade and the demands from groups advocating employment choice and opportunity on the behalf of people with learning disabilities have strengthened. It is likely that less than 10% of people with a learning disability are in employment (Valuing People: 2001, 7.51), although 'Working Lives' (Beyer et al 2004), as part of Valuing People, expressed concerns that estimates of people with learning disabilities in work vary and are dependent on the validity of the definition of learning disability. For example, the source of some figures may refer to people with learning difficulties who have dyslexia. The research by Beyer et al (2004) sought to explore employment from the perspective of people with learning disabilities themselves. Of 158 people interviewed about their work aspirations, 97 had worked in the past. Half of these indicated they wanted paid work, even if they were not working at present. Those respondents 'in employment' (60) wanted to stay in their job or seek better jobs. In the 'never worked' category, the individuals represented did not mention having received help to think about work or develop experience of work. Beyer et al (2004) suggest supporting people who 'have not commonly received help to think about work' would represent a significant extension of job promotion activity.

Work as an option for people with a learning disability

Occupational therapy role

As described for many of the learning disability population, there is limited opportunity for first-hand experience of employment-related opportunities. With this picture in mind, occupational therapists have a distinct role in facilitating an individual with a learning disability to explore the options of employment. The focus of occupational therapy strengths lies in assisting those with more intractable needs or requiring complex management of access to work (Mountain et al 2001). However, in spite of all that has been said, evidence of the current trend suggests that employment in its broadest sense presently plays a marginal position in the role of the occupational therapist (Watson 2006). Few occupational therapy services are taking the challenge and investing their specialist skills in this area. This may be due to the fact that within all areas of practice, occupational therapy managers are faced with a 'chicken or egg' dilemma. Whilst service priorities are informed by consumer demand, decisions are also made because of external factors that place limits on service capacity to 'do everything of which we are capable' (Richards 1998). Occupational therapists need to be aware of the modernization of local services taking place currently and use this as an opportunity. More complex service priorities can be achieved through strong interagency mechanisms and linking with local partnerships to develop supported employment capacity e.g. local authority day services, small supported employment agencies or large specialist organizations such as SCOPE or MENCAP PATHWAY. (See Useful Resources list at the end of this chapter.)

A referral to occupational therapy for assessment of occupation should at least raise the question whether the pursuit of work, with the right options and support to try, is desirable. There is a need to establish both a multi-agency and a multidisciplinary approach to establishing employment. In developing employment as an occupational choice it is important for the occupational therapist to be aware of employment models used to develop employment opportunities by employment agencies.

The work readiness model

Although there are planning and training strategies aimed towards employment for people with learning disabilities, they seldom correspond with real jobs and real work environments or conditions in local areas. Individuals with learning disabilities may find themselves in work preparation and training type programmes with the intention of transition to meaningful work in integrated settings. However, in practice, they frequently never have their aspirations realized. Over the past years, various assessment programmes and tools from a variety of different service models have been developed to determine whether people with a learning disability are employable or not. They establish whether the individual is considered 'ready' for a paid job and are the most widely used approach to accessing employment in both the past and present day. They can include sample assessments, which simulate skills for actual jobs such as assembling tasks and use of tools. Other situational assessments are based on information about the individual's performance

and attitude to work (Cheshire County Council 1997) such as those carried out in day centre projects or vocational training centres. The theory behind 'work readiness' is for the individual to acquire skills to a requisite level (assessed as ready) through work-related programmes and supportive environments, towards becoming eligible to move into the employment market. The limitation of this assessment approach is that it may not consider fully the complex demands and dynamic relationship of the job and the work environment. Although the individual may perform well in a protective environment this might not be how they will perform in the work environment, without careful action planning to accommodate the distractions and stresses that can occur.

Although helping people to establish an understanding of commitment to work (i.e. work ethic) and build a sense of what they want from work is a part of the occupational choice process, Simons & Watson (1999) cite Gardiner (1997) that there is little evidence to support the 'readiness model'. Its effectiveness has been criticized in terms of the low success in facilitating people into employment balanced against the time and financial resources afforded. Additionally, these assessments may not find out the wider extent of skills that have a bearing on the overall success, such as travelling to work, getting there on time, settling into the work place culture, building relationships with colleagues and supervisors etc. Nor do they carry out an analysis of specific jobs and workplaces to match individual requirements.

Self-determination

Self-determination is a recent concept, emanating from the American special educational system, of helping people with learning disabilities to take more responsibility and control about their lives, particularly with regard to transition planning (Wehmeyer 2004). Self-determination is an approach to learning and achieving confidence through which the individual is the locus of control. There is evidence of the effectiveness of 'self determining' techniques, used to enable people with learning disabilities to express preferences about jobs based on real job sampling. Self-determination techniques affect the individual's performance through a process of understanding and believing in their own capabilities, setting and finding their way to personal goals, making choices and advocating them. The results from a structured review by Kilsby & Beyer (2002) on a self-determination programme in job sampling to strengthen informed choice about jobs, showed that individuals demonstrated a high degree of accuracy in reporting factual aspects of their job experience, which also was accompanied by a drop in the rate of trainers' assistance. An essential component of the concept is that self-determined experiences and feedback of the consequences promote the adaptive process. Hagedorn (2002) refers to recent research emphasizing the importance of moving towards experiential styles of learning. When working with adults with a learning disability, occupational therapists need to ensure facilitating client-centred learning and empowerment. To support the development of self-determination capacity for the individual requires the enabler to have skills that are finely balanced to ensure just the right level of opportunity and support is provided.

Supported employment model

Supported employment is a type of employment, not a method of employment preparation, nor a type of service activity. It is a powerful and flexible way to ensure normal employment benefits, provide ongoing and appropriate support, create opportunities, and achieve full participation, integration and flexibility (Mcloughlin et al 1987 p. 27).

The supported employment model holds the social inclusion vision at its heart (BASE 2007) and is rooted in the principle that services assume an individual's right to become employed, with a focus on empowering the individual and providing skilled support resources and mechanisms to access their rights. The remit of the support role using the supported employment model is summarized in Box 7.1. The core of the supported employment process is to enable the individual to think further about their prospective involvement in real work by:

- Taking a positive approach to making available opportunities, training, support and follow up necessary to help the individual become and remain employed
- Assessing suitability of the job and capacity of the workplace to suit the individual's needs

Box 7.1

Supported employment model

Supported employment establishes:
- recruitment by an employer
- real jobs, not makeshift activities
- full employment conditions
- wages at the going rate, not financial incentives
- fully integrated workplaces
- long-term service back up to maintaining support and exploring options for career advancement
- emphasis on provision of natural support by work colleagues

- Ensuring a good match between the individual, the job, workplace and the employer's requirements.

Supported Employment Agencies take the lead in supporting people with learning disabilities into employment. Concepts of the supported employment model, originating in the USA as an alternative to traditional sheltered and competitive employment approaches (Lutiyya et al 1988) were adopted in the UK, emerging and expanding over 20 years under the above service heading. Their emphasis was in contrast to the contract work in 'sheltered' settings (e.g. day centres, hospital industrial therapy service) whose disadvantages were segregation, typically involving rather boring, production line tasks and offering little in the way of pay (Simons & Watson 1999). An over-riding criticism about the effectiveness of this approach was given by Felce et al (1998), cited by Simons & Watson (1999), in that there was no support plan to progress further and by 1991 less than 5% of people attending them had obtained paid work.

There are many Supported Employment Agencies now in the United Kingdom supporting people with disabilities. Their emphasis is on enabling people to link into real community work environments and experience working life to the full. Supported Employment Agencies have partnerships with mainstream employment agencies and government-driven programmes and links with area-based funding initiatives for regeneration.

Occupational therapy and the supported employment model

Assessment

Occupational therapy and the supported employment model share a client-centred focus. Each is influenced by humanistic values and an ecological theory guiding practice, emphasizing the inter-relationship between the person, occupational performance and environments. These concepts are at the core of occupational therapy practice in the development of employment as an occupational choice for people with learning disabilities. The following outline of the supported employment process underpins the role of the occupational therapist in supporting an individual to gain employment by:

- individual vocational profiling
- job development through working with employers and finding out what they need
- job analysis and job matching (i.e. between the requirements of the individual and those of the employers, job performance and productivity needs)
- natural support arrangements from amongst co-workers
- adaptive and training strategies
- recommending sources of benefits advice.

An integral part of 'doing' (i.e. 'work, play, or activities of daily living'), expressed by Keilhofner (2002) to describe occupation, is the cycle of input of information from the environment and the individual's innate ability to process information and apply it to their 'doing'. Using a model of occupational therapy, assessments to ensure a holistic approach will include the individual, activity analysis and environmental factors that are implicit to develop skills towards employment and parallels that used for the supported employment model (see Figure 7.1). Many of the learning disability population have little, or no, first-hand experience of work-related activities and real work environments upon which to base their decisions about work as a potential occupational area. Even before starting a job there are a number of complex tasks to be completed.

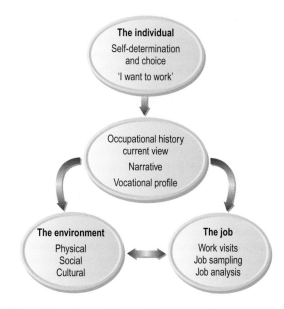

Figure 7.1 • The employement assessment.

Reader activity

Consider the skills you need to do the following:

1. Applying for a job

   - Discerning aspects of the job and how the demands match to your abilities, sense of fulfilment and challenge your capability. You might not find these out until you try a particular job, which therefore requires a self-belief in capability.
   - Recalling your experiences and knowledge and then using handwriting or keyboard skills to sell yourself in the application.

2. Having an interview

   - Competence in communication and interaction skills, that is: clarity of articulation; listening skills, talking about your self; nonverbal communication; comprehension and interpretation of questions
   - Presentation of appearance: personal dress and grooming.

3. Negotiate or agree hours of working

   - Insight into personal capabilities and be able to self advocate needs
   - Appreciate employer's needs, reason logically with him/her, conclude and agree a contract.

4. Arrange to be paid

- Understanding methods of managing money – opening and managing a bank, building society or post office card account
- Awareness of outgoing payments from salary – national insurance, tax, company pension contribution schemes.

Applying a holistic approach right from the beginning and engaging the person with a learning disability throughout the whole of the decision-making process is significant to their learning and adaptation to the prospect of becoming an employee. With this in mind therefore, occupational therapists have a responsibility, as part of this process, to explore with the individual their thoughts and feelings about occupation (or lack of). It is crucial to gather information to enable both the individual and the occupational therapist to build up a profile of both preferences and possibly to options to pursue in terms of employment. Using the supported employment model framework, the occupational therapist can start to assess by opening with an occupational history and current view, developing ideas through narrative and finally vocational profiling.

Occupational history and current view

By taking an occupational history of past and present participation in productivity, leisure and self-care, the information helps the individual focus on the important questions 'Do I want to work?' or 'Might work be an occupational goal?' The range of information to be explored is summarized in Box 7.2. The interaction establishes rapport with the individual and identifies their understanding of 'life world context' (Creek 2004). That is, their experience of 'where they are coming from and where they are going to'. Seeking information to guide an occupational choice must be obtained and presented in a way that is clear for the individual. Recognizing that creativity and investment in time may benefit and profit both the individual, the occupational therapist and later on, the prospective employer is important.

This preliminary part of the assessment process may provide both the individual and therapist insight into whether the individual feels that work is a meaningful occupational option for them to pursue further or not. That is, has work been something the person has

even considered, has it been something they thought they would be able to do, is it something they would like to see themselves trying? From considering all of the above and exploring the occupations as outlined in Box 7.2, the occupational therapist can build a picture of where the individual might need assistance and identify preferences, dislikes or disinterests, as for example:

- In the smaller order of things, what things do they consider they are unsuited to and probably prefer to avoid?
- In the greater order, how many of their life circumstances are depriving them of opportunities to pursue fulfilment?
- What everyday situations and environments sometimes challenge the individual, affecting participation?

For the individual this is an ongoing journey of self-discovery to determine if a future to become employed is the right one or not. The role of the occupational therapist is finely balanced to facilitate that process and not prompt the person towards a decision one way or the other.

Narrative

Further assessment may involve a more in-depth exploration of the individual's level of awareness of the world of work. The occupational therapist may choose to facilitate through narrative (i.e. story telling) the individual's comprehension of the meaning of work (Keilhofner 2002). Narrative does not necessarily require the ability to speak for two people to make a connection. The importance is that the narrator and facilitator are able to comprehend and convey their message to each other. Again, optimizing this relationship relies on creative adjustments that facilitate communication and interaction. In some circumstances, it would be helpful to discuss this with a speech and language therapist. The choice of narrative may promote a subjective or even an imaginary view due to the individual's lack of real experience. Even this is helpful if it orients the person to make more sense of what work is about. Drawing out past and current situations may be useful, for example reflecting how others experience work, such as the work roles of a parent, sibling or other significant people in the community, e.g. a neighbour, newsagent, school staff, postman, gardener, etc.

Box 7.2

Occupational history and current view

Explore with the individual what activities or tasks:

1. are enjoyable, satisfying and thus motivational? For example, taking care of the family pet, making a collection of things of interest.

2. do they consider they can do and do well and are recognized by others? For example, particular domestic skills, hobbies.

3. have occupational and social roles? What personal association do these roles have with others? For example, collecting newspapers for family and neighbours from the local shop, helping out in the neighbourhood allotments, participating in local fund raising events, chairing a self-advocacy group.

4. are important, such as a belief, certain places, ritual activities? For example, maintaining membership within a social club, taking responsibility for assembling the weekly recycling collection, or simply taking turns in making everybody tea at break-time, interest in a particular TV programme.

5. take up everyday occupational use of time, where and with whom? For example, participation in day care centre group projects geared towards production, or tasks which carry individual responsibility to others such as collecting, delivering, emptying, loading, clearing or preparing objects.

6. are involved in educational courses, for example, IT, catering, horticulture, adult literacy, food hygiene.

7. are involved in sporting or creative interests? For example, putting the kit bag together, travelling to sporting fixtures, 'Special Olympics', ceramics, membership of a performing arts group.

8. is there towards recognizing personal achievement and expectancy of developments towards vocational goals? For example, attaining competence based qualifications; has the question been asked *'do you want to work?'*

Vocational profile

The supported employment concept that people, jobs and workplaces are individually distinct, underpins what is involved in vocational profiling and the analysis of all three aspects to make a powerful match. As seen in both 'occupational history and current view' and 'narrative' above, vocational profiling is a process not a form and the important point is to get to know the client (Leach 2002).

The type of information taken in the 'occupational history and current view' or 'narrative' is then encapsulated into the profile with the further generation of the following information relevant to prospective involvement and support in real work:

- specific employment-related strengths and abilities
- preferred work tasks and environments
- employment connections
- benefits information

- related support areas such as money handling and time-telling, personal health or disability issues relevant to potential work activities, routines and environments
- where the individual lives in proximity to local work and access to transportation.

In this way the vocational profile guides the type of job and work conditions that best suit the person's abilities, attributes, interests, and support requirements, which are the basis of finding a good job match.

Observations and interviews with the individual and other people who know the person well take place in a variety of real life settings (e.g. home, neighbourhood, education/workplaces, recreational) and task-orientated situations. Bearing in mind that the way we behave at home with our family or socially with friends is likely to be different or inappropriate to how we should behave at work is

Box 7.3

The job analysis

Conditions of employment

- Wage rates
- Hours of work
- Holiday entitlements
- Sickness and absence policy

Potential support resources

- Is there is a friendly working atmosphere?
- Are there plenty of opportunities for co-worker interactions?
- Are the proposed tasks performed by one person or are they a shared undertaking?
- How do supervisors and managers relate to employees?

Health and safety

- Health and safety policies in place and evidence standards met

Job routines
    Analysis of job patterns into:
- Main: actual regularly repeated job tasks
- Intermittent job tasks: associated with the main job tasks but occur less frequently
- Job related: directly associated to the job, vital to the performance, but sometimes not explicitly required e.g. break times, use of protective clothing, shutting down machinery at break times (Leach 2002)

Job tasks

- Identifying and collecting information (method-the way it is done, sequence, content tools, materials, timing, environment, safety factors, quality/production standard) about the job tasks and skill demands
- A task analysis will show how the task will be performed by breaking it down into teachable sequential actions

---

necessary. Nor is it straightforward to generalize many skills we have learned in one setting to another. The vocational profile is not a tool to determine if a person is employable, rather it is an approach to gathering information by valuing the individual's uniqueness and viewing them as capable of positive development if provided with the appropriate planning and support. Analysis of the vocational profile should result in gaining an impression of the type of job and employer to target.

The work environment – job analysis

An occupational therapist's belief in occupation, the environment and human life as inseparable entities is central to understanding how to enable an individual's development of competent employment performance. Factors in the social and physical environment can enhance or inhibit performance, as can the nature of occupations. A job analysis is an important first step in the occupational therapist making himself or herself familiar with the demands that a job places on a client (Joss 2007).

At this stage, analysis of a potential job may take several visits to the workplace. The aim is to gain a broad picture of the job with a further detailed analysis once the job is offered. Workplace environment designs are generally for efficient production and have properties that can help or hinder performance and purpose at work. It is worth considering how the environment can affect an individual with a learning disability. Summarized in Box 7.3 is an outline of the main areas of a job analysis. To explore this further use the following reader activity to analyse your own work situation environment.

Reader activity

- Does the arrangement of your workplace enable ease of performance, endurance, access and orientation? For example, are there stairs to climb or a lift to manage? Where are tools or stationery stored?
- What social and physical cues are there? For example, how do you know when it is time for tea break and what happens?

- What elements of the socio-cultural environment are conformed to within the workplace? For example, how do people address one another?
- How does the layout allow for contact with workmates and enable a sense of belonging? For example, are offices layouts open plan and busy, or smaller and familiar? Is there a lot of machinery making it difficult to talk?
- How many different varieties of task or activity settings are there: door entry systems, stock rooms, first aid rooms, reception areas etc.?
- How easy is it to access community facilities such as transport routes, newsagent?

Assessing and making judgements and decisions about work may involve other additional techniques, by voluntary working or job sampling, to match the individual with an actual job. The individual may need to acquire more understanding of the concepts and demands of work environments and activities. The individual and occupational therapist might conclude that a further practical exploratory visit is required to help the individual appraise for him or herself if work is the right choice, such as by voluntary working or job sampling. The occupational therapist's role in the everyday natural environment may involve recognizing the individual's chosen way of conveying and understanding information. This can involve establishing the ability to follow verbal or non-verbal task instructions, ability in skill in occupational performance, social interactions with people, ability for performance demands and problem solving in all these areas, and practical and social resources to support the individual (see Box 7.4).

Developing a job

Job development involves the general marketing of the uniqueness of supported employment to employers to gain and maintain successful employment for people with learning disabilities. From here on the person in the role of development and support will be referred to as an employment specialist.

Establishing and maintaining links with Supported Employment Agencies is important to assure an outcome of a positive employment opportunity for the individual. Supported Employment Agencies keep abreast of developing and changing patterns of the local employment market. They are also skilled

Box 7.4

Occupational therapy and supported employment activities

- Promoting the individual's control in identifying employment as an occupational choice
- Assisting an individual to set goals in relation to employment
- Assessment of abilities and needs
- Activity synthesis (building up separate elements of a job and connected activities)
- Analysis and sequencing of tasks
- Analysis of routines
- Analysis of environments
- Ergonomic advice and adaptation
- Grading and training tasks and activities
- Training and support of co-workers.

in accessing additional government employment schemes and programmes that widen the scope of support options (see Useful resources: 'For help and advice on benefits and employment schemes and programmes'). Maintaining awareness of these schemes and types of benefit is also crucial, as frequently they are under review and change. Supported Employment Agencies are practiced at presenting their service to potential employers using materials such as portfolios of high profile businesses who actively employ individuals with a learning disability. They build up databases of companies and employers and recognize other ways to find jobs such as through an individual's network. Agencies tend also to have good relationships with other employment services, in particular the Disability Advisory Service, and local business groups such as the Chamber of Commerce.

The ability to negotiate for jobs to meet both the individual job seeker's and potential employer's needs requires an amount of specialist skill and confidence, particularly when dealing with higher management or handling an employer's concerns. Approaching an employer can be by:

- letter of introduction followed up by a telephone call
- visits by appointment
- drop-in visits.

Prerequisites to visiting include finding out about the company and being prepared with an opening statement and brief. Negotiations aim to identify a job outline and the requirements of both parties and to offer the individual an option to visit the job site if required.

A consideration at this point is that only a few individuals with a learning disability are able to get a full-time job that enables them to come off benefits and become financially independent. For many, the current benefit system provides disincentives to those who would like to work. There are many types of benefits, with different rules, affected by entering work. Understanding how different benefits work together is a complicated and time-consuming business and one that *must* be addressed with extreme caution. Qualified advice should be obtained from the appropriate agencies via a Care Manager, Welfare Rights Service, and Citizens Advice, etc.

Gaining work experience through job sampling

A client-centred focus might be to provide 'tasters' of work prior to making a job choice. Job sampling is the individual's encounter with real employment to help make their own choices from different sorts of jobs, tasks and work environments. It might involve a variety of tasters before being able to eliminate aspects of jobs that are least preferred and identify those with the most meaning for the individual. Job sampling also gives information about what the person is able to do and how they might respond to real workplace problems. There are certain principles to be adhered to in job sampling:

- it must reflect job interests that are identified in the vocational profile
- job sampling must take place in real work situations in the local area
- they are time limited, usually anything between a few hours and a couple of weeks.

In addition to the above aims, job sampling should also protect the individual from abuse of their time and effort and should not slide into work for which they are unpaid. Some individuals work in a voluntary capacity as a legitimate choice of occupation and this may be the impetus to discovering about work, gaining experience and exploring competence. Other methods that have some similar purpose are job site visits and job shadowing.

'Place and train' approach

The phrase 'place and train' characterizes the definition of supported employment, differing from the traditional job readiness model, which is characterized by 'train and place' (Everatt 1999). The supported employment process aims to identify the individual's interests, abilities and needs without setting a minimum criterion of readiness to place them in a job. From the completed vocational profile and job analysis, the focus is upon matching the client to a job with specific tasks, environmental factors and employer expectations. There should be strong emphasis on motivation to work and maximizing a good match between the job seeker and employer. After this has been established, the training and adaptation process commences. This process is referred to as the 'place and train' approach.

Job matching and support

There are two critical stages to the job matching process. The first is to compare the elements of the job analysis to the requirements of the individual's vocational profile. If the match is suitable the second stage is to draw up an action plan devising the practical approaches which will facilitate job performance and fulfil the individual's and the employer's goals. There may be elements that require no intervention strategies, with the individual being able to rely on natural cues in the workplace. Others will require interventions such as structured training or adaptive approaches and techniques. Making changes to a job or environment involves united approach between employer, co-workers, employee and employment specialist, that can help unite the working relationships. The objective in developing the job is to identify the gaps in the individual's current ability to carry out skills needed. Establishing the right supportive environment ensures opportunity to perform to their capability and therefore reach the goal of competent employee. If the employer and individual both accept the job proposal the employment specialist must spend time learning the job and getting to know the co-workers before being able to support and train the individual. Throughout the process there are likely to be refinements, negotiated changes and compromises to maximize productivity and competence. Different employers have different expectations and flexibilities with regard to behaviour and working practices. For example, arrangements may be required for the individual to start and finish at a separate time to their co-workers or to take more breaks. This potential affect on production will need to be discussed at the job negotiation stage. However, the employment specialist needs to be aware of behaviours that will not be acceptable at the workplace. Finally, once the job title, job description and contract are agreed, a start date is arranged.

Starting the job and support strategies

At this initial stage the role of the employment specialist is to facilitate circumstances that enable the individual to become effective at the job, for example by:

- easing relationships with co-workers
- familiarization with the work site and organizational structures
- training to accomplish new skills
- adapting the task performance demand
- improving the physical environment
- altering the routine.

A distinct difference between supported employment and other employment services is that, whilst effort is put into fading the specialist support, increasing the natural support and creating the right atmosphere for the individual to fit in is a crucial element of the employment specialist role. How well the individual settles into the job and then progresses depends a lot on the development of relationships with co-workers. Beyer et al (2004), citing Kilsby & Beyer (1996), suggest that the presence of 'outsiders' (specialist support) can be an impediment to social inclusion. The aim is to assist the employee to access the natural means for learning the job. Evidence shows that assisting people to become more socially competent in the workplace helps them to keep their jobs as well as fit in better (Beyer et al 2004, citing Chadsey & Beyer 2001). Laying these foundations by identifying if there are co-workers with skills who are willing to offer the individual support from the beginning, should ensure the employee, co-workers and employer do not become dependent on the employment specialist.

There are a number of intervention techniques and learning approaches to enable the individual to either develop new performance skills, or enable performance within existing abilities. Although applying the usual methods performed by co-workers in the workplace is the first option when the individual is learning the job, it may be necessary to change some parts to meet the individual's needs. Briefly outlined below are some of the approaches that can be used.

Structured training

Structured training involves teaching the individual to do the task in the order of actions described in a task analysis. Reaching competency in the task is dependent on skilfully applied prompts by the person who is training.

Grading techniques

Grading techniques by decreasing the demand of the task involves:

- leaving a complex part of the task until proficiency has been achieved in the rest
- identifying where there are problems, breaking parts of the task down into smaller steps
- positioning the product components and tools so that they are sequentially linked.

Reinforcement

Reinforcement (reward) as an agent of change is an instrumental factor in learning. It is vital to understand its principles and motivational role in the process of adapting behaviour (Morgan & Chisholm 1990).

Adapting the task

Adapting the task may be achieved by omitting a difficult step and redesigning so that it becomes easier for completion by the individual. Individuals, who may not become independent in an entire task sequence may be able to share a task with co-workers (Hagedorn 2000).

Adaptive tools and equipment

Whilst the support of adaptive devices and special equipment may bring attention to an individual's difficulty, as with some task adaptations, they also may be necessary for improving performance. Referred to as 'trade-offs of competing desiderata' (Wolfensberger 1991), the balance is to enhance competency whilst minimizing risk to image. Adaptive tools and equipment can be categorized into three main areas:

- Examples available generally: e.g. office equipment supplies, copyholders, adjustable chairs, spell checkers
- Suppliers of products specifically aimed to assist people with disabilities: e.g. stool with a special sloping feature enables an individual unable to take weight through their legs for long periods to semi-stand; head switches and voice activators may enable use of computers for an individual affected by limited motor performance skills
- Custom devices: adapting equipment has been a fundamental part of occupational therapy but it is important to keep in mind that any adaptation is within health and safety guidelines.

Environmental adaptation

Environmental adaptation involves improving aspects of information (e.g. signs, clocks), objects (e.g. furniture positioning), or conditions (i.e. noise) in the environment.

Environmental rearrangement

Environmental rearrangement such as moving equipment, furniture or tools around (i.e. higher, lower, at an angle, left, right, nearer, etc.) may reduce the physical aspects demanded, enabling the individual to gain access or subsequently increase their productivity. Likewise, rearrangements may avoid mental interference with concentration. Conversely, structuring seating and table layout can help to promote interaction.

Environmental cues

Environmental cues are the naturally reoccurring cues in the workplace benefiting skills acquisition and maintenance. They may help the individual to understand when things should happen and why, or remember a particular work routine (e.g. signalling break time). An individual may not be able to identify pre-existing cues, therefore providing visual or auditory cues can emphasize particular responses (e.g. colour coding, audible prompt watches, pictorial lists, door symbols, etc.).

Fading, the last stage ... or the first?

Fading, regardless of support need, commences from day one. Support interventions are graded or changed along the way, according to evaluation of progress. Ongoing support must be available to both employee and employer; however, the employment specialist's objective is to enable the relationship between employer and employee to take over so that his or her support can be faded. Individuals are competent when they are consistently adequate in their performance of the job, marking the point when an employer's profitable production begins. Although many individuals may still require one-to-one support throughout parts of their working day, there are also those who with skilled intervention will require minimal support and then later go on to be independently working.

Moving on to unsupported employment

At this stage, the individual will be able to act with confidence about their abilities and contribution to the company's overall performance. However, they may continue to need intermittent support in future matters at different times of their career, such as to move on – recognizing that no job is for life! A strong infrastructure of natural support will have been established amongst co-workers and supervisors and is especially important for adaptation to new demands in the job (e.g. workplace rearrangements, task changes, co-worker moves and changes of business ownership).

Summary

The transition to employment as a competent employee involves a spectrum of experiences. The new employee's confidence and competence grows from the initial exploration of choices, experiencing the first day at work, to spending a portion of time discovering new skills. There is a need to create a climate of opportunity and aspiration towards employment and more focus on employment outcomes as the norm for people with learning disabilities. Getting a job may accelerate a range of additional changes. As well as getting to grips with working, it may mean, for the first time, adapting to new habits and performance areas, for example, travelling alone by public transport, adhering to a strict time-keeping policy and making friends in work. To be effective in responding to these needs requires an understanding of concepts of how human beings are motivated and perform. These skills are all in the professional range of an occupational therapist.

Various reports consistently reflect that the 'lack of access to supported employment is particularly acute for people with greater support needs' (O'Bryan et al 2000). Implied is that many of the individuals who have been supported into working are 'people with relatively low levels of impairment' (Leach 2002). The supported employment model needs to develop the range of skills and techniques to fully include all people.

To remain true to their holistic and client-centred values there are various ways that occupational therapists can act now and in the future, to enable individuals towards the ultimate benefits of a working life. This chapter has explored the issues around supporting people with learning disabilities to achieve employment goals. This is a challenging, stimulating and meaningful area for occupational therapists and the key question is not 'whether' they should be involved but 'how'? Simons & Watson (1999).

Box 7.5

Case illustration: Lee

Lee is a 36-year-old man who has lived in this country with his parents and two older sisters since he was 7 when the family emigrated from the Caribbean. He is 6ft tall and has a moderate learning disability and partial vision. Although he attended a special school for the visually impaired his family is very protective of him and he still lives at home with his parents. Lee has support twice a week from two care workers who have been helping him access the local leisure centre for swimming. However, both at home and when he is out, he is reliant on others to carry out all self-care activities such as dressing and personal care. He is able to speak and enjoys activities that involve interaction with others. Lee has recently taken part in an adult education course focusing on social skills. He particularly enjoyed learning to use the telephone and said he wanted to have a job answering the telephone.

Reader activity

1. How would you assess Lee to explore the vocational aspects of his occupations?

2. Using the supported employment model identify ways in which Lee can be supported towards getting a job of his choice.

3. Outline how you might support Lee using the job matching approach.

Useful resources

Development guidance

Department of Health 2002 Framework for developing an employment strategy. London, HSMO

For help and advice on benefits and employment schemes and programmes

'I want to work' A guide to benefits and work for people with a learning disability: www.mencap.org.uk (accessed 21 May 2008)

Jobcentre Plus: www.jobcentreplus.gov.uk (accessed 4 March 2008)

Directgov-official government website for the public: www.direct.gov.uk/en/Employment (accessed 21 May 2008)

Employers perspective

Hemmings S, Morris J 2004 Employing people with learning disabilities A handbook for employers Joseph Rowntree Foundation www.jrf.org.uk (accessed 4 March 2008)

Employers Forum on Disability www.employers-forum.co.uk/www/index.htm (accessed 4 March 2008)

Further information on supported employment

British Association of Supported Employment Agencies (BASE) www.afse.org.uk (accessed 4 March 2008)

SUPPORTED EMPLOYMENT Website for people involved or interested in the development of supported employment http://www.supportedemployment.net/ (accessed 4 March 2008)

MENCAP PATHWAY: www.mencap.org.uk [accessed 19 May 2008]

Training opportunities

Beyer S, Kilsby K, Leach S 2004 Supported employment survival pack: a job developer's handbook. WCLD SCOPE www.scope.org.uk/work/ (accessed 4 March 2008)

Structured Training Course-Alan Morgan, Dr Mark Kilsby: www.structuredtrainingcourse.co.uk (accessed 21 May 2008)

References

British Association of Supported Employment Agencies (BASE) 2007 www.afse.org.uk (accessed 17 June 2007)

Beyer S, Grove B, Schneider J et al 2004 Working lives: the role of day centres in supporting people with learning disabilities into employment, research report no. 203 HMSO, London

Cheshire County Council 1997 Diploma in Supported Employment. Module 2 Topic 3. Cheshire, Cheshire County Council

Creek J 2004 Occupational therapy new perspectives, 4th edn. London, Whurr

Department of Health 2001 Valuing People: a new strategy for learning disabilities for the 21st century. London, DoH

Department for Work and Pensions 2006a Improving work opportunities for people with a learning disability. Report of a working group on learning disabilities and employment. A report to Ministers and the Learning Disability Task Force Corporate Document Services. HSMO, Leeds

Department of Work and Pensions 2006b Improving work opportunities for people with a learning disability. Report: Working Group. HSMO London

Everatt G, AfSE Co-ordinator 1999 Written evidence submitted to the Education and Employment Select Committee www.afse.org.uk (Accessed 17 June 2007)

Hagedorn R 2000 Tools for practice in occupational therapy. London, Churchill Livingstone

Hagedorn R 2002 Foundations for practice in occupational therapy, 3rd edn. London, Churchill Livingstone

Joss M 2007 The importance of job analysis in occupational therapy. British Journal of Occupational Therapy 70(7):301–303

Kielhofner G 2002 Model of human occupation: theory and application, 3rd edn. Philadelphia, Lippincott Williams & Wilkins

Kilsby MS, Beyer S 2002 Enhancing self-determination in job matching in supported employment for people with learning disabilities: an intervention study. Journal of Vocational Rehabilitation 17(2) 125–135

Leach S 2002 A supported employment workbook. London, Jessica Kingsley Publishers Ltd

Lutiyya ZM, Rogan P, Shoultz B 1988 supported employment a conceptual overview. http://thechp.syr.edu/workovw.htm (accessed 4 March 2008)

Mcloughlin CS, Garner JB, Callaghan MJ 1987 Getting employed, staying employed: job development and training for persons with severe handicaps. London, Paul H. Brooks

Morgan A, Chisholm N 1990 Structured training – a course manual. Publisher not provided. (See useful resources: www.structuredtrainingcourse.co.uk) (accessed 22 May 2008)

Mountain G, Carman S, Ilott I 2001 Work rehabilitation and occupational therapy – a review of the literature. London, College of Occupational Therapists

O'Bryan A, Simons K, Beyer S, Grove B 2000 The Policy Consortium for Supported Employment, a framework for supported employment. York, Joseph Rowntree Foundation Publishing Service

Richards SE 1998 The Casson Memorial Lecture 1998: Occupation for health – and wealth? British Journal of Occupational Therapy 61(7):294–300

Simons K, Watson D 1999 New directions? Day services for people with learning disabilities in the 1990s: a review of the research. Exeter, Centre for Evidence Based Social Services

Watson K 2006 supported employment for people with learning disabilities: the argument for the greater role of the occupational therapist within it. OTPLD Newsletter Spring 2006 Edition 1

Wehmeyer ML 2004 Self-determination and the empowerment of people with disabilities. American Rehabilitation: http://www.ed.gov/news/newsletters/amrehab/2004/autumn/wehmeyer.pdf (accessed 19 May 2008)

Wolfensberger W 1991 A brief introduction to social role valorization as a high-order concept for sustaining human services. USA, Syracuse University

Appendix 7.1 Case illustration: Lee, possible answers

1. How would you assess Lee to explore the vocational aspects of his occupations?

   - Sensitivity to cultural issues and the family belief system is highly important. Lee may need assistance to demonstrate his thoughts about his desire to potentially work and overcome his parents', concerns. Listening to his parents and understanding their needs may be crucial in moving forward with Lee's wishes.

   - The role of the employment specialist is to enable Lee to consider himself as capable of directing his own decision and allowing him time to portray his own past and current experiences and maybe insight to having a job through his sisters' and familiar others', employment situations.

   - Reflecting and finding the right words may not be easy for Lee. With his permission, further information may be gained from people who know him and by observing him participate in his natural routines.

   - His information reveals preferences for employment forms linked possibly to reception or office areas in the leisure industry. There are other factors such as his visual impairment and personal support needs which will present challenges but may be overcome with appropriate training, adaptive strategies and a naturally supportive environment.

2. Using the supported employment model identify ways in which Lee can be supported towards getting a job of his choice.

   - The vocational profile refines the type of job and work conditions that will suit Lee. A crucial element of the assessment is to identify how much vision Lee uses and the non-visual techniques he has developed for interacting within his environment.

   - The job development phase requires liaising with local specialist supported employment agencies to identify suitable jobs and negotiate terms and conditions with the employer. There are also government schemes and services that can assist and advise people with visual impairments into work.

   - Job sampling in real work sites and possibly a voluntary job for a period will confirm Lee's most and least preferred job characteristics and his aptitude. Whilst assisting Lee to build his confidence this may in turn enable his parents to view him with a more positive outlook of attaining employment.

   - Analysis of a potential job match will address tasks, routines and environments including support available and essential conditions such as wage, hours etc. to suit Lee. Health and safety features of the job and environment will be an important aspect of this job analysis because of Lee's visual impairment, and perhaps his height. Elements of a workstation might detract from his independent task performance because of an uncomfortable seating position or incompatible desk height, or inaccessibility to nearby storage systems and electrical points. How far away he is from the rest of his co-workers will have significant bearing on his interactive skills and forming relationships. How much emphasis in the job match should be based on features rooted in his culture should be addressed with Lee and his family.

3. Outline how you might support Lee using the job matching approach.

   - The employment specialist may also be involved in ensuring that Lee receives support from his family and care staff to develop his abilities in the way he dresses for work and travelling to work and directing him towards the appropriate benefits advisory services.

   - In readiness to meet the employer, preparations should guide him on how to express his skills and why he has chosen this particular type of work.

   - Some of the employer accommodations illustrated below would be classified as reasonable under the Disability Discrimination Act 2005 which you would discuss with the employer.

- Once Lee's employment is agreed, the employment specialist will spend sufficient time talking with the co-workers, learning the job, familiarizing with the layout of the environment and the environmental cues that will help Lee to orientate to facilities such as toilets, canteen, fire exits, etc. Identifying other sensory cues, (auditory, tactile, olfactory) will be significantly useful.

- The employment specialist must identify the skills that will initially be a problem for Lee to perform in his job. This includes the awareness he will need of the tools, materials and furnishings within his arms' reach and that of his near environment such as the location of the door and co-workers who share the same room.

- If it may be helpful to identify a co-worker to welcome him at the start of his job.

- It might be necessary to negotiate approval to change the environment or task, or to design some specific environmental cues. How often do you change or add to your work area to make it more comfortable to work in? These changes will probably be only simple features of visual discrimination. For example, lighting adjustments to his work area, colour contrasts and tactile embossing to tools and surfaces. There might be a need for adaptive devices and specialist equipment – there are many innovative tele-communication devices and optical aids available to assist people with visual impairments. It is also advisable to seek the help of a Rehabilitation Worker for the Visually Impaired, if available.

- Training for the job should maximize the natural support in the workplace whether it is the in-house training resources or the identification of co-workers who may take the lead in supporting Lee and ensuring his continued success. The person training will incrementally increase the performance demands of the task as Lee learns and adapts, carefully using physical and vocal prompts. Training is subject to ongoing evaluation.

- The people Lee will be working with may require some information to understand of his visual impairment so that they can assist him to integrate into the workplace and access the work site resources and visual information such as in-out boards, health and safety information, bulletin boards.

- There might be a change in the role of Lee's care workers. In order for Lee to manage his job, he will require personal care assistance at his place of work.

- When Lee has achieved the goal to carry out his job without the employment specialist being around, there must be confidence that Lee and his employer will, between them, problem solve any changes that should arise in the future. The employment specialist will continue to be in touch.

Chapter Eight

8

Leisure

Christine Locke

Overview

This chapter will explore and present some of the perspectives of leisure and client-centred practice for people with a learning disability. Everyday needs are described as a place to live, social and personal relationships, leisure, recreation and work opportunities and security (Scottish Executive 2000). The importance of leisure has been the focus of research generally within disability studies (Di Bona 2000, Aitchison 2003). However, although historically used in learning disability services, there is limited evidence available about both the meaning and types of leisure to meet the individual needs of people with learning disabilities. This chapter will discuss the meaning and complexity of leisure as an occupational performance area. The chapter will also explore the barriers and opportunities of leisure for people with a learning disability. From the professional point of view there is bias towards the perceived therapeutic benefits of leisure activities. Intrinsic attributes of leisure can improve self-esteem, personal growth, increase social networks as well as enhance physical fitness, health and well-being.
The chapter discusses leisure as a

'therapy product' (Neumayer & Wilding 2006) and the challenges of the therapeutic potential to maintaining a client-centred approach ensuring choice and participation for intrinsic benefits – i.e. it should be satisfying. This chapter will enable you to fulfil the following learning outcomes:

Learning Outcomes

- Define leisure as an occupational domain
- Discuss choice, opportunities and barriers in leisure participation
- Explore the therapeutic potential of leisure in present-day social and environmental contexts
- Discuss leisure and occupational therapy client-centred practice.

Defining leisure

A definition of leisure depends on our own view of what leisure is. As a starting point and one to reflect on by the end of this chapter, the question 'How would you define leisure?' should prompt you to identify your own concepts of leisure. Di Bona (2000) suggests 'Further understanding of the potential benefits gained from engaging in leisure might enable therapists to justify their use of leisure to others' (p.50). Leisure is categorized as variably sedentary or active, social or solitary and cultural. It may be relaxing in front of the TV, reading, listening to music, gardening, involvement in sport, taking the dog for a walk or using the computer to contact friends, joining a club, going on holiday or a meal with friends. In other words, we all have our own choice and concept of what leisure is and means to us. It equates with activities involving choice, free from the constraints of self-maintenance or productivity and valued by the individual.

Leisure is defined within occupational therapy as an occupational performance domain such as adult play (Keilhofner 2002), or occupations for enjoyment (Sumsion & Blank 2006) and as fundamental to health and well-being. In the developed world it is often perceived as a foil to productivity. As the third occupation described in models of occupational therapy it is the one area of occupational therapy intervention least often addressed. Suto (1998) p. 272. 'Reflecting the dominant society work ethic, the occupational therapy profession was reluctant to consider adult leisure seriously until recently.' Occupational therapists also need to be sensitive to what are the cultural norms and values of both the individual and family. The emerging Kawa Model (Iwama 2006) further challenges Western cultural norms and values and an occupational therapy culture of 'doing'. This gives an Asian perspective and provokes an awareness of the potential differences in cultural perspectives within a diverse client population.

Neumayer & Wilding (2005) discuss the position of the concept of leisure as a 'therapy product' in achieving therapeutic goals. Historically, in learning disabilities, leisure as a 'therapy product' has been used to generate skills and rewards as a motivating medium for intervention and exploration and can be identified therapeutically in terms of:

- leisure activity to develop social skills
- leisure activities to motivate
- leisure activities to develop skills of choice and participation
- leisure activities to develop/adapt/maintain performance components.

In many instances for people with a learning disability, leisure is aimed at goals of skills establishing social skills, physical fitness or participation to be generalized into other occupational areas rather than as a purely leisure pursuit (Primeau 2003). It may be, however, from the individual's perspective, that activities of productivity (for example doing volunteer work in a woodland project) or self-maintenance (such as baking cakes) can be defined as leisure. The concept of leisure will therefore vary from individual to individual (Passmore & French 2003). Before reading this chapter further take a moment to consider what leisure means to you and ask yourself the following questions.

Reader activity

- What are my leisure activities?
- How and why have I chosen to do them?
- What did I need to have to pursue and carry them out?

Linked with the individual's 'intrinsic need' for self-maintenance and productivity, leisure can provide individual expression and fulfilment in the context of roles and integration into the community. Whilst recognizing these intrinsic concepts, leisure can and does play an important part in maintaining occupational balance and it is often crucial to restoring quality of life balance. In Chapter 5, leisure is also discussed in relation to establishing healthy life routines and occupations. For the occupational therapist, the challenge is to identify the intrinsic and temporal elements of leisure for the individual in a therapeutic context. The context of matching individual preference against therapeutic intervention is succinctly described by Suto (1998) p. 272. 'The complexity of leisure and its place within occupational therapy are complicated by the multiple meanings that the word engenders. Leisure is an occupational performance area, a state of mind, time to be filled and a tangible activity through which therapeutic goals are met.' The inherent individual basis, value and complexity of leisure and its importance to quality of life for people with a learning disability as therapeutic potential can be summarized as follows:

- Intrinsic motivation leading to overall aim of satisfaction of enjoyment or pleasure
- Linked to learning and development of social skills and social behaviour including relationships and community integration (e.g. sport, drama groups)
- Perceived freedom and positive self-esteem and different role value from other occupations such as productivity
- Done in free time but could have 'gain' (e.g. bingo – fun, monetary).

Leisure can be summarized as involving those activities usually associated with enjoyment, recreation and individual preference. However, the opportunity to fulfil any one of these is limited for an individual with a learning disability. The move from large institutions and community living for people with a learning disability places an emphasis on what leisure means in the present-day community context. Many studies of leisure have identified that opportunity for access to leisure activities is much less for people with learning disabilities than for the general population (Beart et al 2001).

Leisure opportunity and barriers for people with a learning disability

By exploring leisure as a 'therapy product' this next section will explore choice, opportunity and barriers to leisure and the role of the occupational therapist. Occupational participation, including leisure opportunities, is identified in Valuing People (DoH 2001) which advocates the need for leisure as important to enable people with a learning disability to lead 'full and purposeful lives'. Whilst this acknowledges the importance of a balance of occupations for people with a learning disability, there are factors that limit both the choice and opportunity for leisure activities. The role of the occupational therapist in establishing leisure needs is often in the context of multidisciplinary and multi-agency working. However, identification of leisure as an opportunity for social integration as well as contributing to improving quality of life is very often minimized in care plans and seen as a low priority within a service provider's limited resources (DoH 2001, McConkey et al 2006). The occupational therapist, through using holistic client-centred assessments, can identify the need as well as the barriers and the benefits of leisure pursuits in relation to the individual's ability and choice. The factors that have an impact on leisure opportunity will now be discussed further in the contexts of:

- occupational balance of leisure, self-maintenance and productivity
- meaningful, positive roles
- social segregation and integration
- environmental factors
- development of competency and fun.

Context of occupational balance of leisure, self-maintenance and productivity

Research indicates that there is a limited range of activities for people with a learning disability and often they do not take part in community leisure activities (Abbott & McConkey 2006). The literature indicates several external and internal factors that influence the choice and use of leisure. External factors may include age, gender, culture, finance, living situation and society, that dictate both type and use of recreational facilities. When considering external factors the occupational therapist also needs to identify the accessibility of leisure opportunity in relation to the individual's daily and weekly routines. Internal factors include variables such as:

- limited personal meanings of leisure or choice
- poor motivation, low self-esteem or lack of confidence
- poor physical or cognitive skills.

Choice or opportunity can be limited by high level of dependency in self-care (i.e. dressing, bathing) or availability of support for home or community based activities at appropriate times. Daily or weekly routines (i.e. shopping, housework) established through person-centred planning and care plans are often prioritized to enable the individual to develop skills rather than necessarily to have an opportunity for enjoyment or intrinsic satisfaction. Also, changes to routines, very often during transition, or changes in health status can provoke behaviours that reduce or remove the opportunity for leisure pursuit. High levels of dependence in areas of self-care mean that the individual, even if they are able to make a choice, is reliant on others for transport and accessing facilities such as the swimming pool or going to the local pub. To explore these aspects further reflect on the questions asked in the case study presented at the end of this chapter.

Identifying needs and preferences

By using a model of occupational therapy in which leisure is a key component, assessments such as the Model of Human Occupation (MOHO) interest checklist, volitional questionnaire, role checklist or other standardized assessments of performance components such as assessment of motor and process skills (AMPS), will identify performance skill, balance of occupations, preference and opportunity for choice. The individual with a mild or moderate learning disability can identify both balance of occupations and choice through appropriate non-standardized assessments such as a self-rating leisure questionnaire, routines or leisure patterns checklist, satisfaction or interest checklist, all of which can be custom made. There can, however, be difficulties for clients in acknowledging their own leisure goals or needs as well as understanding a rating scale unless its design incorporates appropriate symbols, pictures or actual situations. The process of assessment can include trying alternative activities such as bowling, gardening or attending a relaxation group over a period of weeks or months before completing a rating scale. For an individual with profound or multiple learning disability, observation and using an occupational analysis of daily routine activities or a sensory inventory can give an indication of preferences or negative reactions. Assessment of preferences can also include recording narrative or life history or gathering information from parents or carers to indicate their perception of the domains of self-help, interpersonal, social skills and cognitive abilities. An assessment may identify that the individual will have had little opportunity to explore different types of leisure and have only experience of solitary or sedentary activities (Beart et al 2001). By determining the categories of leisure occupations listed in Box 8.1, occupational therapists can identify appropriate areas for assessing preference. As mentioned above, in carrying out an initial assessment the occupational therapist can also identify preference through 'taster sessions' to enable the individual to experience the activity and therefore make an informed choice. A risk assessment should be carried out prior to the taster sessions and during a leisure activity to ensure that planning and intervention can be put in place to minimize risk for the individual and/or carer. Risks can include the social context where there is a chance of harm to the individual, such as vulnerability or of abuse to others due to behavioural concerns. It may be a physical or functional risk for the person supporting the individual such as, for example, a manual handling risk when using a car or supporting a wheelchair user to get to a leisure centre.

The context of meaningful, positive roles

A barrier to both individual choice of activities and development of positive roles through leisure pursuits

Box 8.1

Assessment areas of leisure occupations

- Therapeutic (snoezelen)
- Physical (e.g. walking, gardening, sport)
- Creative (e.g. art, pottery, drama, music)
- Solitary (e.g. reading, sewing, computer, watching television, listening to radio)
- Cognitive/psychological (e.g. meditation, relaxation, computer)
- Entertainment (theatre, concerts, bingo)
- Hobbies (e.g. collecting, pets)
- Social (e.g. meeting/making new friends, eating out, shopping day trips, holidays)
- Voluntary (e.g. club, organization)

Adapted from Leisure Interest Checklist (Baxter et al 1995).

is often the compliance of the person with a learning disability with the goals of service providers or carers. As occupational therapists, why do we need to define leisure interests or needs in relation to developing a positive role for people with a learning disability? When discussing leisure in relation to social images, Taylor (2003) discusses the relevance of 'symbolic interactionism', 'social identity theory' and 'stereotype theory' to provide an understanding of personal and social identities in leisure (refer to Box 8.2). The perception of leisure as an occupation for people with learning disabilities is often as a substitute for employment or productivity. In some instances, for example being a participant in competitive sporting activities such as swimming or athletics, leisure could and does substitute a productivity role for people with learning disability. Some leisure activities have a gender-specific image shared by the individuals and by society. Leisure activities as defined by Law et al (1996) are necessary to meet the person's 'intrinsic need' and it is important to determine both the characteristics of the leisure activity and what the outcome is for the individual to develop positive age appropriate roles or for gender preferences. Occupational therapists can start to address these needs by matching the individual's abilities and goals within the context of leisure roles and the environment. For those individuals with emotional and behaviour problems or attention deficits, grading can enable them to develop both skill and preference, with an aesthetic reward immediately

Box 8.2

Leisure theory (Taylor 2003)

- *Symbolic interactionism theory* – engagement in a leisure activity in which shared symbols or dress code make a statement about a leisure role and identity that have both personal and social meaning for those the individual interacts with (e.g. club stickers on wheelchairs, wearing a club cap).
- *Social identity theory* – explains that being a group member results in shared attribution of social image by the individual and by others (e.g. Scrabble club members are cerebral and quiet, rock climbers are adventurous).
- *Stereotype theory* – a set of beliefs by others of the personal attributes of a group which group members may not have but result in the creation of 'self-fulfilling prophecies' (e.g. perception of gender difficulty for a women joining a football club and the social image that is associated with football clubs).

or over time. For example, an activity such as gardening can be graded from a visit to and exploration of a sensory garden or graded tasks in gardening activities such as potting, planting or weeding. This can enable the individual to identify and explore opportunities for individual expression and fulfilment.

The development of 'normal' life roles for people with a learning disability is intrinsically linked to not only work roles but also social or leisure roles, to provide opportunity to develop positive self-image, appropriate stimulation and practice of social skills and choice (Reynolds 2002). The importance of social networks and relationships has been recognized philosophically in policy documents for people with learning disability, including normalization theory as discussed in Chapter 2. These emphasize that people with a learning disability have the same rights as everyone else (DoH 2001). Tyne & O'Brien's (1981) five accomplishments included valued relationships towards good qualify of life. Although it is not the purpose of this chapter to discuss aspects of friendships, relationships and sexuality in depth these are relevant when considering the potential for developing positive roles of friendships and valued relationships through leisure opportunities. People with a learning disability lack opportunities to meet

people to allow relationships and friendships to flourish (Knox & Hickson 2001) and to build social skills for developing friendships and relationships. This may be due to a lack of supportive social networks, lack of privacy or exclusion from participation in community-based activities. Poor social skills or actual disability or lack of fitness can lead to rejection and social isolation. There is a need to question the appropriateness of traditional approaches to social skills training which may be segregated and isolating. The focus on using integrated peer groups, clubs or resources within the community to empower an individual with a learning disability in developing and maintaining friendships will involve identifying the type of support needed. Training of support staff to support individuals can also augment a multidisciplinary approach using social skills programmes, sex education, creative medium group or transition group or on an individual basis to enable the individual to develop social skills towards a valued role. Participation in sport or exercise establishes levels of competency but also positive roles and friendships. A graded approach to sport and exercise can improve and develop good physical health status, weight loss, motor skills and coordination. However, the demands of any activity can produce negative effects, such as exhaustion when carrying out a sporting activity, nervousness when meeting new people, limited ability to acknowledge being a member of a team, disappointment or poor behavioural responses when losing in a game. Identifying the type of support either on a one-to-one basis (e.g. access to go to a concert), using peer support (e.g. in a bowling group) or providing/adapting equipment (e.g. to play in a darts match) can provide achievable goals, reducing failure and developing positive self image. To consider the context of meaningful roles further, reflect on the questions in the following reader activity.

Reader activity

- What roles does your leisure activity give you?
- In what way are the leisure roles different from self-care and productivity?

The context of social factors

Whether the individual lives on their own, in a family, a small group home or institutional setting, opportunity for leisure activities can be variable in terms of choice and value. Leisure for people with a learning disability can also be frequently solitary with little or no physical demand (Messent et al 1999). Individuals are reliant on family or relationships that often diminish once they have left school or college (Carr 2004). Changes to the individual circumstances, as discussed in Chapter 9, can either remove or limit the opportunity to pursue leisure that has a real meaning for the individual. An illustration of the possible causes and issues of segregation and isolation is given in the end of chapter case illustration for Andy. Although he is a sociable person, due to his complex needs his opportunities are reduced to a segregated, passive role at the day centre and isolation in his bedroom at home.

For people with a learning disability the identification of leisure is often based on limited past experience, significantly dominated by participation in group leisure activities or outings with the family rather than on individual need. Although participating in a group may have been one of the individual's choices, the actual activities undertaken are chosen by group consensus or by the facilitators. Alternatively, leisure activities instigated and undertaken for a number of years do not offer opportunity to explore alternatives. Equally, communication difficulties or reliance on non-verbal skills and behaviours limits the opportunity to express oneself. Thus establishing an informed preference for new experiences may be overlooked. Optimizing leisure opportunities is possible by using occupational or task analysis linked with a graded approach and appropriate support to develop leisure pursuits over a period of time. Referring to the end of chapter case illustration for Andy, it was identified that he is able to communicate adequately through a communication board on a day-to-day basis with family and day centre staff mainly in relation to his self-care needs (i.e. symbol for drink). However, the board did not give flexibility to communicate leisure needs in new situations or with unfamiliar people. The importance of allowing the individual to communicate by appropriate methods either by verbal or non-verbal means is discussed comprehensively in Chapter 4.

Other people in the social context may negatively influence the individual's expression of choice if they believe it to be inappropriate in terms of age appropriateness, perceived risks or challenges in the social environment. Unfortunately, identified barriers to social inclusion still prevail in societal attitudes and parental concerns. For parents especially, concerns about the individual's lack of skill, behavioural issues,

vulnerability or fear of failure, exploitation and rejection can present real barriers to them taking part in community leisure activities. These are realistic concerns mirrored by attitudes of the wider community and result in emphasis on participation that is limited to activities that are statistically normative rather than freely chosen by the individual. There can be a bias towards therapeutic or health benefits of the leisure activity, such as social skills development in a drama group or health benefits from a women's group or relaxation from a yoga group rather than the intrinsic or social value of the activity itself. Implied segregation in policies and procedures suggested by Abbott & McConkey (2006) presents other barriers such as limited financial resources or insufficient levels of support, preventing opportunity to explore community leisure venues outside of the nine to five working day. The occupational therapist can help by identifying resources at a local level requiring minimal financial resources, including websites (useful websites are listed at the end of this chapter), libraries, local health and leisure groups, leisure centres and voluntary organizations. In this way access to community, leisure facilities and environmental aspects may be optimized for the individual.

The environmental context of leisure

The closure of the large institutions has removed, in many ways, the 'group' emphasis of opportunity for leisure, with greater access to community resources and integration. However, community integration and leisure opportunity is still limited compared to the general population (Beart et al 2001). For the individual with a learning disability accessing any leisure facility may pose a major barrier outside of the home. Barriers can include architectural layout, adaptation and equipment needed, cost and availability of appropriate transportation, access for wheelchair mobility or need for special equipment or clothing. Carr (2004) states that 'people who may not normally need help at home will often require assistance outside to negotiate a hostile physical and social environment'. Utilizing a model framework such as the person–environment–occupational model (Law et al 1996) provides a useful theoretical framework for the occupational therapist to establish what the demands of the environment are.

Environments can potentially be stimulating or relaxing and the sensory context can be challenging for the individual. For instance, consider the sensory impact of entering a crowded room with music and strobe lighting compared to listening to music in a quiet room at home. The case illustration for Andy illustrates how the level of stimulation at the day centre resulted in passive, withdrawn behaviour whereas at home, albeit isolated, he had control over his environment using an environmental control system. There is a challenge, however, to adapting the physical environment at home to promote lesser or greater sensory stimuli without developing a mini institutional environment. Sensory equipment used in multi-sensory rooms can be available either through leisure centres, day centres or in a room in the home to give the individual opportunity to control and explore an environment for relaxation or for stimulation in a different environment (Baillon et al 2002, Urwin & Ballinger 2005). Computer technology offers elements of fun, exploration and recreation that can be shared or solitary in the home or club. Creative leisure activities, such as listening to music or art classes, are commonly available and have the potential for social integration or to be developed as a hobby in the home. Separate social skills training can simultaneously be incorporated and practised within the community. The important consideration is what type of environment best meets the individual's need for leisure participation.

Acquiring resources and adapting leisure environments can be costly. An alternative to changing the environment could be to adapt the process of how the activity is carried out. For instance, it is important for an individual with profound disability not to have too much happening at any one time as this may confuse them or increase anxiety or agitation. For example, to attend a community music group the impact of the car journey needs to be considered and the establishment of strategies to familiarize, relax and integrate people into the group. Equally, anticipation and limitation triggers to challenging behaviour, such as light, noise or movement, can help to reduce distress. By assessing the ergonomic aspects of the environment, occupational therapists can identify the negative or enabling environmental impact on the individual's performance and ensure that the activity retains both meaning and value for the individual. To encourage appropriate behaviour and success in new social settings the role of support staff may be vital in role modelling, consistent use of prompts and cues and encouragement to participate.

The context of development of competency versus the context of fun and play

How can we ensure that the context of fun and play is achievable for the individual with a learning disability whilst ensuring development of skills? The personal context of feeling and satisfaction leading to quality of life is one that is inherent in leisure, but there can be a danger that leisure as something therapeutic can diminish the personal gain. It is important to consider the intrinsic purposes of leisure occupations as personal goals and how the individual can attempt and successfully achieve leisure through therapeutic means. Baxter et al (1995) discussed the benefits and categorized leisure into the following taxonomy:

- pleasure
- educational
- psychological
- social
- relaxation
- physiological
- aesthetic
- challenging.

Any leisure activity can involve one or more of the above and the following Box 8.3 Case illustration: Peter will illustrate the concepts of leisure benefits.

Box 8.3

Case illustration: Peter

Peter has a moderate learning disability and has been referred for an occupational therapy assessment due to his agitated and unmotivated behaviour at home. Although Peter has limited verbal communication and is reported to be uninterested in doing anything, he is a friendly individual. At the initial assessment, he persistently indicated an interest in a book of cars, insisting the occupational therapist look through it with him. The occupational therapist was able to use this initial interest to start to build a picture of Peter's personal goals for leisure. By exploring opportunities for accessing leisure pursuits through a graded approach Peter was eventually introduced to a peer mentor of the same age

(Continued)

Box 8.3 (continued)

and started to attend a local car club with him. This became a valued weekly routine. Although as professionals we need to identify skill deficit and the impact of limited ability, control and choice, we do need to maintain a client-centred approach to identifying skill potential. This potential is illustrated by Peter's acceptance by others of his perceived friendliness despite limitations to his skill level whilst sharing an enthusiasm and common interest in cars. On the face of it, he was very dependent on support to get to and from the club and had poor verbal communication skills. By exploring his interest in cars and friendliness as potential strengths, facilitating his non-verbal communication skills and overcoming environmental barriers, he increased his independence to access a leisure opportunity of his choice. This improved his motivation, participation and enjoyment.

Many areas of leisure activity may, however, appear initially to be unsuitable for those with severe and multiple physical and cognitive limitations. Establishing recreation or leisure activities that are age-appropriate and have those elements of personal interest and fun is challenging. As discussed previously within the environment context, multi-sensory rooms can be used for an individual with a learning disability to explore and control an environment in a safe controlled way. Therapeutically the goal may be towards reducing anxiety and relaxation. It is also a shared environment enabling a social experience with others (Baillon et al 2002). Assessment of responses and preferences to graded stimuli can form the basis of adapting a home environment for relaxation purposes. Using switching to enable someone with a profound learning disability can also give a sense of empowerment and satisfaction.

Summary

The value and choice of leisure pursuits is based on personal preference. Historically, leisure has been used as a therapeutic product aimed at developing skills for people with learning disability. Leisure participation can give an individual with a learning disability the opportunity to acquire, maintain and generalize skills and behaviour into other settings

(Buttimer & Tierney 2005). The challenge, however, in the present day context of community living and limited resources, is to enable both opportunity and choice towards a leisure outcome that is satisfying for the individual. The occupational therapy role in the leisure domain is to provide effective therapeutic intervention to enable the individual to gradually develop skill through short- or long-term participation in leisure pursuits of their choice. Utilizing an appropriate model and assessment tools occupational therapists can explore with the individual the range of opportunities, their context and barriers that may prevent them from achieving leisure activities of their choice. Overcoming these barriers through skill training, environmental adaptation, additional support or changing the way the activity is presented can result in a successful outcome for the client. This is demonstrated finally by a few words from a service user: 'On trampoline ...I like to do it because I like doing it ...It makes me laugh'.

Reader activity

1. How would you establish Andy's leisure needs?
2. How could you establish his choices?
3. How would you identify the barriers and opportunity to access leisure?

Box 8.4

Case illustration: Andy

Referral

Andy was referred by the case manager for an occupational therapy assessment to identify preferences for day and evening activities. The referral also requested a risk assessment to access community facilities. Andy is 29 years old and has cerebral palsy with spastic quadriplegia, windswept hips and painful dislocation of the left hip. Dependent on an indoor electric wheelchair with lateral support, it was reported that Andy did not explore any of the facilities in the day centre unless prompted by staff. He appeared withdrawn, sleepy and reluctant to take part in activities within the day centre (e.g. painting). His day is mainly dictated by the routine at home and attending the day centre as he is fully dependent for all aspects of personal care.

Useful resources

Baxter R, Friel K, McAtamney A, White B, Williamson 1995 Leisure enhancement through occupational therapy. London, College of Occupational Therapy

College of Occupational Therapy 2003 Principles for education and practice: occupational therapy services for adults with learning disability. London, COT

Leitner MJ, Leitner SF 2008 Leisure in later life. A sourcebook for the provision of recreation services for elders, 3rd edn. NY, Haworth Press

London Sports Forum for Disabled People: www.londonsportsforum. org.uk a useful website with links to recreation and leisure material and information (accessed 4 March 2008)

Foundation for People with Learning Disabilities: www. learningdisabilities.org.uk (accessed 4 March 2008)

NHS Library: www.library.nhs.uk (accessed 4 March 2008)

OT Seeker: www.otseeker.com/ or ingentaConnect (minimal abstracts and systematic reviews randomized trials in relation to leisure) and people with a learning disability (both accessed 4 March 2008)

References

Abbott S, McConkey R 2006 The barriers to social inclusion as perceived by people with intellectual disabilities. Journal of Intellectual Disability 10(3): 275–287

Aitchison C 2003 From leisure and disability to disability leisure: developing data, definitions and discourses. Disability and Society 18(7):955–969

Baillon S, van Diepen E, Prettyman P 2002 Multi-sensory therapy in psychiatric care. Advances in Psychiatric Treatment 8:444–452

Baxter R, Friel K, McAtamney A, White B, Williamson 1995 Leisure enhancement through occupational therapy. London, College of Occupational Therapy

Beart S, Hawkins D, Stenfert Kroese B, Smithson P, Tolosa I 2001 Barriers to accessing leisure opportunities for people with learning disabilities. British Journal of Learning Disabilities 29: 133–138

Buttimer J, Tierney E 2005 Patterns of leisure participation among adolescents with a mild intellectual disability. Journal of Intellectual Disabilities 9(1):43–57

Carr E 2004 Leisure and disabled people. In: Swain J, French S, Barnes C, Thomas C (eds) Disabling barriers – enabling environments, 2nd edn. London, Sage

Department of Health 2001 Valuing people: a new strategy for learning disabilities for the 21st century (Chapter 7). London, HSMO

Di Bona L 2000 What are the benefits of leisure? An exploration using the Leisure Satisfaction Scale. British Journal of Occupational Therapy 63(2):50–58

Iwama M 2006 The Kawa Model: culturally relevant occupational therapy. Philadelphia, Elsevier

Kielhofner G 2002 Model of human occupation – theory and application, 3rd edn. Baltimore, Lippincott, Williams & Wilkins

Knox M, Hickson F 2001 The meanings of close friendships: the views of four people with intellectual disabilities. Journal of Applied Research in Intellectual Disabilities 14:276–291

Law M, Cooper B, Strong S et al 1996 The person-environment occupation model: a transactive approach to occupational performance. Canadian Journal of Occupational Therapy 63(1):9–23

Neumayer B, Wilding C 2005 Leisure as a commodity (Chapter 19). In: Whiteford G (ed.) Occupation and practice in context. Australia, Elsevier

Messent PR, Cooke CB, Long J 1999 Primary and secondary barriers to physically active healthy lifestyles for adults with learning disabilities. Disability and Rehabilitation 21(9):409–419

McConkey R, Abbott S, Noonan-Walsh P et al 2006 Variations in the social inclusion of people with intellectual disabilities in support living schemes and residential settings. Journal of Intellectual Disability Research 10(3):275–286

Passmore A, French D 2003 The nature of leisure in adolescence: a focus group study. British Journal of Occupational Therapy 66(9):419–426

Primeau LA 2003 Play and leisure. In: Crepeau EB, Schell BAB (eds) Willard and Spackman's occupational therapy, 10th edn. Philadelphia, Lippincott, Williams & Wilkins

Reynolds F 2002 An exploratory survey of opportunities and barriers to creative leisure activity for people with learning disabilities. British Journal of Learning Disabilities 30:63–67

Scottish Executive 2000 The same as you? A review of services for people with learning disabilities. Edinburgh, Scottish Executive

Sumsion T, Blank A 2006 The Canadian model of occupational performance. In: Duncan E (ed.) Foundations for practice in occupational therapy. London, Elsevier, pp 109–124

Suto M 1998 Leisure in occupational therapy. Canadian Journal of Occupational Therapy 65(5): 272–277

Taylor J 2003 Women's leisure activities, their social stereotypes and some implications for identity. British Journal of Occupational Therapy 66(4): 151–158

Tyne A, O'Brien J 1981 The principles of normalisation: Campaign for Mentally Handicapped People. London, Campaign for Mental Handicap Education and Research Association

Urwin R, Ballinger C 2005 The effectiveness of sensory integration therapy to improve functional behaviour in adults with learning disabilities: five single-case experimental designs. British Journal of Occupational Therapy 68(2):56–65

Appendix 8.1 Case illustration: Andy, possible answers

1. How would you establish Andy's leisure needs?

Assessing needs

An appropriate model such as MOHO or CMOP can be used as an assessment framework to maintain a client-centred holistic approach. Observation of his activities in the day centre would identify a number of strengths. Using a volitional questionnaire at the day centre identified that Andy showed most interest in watching others working on the computer and meal times. He was least interested in the creative activities on offer. Andy is sociable, with good eye contact, and enjoys being with people and interacting but did not appear to have any close friendships. A home visit identified that he lives with his elderly parents and his evenings are mainly solitary as he spends most of the time in his bedroom.

2. How could you establish his choices?

Strengths and needs

Assessing his ability to use the environmental control identified that he is able to make choice/preferences for programmes and will turn the TV/music on or off when he wants. He is capable of developing and making his own choices and pursuing interests by using his right hand. By pointing, pressing and gripping with both hands he communicates likes and dislikes (i.e. music preferences, animal programmes on TV). It was also identified that Andy is able to communicate needs by pointing to a communication board or verbalizing when unhappy and understands cause and effect, and has object, colour and shape recognition. He has some recognition of familiar names, of objects and some number recognition. However, this was a slow process and he needed to develop a more effective form of communicating his preferences.

Communication

A joint upper limb assessment and communication assessment with occupational therapy and the speech and language therapist identified that Andy wanted to continue to use his communication board but required different cards to use when communicating at the day centre and in the community. His keyworker helped Andy to develop his own symbol board. Using his board and adapted pointer Andy started to participate in activities offered to him such as computer games with 1:1 support, some physical assistance and verbal prompting. By using a leisure checklist in conjunction with the communication board he was also able to identify what he would like to do both at the day centre and at home. He identified that he wanted to try the computer and maybe have one at home. He also wanted to go out in the evenings but not with his parents!

3. How would you identify the barriers and opportunity to access leisure?

Physical environment

A manual handling assessment identified that he is dependent for all aspects of self-care and transfers with one person using a changing bench and hoist. To get to the day centre Andy is assisted in and out of his adapted car but this is not used in the evenings. A wheelchair assessment was carried out to review his seating and ability to control his powered wheelchair. As Andy could safely use the powered wheelchair the occupational therapist set up a daily practice session with Andy and support worker to manoeuvre around independently in the day centre and in and out of his adapted vehicle. After a 2-week period he was able to achieve both with minimal verbal prompting.

Social environment

Working jointly with Andy, his parents, and case manager, a support worker was employed to support Andy twice a week to go out in the evenings. By establishing his independence in communicating and using his car Andy started to access a local pub where his older brother and friends met with him once a week. He also started to visit computer shops to look for a computer for home use. At this point it was agreed with Andy that he had achieved what he wanted and that the occupational therapist would no longer see him.

Section **Three**

This section of the book looks at some of the transitions that can occur in everyone's life. In planning and contributing to this section the authors reflected on the personal transitions they have experienced and the impact of those experiences from an individual and family perspective. However, people with a learning disability very often have their rights to these personal life events questioned in a way that others would not. The section is structured to explore the perspectives of life changing events across the life span that sometimes can go unnoticed unless a problem occurs for the individual with a learning disability.

The complex narrative of transition from childhood into adulthood for a young person with a learning disability is often one which challenges parents and service provider. Chapter 9 explores the context of transition for a young individual with a learning disability and their carers. Examples are given of the ways in which the occupational therapist can address some of the issues through occupation to support the individual to make the transition successful.

Parenting is another skill that many of us manage to acquire as we go along but possibly many of us would not ask for a reference from our offspring. Chapter 10 explores the occupational therapist's role in the context of multidisciplinary and multi-agency working in the assessment and legislative framework in relation to the issues of child safety. Case scenarios illustrate perceived needs and abilities of parents and the impact of the environmental demands on parenting and families. A parenting model is discussed in relation to the current and future trends for supporting parents with a learning disability.

For Jenni Hurst, her experience and interest in bereavement counselling arose because of her clinical work in both mental health and learning disabilities. In Chapter 11 Jenni Hurst sensitively explores the issues of loss and bereavement, which can leave any one of us vulnerable. Her chapter discusses the particular issues for people with a learning disability and the need for acknowledgement and expression of grief. The actual experience of what can happen when someone dies involves difficult abstract concepts, including the rituals around funerals and coping with the loss afterwards. These are explored with examples and suggestions on the type of approaches that can help to support clients, relatives or carers by the occupational therapist and other members of a specialist learning disability team.

Older people have a higher profile and voice in the community and are more able to articulate their needs. However, the increasing numbers of older people mean that we need to ensure that older people with learning disability also have the right to suitable community services. Chapter 12 discusses the implications of government policy, such as the NSF for Older People, and assessment of need for older people with a learning disability. The role of the occupational therapist in screening and support for people with Down's syndrome and their increased risk of Alzheimer's disease is also explored. Case scenarios illustrate the importance of maintaining occupation through the changes to physical and mental health by identifying supportive environments and meaningful occupations.

We hope that this section will help you reflect on your own transitions and to recognize that people with a learning disability need support to negotiate these potentially difficult times in their lives.

Chapter Nine

9

The challenges of maintaining occupation at times of transition

Jenni Hurst

Overview

This chapter looks at the variety of transitions that occur for people with a learning disability when they wish to assume adult roles and relationships. It will also explore how people with a profound and multiple learning disability may be seen by others as unable to assume adult relationships. This transition does not naturally occur for people with a learning disability when they leave school.

Occupational therapy contributes to this transition by assisting both young adults and older people with a learning disability to transfer their existing occupational performance into a different setting. Using occupational performance analysis they can also help them identify and acquire the skills that will enable them to improve their occupational performance and demonstrate occupational competence in the new setting.

Initially parents have to accept that the child they expected is different and then cope with the stigma that accompanies this. This in turn may influence the attachment experienced by the child with its parents. As part of the maturation process from child to adult each individual learns to adapt to change and for some adolescents this can be a turbulent period of their lives. This leads to some people with a learning disability being identified as difficult to support because of their behaviour. Difficulties in developing adult relationships may be a reflection of their early attachment experiences (Dallos 2006). For a variety of reasons people with a learning disability have to cope with different expectations and may not have had opportunities to develop secure attachments and this can influence what happens to them as adults.

Listening to and trying to understand the complex narrative of transition gives additional information which will assist the occupational therapist to work with the service user and significant others in their life. While education will bring its own challenges the transition to adulthood contains additional challenges as service provision and service expectations may differ. At this time people with a learning disability can become aware of the expectations of society for adults. This includes both society and the law's view on adult relationships and their vulnerability to people who offer friendship. Sometimes

even the most carefully planned and anticipated change will alter the direction of their lives in ways that had not been considered.

Learning Outcomes

By the end of the chapter you will be able to:

- Understand the significance of transition from childhood to adulthood for a person with a learning disability and their parents
- Be able to support the person with a learning disability to transfer existing occupations and acquire new occupations that they will need to make the transition successful
- Be able to explain the contribution of occupational performance to successful transitions to service users and providers.

Being a family member with a learning disability

Parents in the developed world expect that their children will grow and thrive and outlive them; this is due mainly to public health measures, which include health education, management of water supplies and immunization of young babies, that may not be available in other countries. Medical science has improved the viability of preterm delivery babies, which is also leading to an increase in children with multiple disabilities; understandably parents may often strive to keep alive a child that requires intensive medical support. Some of these babies will have difficulties because of their early experiences and the medical interventions necessary to keep them alive and this will continue to influence their development.

When parents are told that their child has a learning disability many of them will need to grieve the loss of a 'normal' baby. They will also have to communicate this news to family and friends and this may be influenced by the way that the news is given to them by the professionals they meet at this time. This first interaction with the professionals in these services may influence subsequent relationships, especially if it increases the trauma and loss already being experienced (Grant 2005, Bloom 2005). How parents see the future of their child will have significance for the whole family as that child grows up. Koontz-Lowman (2005) suggests that considering the key components of a family systems model will put the young person into context. Components of the model consist of the family structure, the family functions and family interactions, and this should be set in the context of the family life cycle. Use of this structure will enable the occupational therapist to understand how their family perceives the person with a learning disability and whether they consider them able to assume adult status. At some stage a young person who has a mild learning disability can become aware of the fact that they are different and perhaps not the child that their parents wanted. If they have siblings, as they all reach teenage years the differences in expectations and opportunities will be more apparent (Koontz-Lowman 2005). Difficulties can arise as they become viewed by adult services as 'service users'; this provides a different route to becoming an adult than that available to their siblings and they will want to understand their options. It is important that the opportunity to be able to articulate this is appreciated (Flynn & Russell 2005). Differences in culture and ethnicity will also affect the view that society has of them and the way they view themselves (Mir & Raghaven 2005, Pawson et al 2005).

While some people with a mild learning disability will become independent, people with profound and multiple disabilities will be dependent on either their parents or carers for all of their lives. Smyth & McConkey (2003) found that people who had been identified by the educational system as having severe learning disability were still able to identify what they would like the transition to adulthood to include. As can be seen in Figure 9.1, while the person with a learning disability will be asked what their needs are the family will also have an influence and even more of an influence will be the resources available.

Service expectations rather than service requirements are set out in a range of transition guideline documents with a clear pathway to adult services. Smyth & Bell (2006) express concerns about the choices offered to people with a learning disability and the ability of the services supporting them to assist them with these choices. Their discussion explores the difficulty of promoting choice with regard to a balanced diet and the need to eat healthy food to prevent obesity. The implications of their paper have a wider perspective as choice and cognitive ability and occupational performance may not always result in a healthy lifestyle.

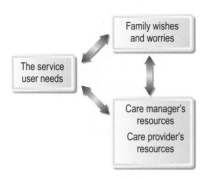

Figure 9.1 • Choice versus resources.

The contribution of attachment to developing occupation

An understanding of the influence of attachment theory on people with learning disabilities is important for the occupational therapist if they are working with someone who is having difficulties in managing to cope with a transition. Bowlby (1990), in a collection of earlier work, suggests that a child or adolescent needs a secure base provided by both parents, which means that they will be available to support them and provide comfort and reassurance when they are troubled or afraid. Difficulties in forming a secure attachment will alter the relationship that a child forms with its parents or significant others and will subsequently influence future relationships. Byng-Hall (1995) has more recently formed the opinion that attachment behaviour does not relate to the entire parenting relationship but the aspect of the relationship that is important in times of stress. As part of development a child gradually learns to manage away from the individuals who give support and the primary attachment made with the parent or caregiver, as they have learnt that they will be available if they feel threatened. If this pattern is threatened then developing any further occupational skills may be disrupted as the individual struggles to put the physical and social environment into context.

For most people growing up and leaving home is part of a process that they and their parents have been expecting as part of growing up and signifies a level of functional independence and maturity. Recent research on attachment theory suggests that the way that people develop relationships can be a reflection of their early attachment experiences (Feeney 2000, Dallos 2006). This research explores the importance of communication to attachments and identifies the difficulties that can arise when a child fails to form a secure attachment with their parents. People with a learning disability who have additional behavioural needs may have learnt to be fearful of close relationships or be unable to communicate their need for a relationship in a culturally appropriate way. For people with a mild learning disability, listening to the narrative by inviting them to talk about the people they are close to can enlighten the team working with them. These ideas are relevant to occupational therapists as they also focus on the narrative experiences of their clients' lives; this helps them to interpret the way that the client views the importance of significant occupations. When growing up, people with learning disability have a range of additional communication difficulties that can affect their ability to interpret the meaning and importance of both child and adult attachments. A significant number of service users will have been separated from their parents at a younger age and this applies to many older people who were separated from their families at an early age. Stuart (2002) recorded the experiences of a group of services users who had had this experience so that their stories would remain to illustrate the occupational disruption of their lives.

To explore the impact of the process of transitions, complete the following reader activity and spend some time reflecting on the transitions you have already experienced, negotiated and overcome. Refer also to Table 9.1, which although does not cover all, does list some of the transitions that most individuals may experience during their lifetime.

Reader activity

- How many of the transitions listed in the table have you already experienced?
- How many have been experienced by people close to you?
- Reflect on your experience of these transitions; who gave you the support you needed?

These transitions have resulted in you adapting to changes as you absorbed them within your occupational form. At a new school you had to learn how to cope both in a new physical environment and with new relationships. On entering higher education

Table 9.1 Transitions during the lifespan

Childhood and adolescence	Adulthood	Older adult
Nursery school	Leaving home	Retirement loss of employee status
Primary school	First job and career	Becoming a grandparent
Secondary school	Meeting a partner	Voluntary worker
Gap year	Buying a home	Moving home
Further or higher education	Moving home	Moving into residential or nursing care
First boy/ girlfriend	Death of significant others	Death of significant others

you may have started to form new significant adult attachments. Now take a moment to reflect on how many of these transitions are available to a person with learning disability. Some people with a learning disability will not transfer from primary to secondary education in any meaningful way if they remain at the same school. They may also have limited opportunity for paid employment, choice of accommodation and leisure activities.

Leaving school: transferring occupational performance

Clear guidance is given in Valuing People (DoH 2001) Chapter 3, on how services need to develop. As an occupational therapist working in adult services you will need to understand the transition process used by service providers and regional differences and how this fits into the statutory framework. Tarleton & Ward (2005) completed a study at the Norah Fry Research Centre, that examined what young people and those associated with them needed when they were due to leave school. Using focus groups, they found that people wanted to know who was involved and what funding was available. They also wanted detailed information on the local processes and how they viewed the family member in the context of adult rights and responsibilities.

All children who have been identified as having special educational needs (SEN) have a clearly defined transitions process and it is the responsibility of the head teacher to initiate the transition plan, which should be written when the student is in year 9 (SW Regional Partnership). They will also need to involve others in this process, including the local Connexions Personal Advisor and professionals from other appropriate agencies. At the end of this chapter you will find some links to useful resources that are currently available on the internet, which will help you with further reading.

It is important to note that people with a learning disability are only a proportion of the people identified as having special educational needs who leave school in any year and there will only be limited resources available. In the report produced by the Select Committee on Education and Skills (Third Report, 2006) it is noted that the proportion of children in segregated education has decreased to 1% in the context of 18% of children with SEN, of which 3% are children with statements. They also express concern that the current framework still has not moved significantly from the one introduced in the 1981 Education Act, which follows the Warnock Framework. The SEN and Disability Act (SENDA) of 2001 and the SEN Strategy Removing Barriers to Achievement (2004), while seeking to improve services, still use the dated framework (UK Parliament 2006).

As the majority of children with learning disability now live at home they have experience of their siblings growing up and leaving home. The relationship established with the specialist team and the contribution they can make to the needs identified by the young person and their family will be crucial at this point. If there is an occupational therapist involved with the child they may contact the specialist team at this point to discuss the transfer of therapist involvement. The needs of the children who still attend specialist boarding schools will vary as they will involve moving from a known environment and the ability to transfer or acquire a range of occupations and relate them to the new setting. George is going to have to manage this type of transition when he leaves his boarding school and moves back to his hometown. Read about George in Box 9.1 and answer the questions in the following reader activity. Some of the issues surrounding his transition are then discussed in the context of his transition and assessment in his new setting.

Box 9.1

Case illustration: George

George is 19 and because of the complexity of his special educational needs he has been at a segregated boarding school since he was 11. He has a mild learning disability and cerebral palsy and in addition is registered as partially sighted. While George has been happy at his school he now wants to return to his hometown. Using his transition plan he has identified that instead of living with his parents he wants to live independently and attend a horticultural course at his local college and he has already been offered a place. For the past year he has been adding to his knowledge and skills at school by living in a flat with two other students. His parents are expressing concern as George has never lived alone and yet he is adamant that he can do this.

The report from the occupational therapist at the school is detailed and it is clear that George is not yet managing his own budget and frequently asks other students for food at the end of the week. As part of his time in school he has learnt techniques which enable him to be independently mobile from school into his local community. During school holidays he has been able to practise applying these techniques at home. He has also learnt to use the bus services at home when on holiday and has been accepted on the course. George is friendly and outgoing and has made friends at school so he is expressing concern that he has no close friends at home. While he has no problem communicating his needs he finds complex instructions difficult to follow. He has difficulty with shopping unless he knows the layout of the shop and avoids large supermarkets because they 'change everything'. He has enough insight to recognize money, he has limited abilities when he needs to pay or check his change.

Reader activity

Focus on the fact that George is 19 rather than his mild learning disability and other physical difficulties and think about the following questions:

- Does every young person who leaves home to live independently know how to manage his or her money?
- What are the barriers to George leaving home?
- List the skills that are essential for George to manage independently.
- List the skills that he can acquire as he goes along.

Depending on your ability to manage your own money, the first question has made you think about how difficult coping with a limited budget can be. With the changes in the cost of higher education in the UK increasing numbers of students remain living at home and are relying on their parents for financial support. One of the barriers to George leaving home is the limited choices that may be available to him. Harris (2003) suggests that the way choice is interpreted for people with a learning disability has its limitations. For instance, although George has indicated his preference there are many factors that affect his occupational form and these may mean that he has no choice and has to return to live with his parents (Tarleton & Ward 2005). George has a Connexions Advisor allocated to support him during his transition but his special educational needs may not be given a high priority as he has managed to identify an appropriate vocational education course. He will not get a high priority on the housing list unless his local housing association specifically caters for school leavers. Cost of accommodation in the private sector may present another barrier to him developing his independence. He may have no choice and will have to return home to live with his parents and this will be a disappointment to him.

From an occupational therapy perspective, the Model of Human Occupation Screening Tool (MOHOST) is a useful assessment when gathering information from and about a person with a learning disability. If there is an occupational therapist at George's school they will be able to pass on their assessment but this will relate to his occupational performance in the familiar environment of his current community (Forsyth & Kielhofner 2006). By using the MOHOST and working with George, his parents and the FE College, the occupational therapist can support George to transfer his existing skills and learn the new ones needed.

The next section of this chapter uses the MOHOST framework to present the information available systematically. While this information does not allocate a numerical rating, it serves to highlight the areas where he will have difficulty. This will help the occupational therapist to work with him to produce a person-centred intervention. The MOHOST frame-work can be used again if further assessment is needed once George has returned home and has started college.

Motivation for occupation

- Appraisal of ability

George rates himself as very motivated but the indications from school are that he cannot plan how to manage his budget so that his food lasts the week. So far he has declined support in this area, preferring to scrounge from others in the flat. You may have decided that not being able to manage your money is within the normal range for a young man of his age.

- Expectations of success/interest/commitment

George is clearly optimistic as he has already identified a career choice and obtained a place on a suitable course. He is very committed to continuing with the vocational aspects of his education. He also wants to be nearer his parents as they have a good relationship and he wants to make new friends.

Pattern of occupation

- Routine and adaptability.

This will be a challenging area for George as he is well adapted to his current social and physical environment apart from annoying the other people in the flat when he runs out of food. How he adapts to new roles and routines will make a significant difference to this transition especially as he can have trouble being on time.

- Responsibility and roles.

There are going to be challenges for George and one of his parents' worries is that he is not yet ready to take on the responsibility of running his own home. George is also having to come to terms with the idea that he will need to budget to rent a flat in the private sector and the local Housing Agency does not provide homes for young single men. He may therefore have to move back home, which will impact on his view of the adult independent role. He will also have to discover what the role of student in an FE horticulture course will require.

Communication and interaction skills

George has some difficulty in articulation but because he has been to a specialist school he has learnt techniques with the help of a speech and language therapist. He can communicate effectively but has difficulty with complex questions or instructions. One of his problems is that like some other young people he needs to ensure that his non-verbal interactions are appropriate when he is bored or frustrated.

Process skills

Feedback from school indicates that George can apply his knowledge in that setting although he can sometimes have difficulty transferring the skill. For example, while he can use the cooker at school he has difficulty with the one at home. He also needs to learn each new bus route but it is difficult to establish if this is to do with his eyesight or his learning disability. Once into his routine he can plan ahead and with support he can work out ways of solving problems.

Motor skills

George does have some problems with his balance and mobility. Because of his physical problems, he uses a white stick outside and avoids uneven ground and long flights of stairs and escalators. He can manage in a lift once he has used it a few times with support and can manipulate the majority of objects. One of his concerns for his course is how he will handle delicate plants and his parents have already helped him find pruning shears that he can use. George also needs to learn to pace himself otherwise he can become very tired at the end of an active day.

Environment

George will initially be returning home to live although he is still planning to move out as soon as possible. This will affect his social life and while his parents live close to the bus route the service ends in the early evening. His family are keen to offer him support but he will need assistance in identifying a range of leisure activities. As the course will require physical activity this will need a review to ensure he has all the resources required. There will also be a lot of walking at the college between teaching rooms and the student canteen.

George will need support in adjusting his occupational demands to his new lifestyle and it is important that he is encouraged to work at a balanced healthy lifestyle. As he will be living with his parents he will not have difficulties with food preparation and other daily living tasks while he settles into the college routine.

Having accepted that he will have to return home in the short term George, with the support of his parents, can maintain and improve his self-care and homemaker productivity skills and learn how to manage a budget. He has the security of knowing that he will have meals available and can concentrate all his energy on managing the new college environment. Meininger (2006) suggests that life story work can be an aid to self-advocacy and with an occupational therapist's support George can gather the evidence to demonstrate his ability to improve his occupational performance and his level of independence. This narrative will enable him to reflect on his achievement and can be goal orientated and structured to ensure a person-centred approach that includes his health needs and social needs. George will also have the opportunity to establish new friendships within his peer group, which will provide additional support for him settling into a new course and when he eventually leaves home (McVilley et al 2006, Moore 2005).

Leaving home

The second half of this chapter will focus on a different group of people in transition. These are people with a learning disability who have remained at home within their family unit until the time comes for them to leave home. Often people leave home because they want to see themselves as independent of the family structure or their family are no longer able to provide support for them. Increasingly, leaving home is a challenge for all adult children, who are faced with economic realities as the cost of buying or renting housing increases throughout the UK. As mentioned earlier in the chapter, the majority of people with learning disability now grow up at home and may continue to live there into middle age. People with a learning disability are subject to an additional range of economic pressures, as they are not always viewed as productive members of society. As you have seen with George, aspirations for living independently can be limited by social policy and availability of social housing provision in the postcode area.

Thomson & Pickering (2001) identify the importance of understanding the process that underlies an individual's approach to transition. They suggest that this is a process that can be understood by using a model with the following sequential stages. They also acknowledge that someone may not be aware that a transition is beginning or how complicated it will be until they start to reflect on their confusion:

- beginning
- confusion
- reflection
- engagement
- action planning
- resolution.

It is important to remember that while this approach may be useful in interpreting the stage of the transition, the service user is experiencing in a period of change. As with all life changes it can be difficult to define and communicate clearly to a service user who has limited communication skills. People with a learning disability have limited opportunities for social interaction and can find it difficult to meet a new girl or boyfriend. They also may need support to understand the concept of the responsibilities that come with a relationship. Due to this lack of opportunity and limited social networks, and can find it difficult to meet a potential partner. In Box 9.2 Sally and Paul have reached a stage in their lives where they want to set up home together and are looking for help and advice on how to do this.

Reader activity

Sally and Paul (in Box 9.2) come to the specialist team asking for help with finding somewhere to live together and it quickly becomes apparent to the social worker that this is a complex transition.

- Which members of the team do you think will need to be involved?
- What are the key points that will need attention?
- Sally and Paul are offered a support worker when they move into their flat. How can an occupational therapist work with them all to assist in the development of the necessary knowledge and skills to manage independently?

Sally and Paul's parents were worried at this new development and this is adding to the confusion about the change. Asking them to support the change by contributing to their son and daughter's role development helped to reassure them. Assessing and identifying the essential skills and identifying how the learning can be supported means that

Box 9.2

Case illustration: Sally and Paul

Sally (30 years) has Down's syndrome and she met Paul (33 years) who has Fragile X syndrome 3 years ago when she went to the local social group disco. Both Sally and Paul still live at home with their parents although Paul's mother is divorced. They live in a large town and are able to manage transport and they have a wide range of different opportunities available during the daytime. Sally and Paul have never looked after themselves. They are able to make a hot drink and a snack but have only ever had 'pocket money', with their parents managing their allowances. Recently, Sally and Paul have surprised their parents as they announced that they want to get married. They want to have a flat and live together although they have no clear idea how they can achieve this. Paul is upset and annoyed with his mother who refuses to discuss them getting married, while Sally's parents are prepared to see what can be done to help the couple.

considerable preparation can be achieved before they both leave home.

While they both have personal self-care skills, they need to work out how to manage their home and their budget. Negotiation to release their allowances so that they can learn to manage them can be a difficult issue to discuss with parents who have been using the income. Sally and Paul had the support of an occupational therapy assistant to assist them to adapt to managing together as a team. The occupational performance skills that they needed to learn included basic skills such as preparing simple meals, using a washing machine and cleaning the home. Sally was already more independent as her parents had encouraged her to look after her own bedroom and cook simple snacks, so she was able to teach Paul.

One of the important factors that emerged from the assessment was the significance of the differing occupational performance levels for a specific task between the couple. For example, Sally was happy to cook the supper while Paul discovered that he was good at ironing, something that Sally hated. This meant that the intervention was planned with Sally and Paul to build on their existing strengths.

While life changes do not necessarily cause confusion, this change was complex and needed time for reflection and planning because of the number of people involved in the network that surrounded the couple. Good communication was essential and also for the team to acknowledge Sally and Paul's right to decide what to do with their lives. It was also important to involve the parents so that they continued to offer support rather than expecting failure. Sally and Paul were further supported by the network with assistance to apply to the Housing Association and support from the specialist nurse to explore all the health issues, including family planning services.

For individuals with profound and multiple disabilities the situation post Valuing People (DoH 2001) will either depend on their parents or, when they move into residential care, the skills of the paid carers. The right to be seen as part of society can become an issue when they move into residential care and is dependent on the skills of the paid carers (Gilbert et al 2005). A lack of communication skills and difficulties in interpreting non-verbal communication will increase the difficulties in identifying the emotional implications for the client during a transitional period (Arthur 2003). Difficulties can arise because they are adults, but they may be used to a close and loving child–parent relationship, which will not be appropriate with paid carers (Hewitt & Nind 1994,1998). The framework proposed by Thomson & Pickering (2001) will still work in supporting the family during transition; however, you need to remember that reflection, engagement and action planning are all areas that not only require a level of cognitive functioning, they also require available choices. If an individual with profound and multiple disability does not have a choice because of overlying socio-economic factors, for example limited choice of homes offering the level of care they require, then this part of the process will have little meaning for them. People with profound and multiple disabilities will need additional support to be able to understand and communicate their wishes and often family or support workers will reach the transition decisions for them. Sheehy & Nind (2005) discuss the importance of 'becoming a person' and identifying meaningful occupations for someone with profound and multiple disabilities is a challenge for an occupational therapist. Even something as simple as changing individual clothing to something more colourful and age appropriate can cause distress to parents and confusion to the support worker who thought it a 'good idea'. Spending time interacting with the individual is one way to establish what these occupations are by offering different opportunities for engagement and noting their response. Sheehy & Nind (2005 p. 37) also highlight the importance of being seen as a person with emotional needs and suggest that the key issues might include:

- What kinds of environments help people's emotional well-being?
- What kinds of environments are bad for people's emotional well-being?
- How can we know when a young person with multiple learning disabilities has mental health difficulties?
- How can the people who know the person well act as a kind of 'interpreter' for mental health professionals?

Often mental health issues are not identified for people with learning disability and this can be significant issue during the transitional process for people with multiple disabilities who lack the ability to communicate their distress. Emily (Box 9.3) is now faced with a move that will mean a major change in her life. Read about her life so far and complete the reader activity.

Reader activity

- How can the occupational therapist identify the important factors in Emily's occupational form that need to be replicated in her new home?
- Emily is very dependent on her mother for all her care needs so what can the occupational therapist do to ensure that these needs are communicated effectively to the new carers?
- What emotional implications may arise for Emily and her parents?

The issues for Emily cover two main overlapping areas that will both influence how happy she is in her new home. They are important as well for her mother who will have to cope with her role loss as main carer for Emily. If she sees that her daughter is unhappy and perhaps losing weight she may, as other parents have, want to take Emily back to live at home again.

Box 9.3

Case illustration: Emily

Emily (40years) has profound and multiple learning disability including epilepsy and has remained at home with her parents. Her mother has recently been ill and her father is due to retire from work and he decided that the time has come for Emily to leave home. Her mother has reluctantly agreed to this. Although Emily and her parents have used respite care services for several years this will be a major transition for both her and her mother and loss will be part of the change. The specialist team occupational therapist knows Emily well as she was involved in the provision of equipment, working with the social services adult team and sensory input, working with the speech and language therapist to ensure that she has some leisure activities for home. Emily is hoisted for all transfers and her parents' bungalow has been adapted to meet her needs so she can transfer from her bedroom to bathroom.

Emily needs 24-hour support and assistance with all self-care routines including having her food pureed and being fed. She relies on a specialist wheelchair for her seating and has a specialist easy chair for when she wants to relax. While she has no verbal communication skills she has developed effective non-verbal skills and is very successful at communicating distress or annoyance. Her bedroom at home has been fitted out with sensory devices that she uses when she wants to relax and spend time alone.

The physical environment

The environment will need to meet Emily's needs and if possible mirror the physical home environment; as she is leaving home for good her sensory equipment can move with her. The space in the home environment needs to give staff space to move equipment easily as this will ensure that they use it appropriately. Limited space means that staff will not always use the correct equipment, leading to increased risks for all concerned. Transport can also be a major issue for people with the level of physical need experienced by Emily, which will restrict her opportunities for leisure. Emily's mother will still be able to transport her to her weekly swimming session if a home is found near her parents. Long-term, the home will need to provide transport as an essential need for Emily if she is not to be confined to her home.

Communication and the emotional environment

Emily needs to be able to communicate with her new carers and time spent working with both her and her mother will help the new keyworker understand their communication system. If this is not possible then encouraging her mother to list the subtleties that indicate her preferences will be useful. Staff should be encouraged to maintain the routines that underpin Emily's day. Support staff can be keen to promote what they see as more choice and independence and there may well be a time for this when Emily is settled into her new home.

Forming relationships

People with learning disability are potentially more vulnerable than the rest of the population when forming adult relationships. This can mean that people with a learning disability are perceived at greater risk. Those supporting them are understandably risk averse when faced with some situations. It is important to remember that all adult relationships have the potential for abuse, otherwise women's refuges would not exist. Abusive relationships do not necessarily correlate with cognitive function. The occupational therapist as a member of the specialist team must be aware of the potential for these situations and understand service guidelines if a service user confides in them. The nurse working as part

of the specialist team will be able to give advice to service users to help them understand the risks of engaging in sexual activity. Occupational therapists also work with other members of the specialist team using individual sessions of group work to allow people with a learning disability to explore the potential of adult relationships. While this is not usually an area of expertise for a newly qualified occupational therapist, ensuring that any problems mentioned by service users are dealt with in an appropriate way is important.

Summary

This chapter has looked at the significance of the transition from childhood to adulthood for people with a learning disability. It has highlighted the importance of attachment theory and how this can influence the process of transition. It then identified how occupational therapists have a significant role in working with people with a learning disability who are making transitions at this time and wish to leave home or set up home together. One of the difficulties with this transition is the development of new roles and for a couple, how to share the tasks that need performing. Assessment and planning the occupational performances required within a client-centred frame of reference can achieve this. When working with people who have profound and multiple disabilities occupational therapists can contribute to ensuring the physical environment meets the needs of the individual. By carefully mapping the service user's preferences they can also minimize distress when the main carer changes.

Further reading

Forsyth K, Kielhofner G 2006 The model of human occupation: integrating theory into practice and practice into theory. In: Duncan E (ed.) Foundations for practice in occupational therapy. Edinburgh, Elsevier

Thompson J, Pickering S 2001 Life transitions and personal change. In: Thompson J, Pickering S (eds) Meeting the health needs of people who have a learning disability. Edinburgh, Bailliére Tindall

Useful resources

The Connexions site has useful information on disability – Connexions-direct: information and advice for young people – click on disability section: http://www.connexions-direct.com (accessed 14 March 2008)

The Valuing People support team has produced a useful site with a wide range of resources you can download: http://valuingpeople.gov.uk/index.jsp they have a produced the Transitions Champions pack at http://valuingpeople.gov.uk/dynamic/valuingpeople103.jsp (accessed 5 March 2008)

Department of Constitutional Affairs has produced a document titled: Making Decisions: helping people who need support to make decisions for themselves. This can be found at http://www.dca.gov.uk/legal-policy/mental-capacity/guidance.htm (accessed 5 March 2008)

References

Arthur A 2003 The emotional lives of people with a learning disability. British Journal of Learning Disabilities 31:25–30

Bloom J 2005 Breaking bad news. In: Grant G, Goward P, Richardson M et al (eds) Learning disability: a life cycle approach to valuing people. Maidenhead, Open University Press

Bowlby J 1990 A secure base: parent child attachment and healthy human development. New York, Basic books

Byng-Hall J 1995 Creating a secure family base: some implications for attachment theory for family therapy. Family Process 34(91):45–58

Dallos R 2006 Attachment theory therapy: integrating narrative, systemic and attachment therapies. Maidenhead, Open University Press

Department of Health 2001 Valuing People: a new strategy for learning disability for the 21st Century. London, HMSO

Feeney JL 2000 Implications of attachment style for patterns of health and illness. Child Care, Health and Development 26(4):277–288

Flynn M, Russell P 2005 Adolescents and younger adults: narrative accounts. In: Grant G, Goward P, Richardson M et al (eds) Learning disability a life cycle approach to valuing people. Maidenhead, Open University Press, pp 289–305

Forsyth K, Kielhofner G 2006 The model of human occupation: integrating theory into practice and practice into theory. In: Duncan E (ed.) Foundations for practice in occupational therapy. Edinburgh, Elsevier

Gilbert T, Cochrane A, Greenwell S 2005 Citizenship: locating people with learning disabilities. International Journal of Social Welfare 14:287–296

Grant G 2005 Experiences of family care. In: Grant G, Goward P, Richardson M et al (eds) Learning disability a life cycle approach to valuing people. Maidenhead, Open University Press

Harris J 2003 Time to make up your mind: why choosing is difficult. British Journal of Learning Disabilities 31:3–8

Hewitt D, Nind M 1994 Access to communication. London, David Fulton

Hewitt D, Nind M 1998 Interaction in action: reflections on the use of intensive interaction. London, David Fulton

Koonz-Lowman D 2005 Family and disability issues through infancy. In: Cronin A, Mandich M (eds) Human development and performance throughout the lifespan. New York, Thomson

McVilley K, Stancliffe R, Parmenter T et al 2006 'I get by with a little help from my friends'; adults with intellectual disability discuss loneliness. Journal of Applied Research in Intellectual Disabilities 19:191–203

Meininger H 2006 Narrating, writing, reading: life story work: life story work as an aid to (self) advocacy. British Journal of Learning Disabilities 34(3):181–188

Mir G, Raghavan R 2005 Culture and ethnicity: developing accessible and appropriate services for health and social care. In: Grant G, Goward P, Richardson M et al (eds) Learning disability a life cycle approach to valuing people. Maidenhead, Open University Press

Moore T 2005 Friendship formation in adults with learning disabilities: peer mediated approaches to social skills development. British Journal of Learning Disabilities 33:23–26

Pawson N, Raghavan R, Small N 2005 Social inclusion, social networks and ethnicity: the development of the social inclusion interview schedule for young people with learning disabilities. British Journal of Learning Disabilities 33:15–22

Sheehy K, Nind M 2005 Emotional well being for all: mental health and people with profound and multiple learning disabilities. British Journal of Learning Disabilities 33:34–38

Smyth C, Bell D 2006 From biscuits to boyfriends: the ramifications of choice for people with learning disabilities. Journal compilation @ 2006 Blackwell Publishing Ltd. 34:227–236

Smyth M, McConkey R 2003 Future aspirations of students with severe learning disabilities and of their parents on leaving special schooling. British Journal of Learning Disabilities 31:54–59

Stuart M 2002 Not quite sisters: women with learning difficulties living in convent homes. Kidderminster, British Institute of Learning Disability

Tarleton B, Ward L 2005 Changes and choices: finding out what information young people with learning disabilities, their parents and supporters need at transition. British Journal of Learning Disabilities 33:70–76

The United Kingdom Parliament 2006 Select Committee on Education and Skills (Third report) House of Commons, London

Thomson J, Pickering S (eds) 2001 Meeting the health needs of people who have a learning disability. Edinburgh, Bailliére Tindall

Working with parents with learning disabilities

Christine Locke

Overview

Parenting is a contentious role and one where there are many experienced, but few skilled experts. At some point during a child's upbringing, the parents will experience a sense of failure. Consider the challenge of getting a child to bed when they do not want to sleep, or a child refusing to eat anything except chips and baked beans. Children are adventurous and prone to accidents such as falling off the swing and injuring themselves the minute the parent's back is turned. This is normal parenting and, ultimately, the parental role is one of responsibility of care. Embedded in parenting skills is the complexity of the need to recognize both a child's emotional and developmental requirements in a safe and engendering manner. However, for parents who have learning disabilities, the natural consequence of failure to parent adequately is involvement of both the legal process and of statutory agencies for parenting assessment (Booth et al 2006). For occupational therapists, psychologists, social workers, community nurses and health visitors working within a multidisciplinary context it is important

to be aware of the factors and issues surrounding the needs of both the child and the parent(s) with learning disabilities.

It is likely that the occupational therapist working within the learning disability field either in a community learning disabilities team or as specialist occupational therapist may receive a referral involving a parent with a learning disability. The actual number of parents with a learning disability is unknown although there is an indication of an increase in the number of parents referred for assessment, placing a challenge on service provision (Booth et al 2006, Woodhouse et al 2001, Guinea 2001). Whilst not taking any definitive perspective on all parenting models it is hoped that this chapter will enable you to reflect on both your knowledge and understanding of the current and future trends for supporting parents with a learning disability. The focus of this chapter is therefore to discuss what the role of occupational therapy is in this emotive and challenging area.

The chapter will first outline the complex issues of child safety and implications for services within the assessment and legislative context. Case scenarios are used to illustrate perceived needs and abilities of parents and to identify the impact of the environmental demands on parenting and families. The occupational therapy assessments and interventions of parental skill ability will be discussed in the context of multidisciplinary and multi-agency working.

Learning Outcomes

By the end of this chapter you will be able to:

- Explore the complex issues of child safety and assessment of parents with a learning disability
- Identify the legislative implication of services for parents with a learning disability
- Discuss the factors which can impact on parents with a learning disability
- Identify the role of the occupational therapist in a multidisciplinary context.

What are the issues?

We need to acknowledge that the majority of parents with learning disabilities are referred to the statutory agencies for issues of child protection when they are in crisis. Very often, statutory processes and the complexity of the legal framework increase parental difficulties to advocate for themselves. The legislative framework, whilst recognizing the rights of choice and empowerment of the individual with a learning disability, has a legal obligation to ensure child safety (McGaw 1997). From the point of view of local authority and health practitioners the issues of inadequate parenting and risk of abuse to the child are paramount. Risks are those attributes of the parent(s) that incorporate lack of providing opportunity to learn, lack of knowledge of child development, poor understanding and support for emotional needs for the child to safely develop. The definition of assessment and criteria for referring a child in special circumstances are described by Framework for the Assessment of Children in Need and their Families (Box 10.1, DoH 2001a). The knowledge and skills needed in child care involve not only substantial attributes of 'caring' but also cognitive processes in terms of attention, memory, working memory, abstract thinking, generalization, and problem solving. Lack of planning ability, problem solving and anticipation or awareness of safety factors can lead to inability to identify and generalize risk

Box 10.1

Assessment of children in special circumstances

Framework for the assessment of children in need and their families (DoH 2001a) Section.3.62

They are children whose problems or those of their parents are not sufficiently serious to receive services under social services priorities. These children's health or development may not be considered to be impaired but an analysis of the risk factors and stressors in their lives would suggest they are likely to suffer impairment in the future. What is required is recognition of the interaction of child and/or parental problems on a child's health and development and the cumulative effect of such problems over time. For example, a mother with a mild learning disability may not reach the criteria for help from an adult services team and her child's standard of care may not be sufficiently poor to meet the criteria for children's services intervention. However, the failure to recognize the need for early intervention to provide support to the child and family on a planned basis from both children's and adult's services may result in the child's current and future development being impaired. (p. 50)

factors for different contexts and environments. For example, poor reading and writing skills can influence everyday tasks such as management of budgeting, shopping for appropriate foods or dispensing medicine for a child. The lack of understanding of appropriate nutrition for a child can lead to a poor dietary intake affecting a child's development. The inability to set routine and boundaries to meet a child's developmental needs and behaviours can often result in unrealistic expectations of the child. Poor communication skills can be perceived as negative parental attributes and are often perceived as non-compliance by practitioners (Booth et al 2006, James 2004, Guinea 2001).

Research both nationally and internationally (Booth & Booth 1996, James 2004, McConnell et al 2003) indicates that parents with learning disabilities may demonstrate a failure of responsibility and adequate parenting skill, often resulting in the child being put at risk. Risk can be defined as 'neglect' or omissions of care that might produce harm and 'abuse' as actions that hurt children. Someone may abuse or neglect a child by inflicting harm or failing to act to prevent harm (National Assembly for Wales 2000), while harm is perceived as that which negates the normal development of a child. Risk to development can present in many ways; physically, psychologically and socially in those families who are unable to provide, for example, an adequate stable diet for normal and healthy physical growth or give punitive or inconsistent responses to meet the child's emotional and psychological needs. Guinea (2001) describes factors that contribute to risk as poverty, debt, housing problems and poor living conditions which 'overwhelm' the daily lives of the family. The precursors to a child being at risk or parents who injure their children are identified as more likely to be of lower social status, of low or average intelligence, to have children at a younger age and to have large families (McGaw 2000). Other factors include:

- parents with a premature baby
- low income
- headed by a single teenage parent
- an adult or child who has a learning difficulty or disability
- mental health status of the parent
- poor parenting history.

Inadequate parenting skills can present in those individuals who have spent a considerable part of their own childhood within a large institution or in circumstances where they have not experienced positive parenting or had contact with a good parent role model. Literature on parenting skills of adolescent mothers reveals a number of similarities to the antecedents of poor parenting skills of mothers with learning disabilities (Coren & Barlow 2001). For example, ex-care mothers showed less sensitivity in handling or playing with their children and were more prone to irritable and aggressive responses in disciplining. Parental neglect or abuse appears to result when any one or more of the following individual attributes are in evidence:

- low self esteem
- self-fulfilling prophecy of failure
- lack of knowledge of developmental stages and needs of the child
- stress.

Other factors common to both sets of parents include poor mental and physical health, overcrowding

or inadequate housing, marital discord and insufficient support. The capabilities of parents will vary greatly in terms of general life skills as well as parenting skills. Examples of the types of issue that can arise are presented below in Box 10.2, Case illustration: Kate, where monitoring by the health visitor has identified risk of the child's developmental needs not being met resulting in developmental delay. The issue of the type of support needed and the importance of effective information will be touched on later in relation to Kate.

Legislative implication of services for parents with learning disabilities

The Disability Discrimination Act (DDA) (1995) defines a disabled person as someone who has a physical

Box 10.2

Case illustration: Kate, 'issues of harm'

Kate is the single mother of a daughter of 18 months referred by the Child and Family Team (CFT) to assess her parenting skills in response to a child protection order, to be reviewed in 3 months. The health visitor identified that the child had not achieved the milestones in both physical and psychological parameters. Working jointly with the psychologist, the occupational therapy assessment included self-care, routines, play and accessing shops and public transport. Although able to carry out basic care for her child including feeding, washing and dressing, the areas of risk included difficulty in planning (e.g. inability to dress her child in warm clothing when going out on a cold day), difficulty in maintaining established routines including sleep and play. She had little knowledge of child development and her expectation of her child's abilities was unrealistic of an 18-month-old child. A weekly programme was agreed with Kate including individual sessions on child play, nutrition and shopping. A support worker was to continue the sessions. However, through the court proceedings the child was taken into care at the end of the assessment period and subsequently put forward for adoption. Members of the Community Learning Disabilities Team (CLDT) gave support to Kate during the adoption process.

or mental impairment that has a substantial and long-term adverse effect on ability to carry out normal day-to-day activities. As defined by the DDA 1995 parents with learning disabilities are 'disabled' parents. Such parents are more likely to come within the jurisdiction of child protection systems as well as health and welfare statutory services (Booth & Booth 2000, Gender 1998). A number of organizations are involved in the assessment and intervention with parents with learning disabilities including primarily family and child teams, community learning disability teams and child and adolescent mental health teams. Others involved include health and education professionals, police, advocacy and voluntary agencies. The importance of inter-agency working and communication is crucial. All of these agencies are under the auspices and remit of child law, primarily the Children Act 1989. Box 10.3 lists some of the key legislation and policy documents for further reading and clarification. The Framework for Assessment of Children in Need and their Families (DoH 2001a) acknowledges the challenge of working towards success with families and children and highlights the need for collaborative working as follows:

Effective collaborative work between staff of different disciplines and agencies assessing children in need and their families requires a common language to understand the needs of children, shared values about what is in children's best interest and a joint commitment to improving the outcomes for children. (Page x.)

The Framework highlights the need for a more flexible approach to health and social support services as well as the development of empowerment and self-advocacy. It is required that professionals are familiar with legislation and policy documents, which formulate the legal and procedural requirements of child protection.

The complexity and legal demands of interagency and service organizations can and do undermine supporting parent(s) with a learning disability. There is indication that the dilemma between statutory child protection proceedings and the process of intervention can lead to these parents being disadvantaged and discriminated against. Perceptions of professionals of the limitations rather than abilities of the parent have been well documented recently. Booth & Booth (2000 p.3) identifies that often family and child care problems are singularly focus on the

limitations of the parents instead of environmental pressures or deficiencies in the support services. The initial contact with Kate at a case meeting identified different perceptions of the issues between Kate, the CFT and the CLDT. The differences in perceptions of issues between the parents, child and family teams and learning disability teams are illustrated in Box 10.4, as an example of how the process resulted in identifying and limiting an effective, holistic approach towards support for both Kate and her child. Ultimately, negative contact and outcome with service providers can result in a lack of

Box 10.3

Legislation and policies

Legislation

Children Act 1989

Child Protection 1995

Community Care (Direct Payments) Act 1996

Disability Discrimination Act 1995

Education Act 1996

Human Rights Act 1998

Health and Social Care Act 2001

National Health Service (NHS) and Community Care Act 1990

Key documents

Department of Health 2001a framework for the assessment of children in need and their families. London, HMSO.

Department of Health 1989 Children's Act. HMSO, London

Department of Health 2001b Valuing People: a new strategy for learning disability for the 21st century. HMSO, London

Department of Health 2001c National service framework for children, young people and maternity services. Published on 15 September 2004

Social Services Inspectorate 1999 Inspection of services to support disabled parents in their parenting role (e.g. Manchester, Bristol, Northampton, etc.)

Department of Health 2006 Working together to safeguard children. HMSO, London

Every Child Matters (2003) The every child matters: change for children programme

Box 10.4

Perceptions of issues for Kate: adapted from joint meeting with parent with a learning disability to highlight issues

Kate

- Has been in several foster homes during her childhood
- Has few experiences of child care to draw on
- Experiencing confusion of roles of mother/partner/worker
- Inflexible in her approach to child care
- Unrealistic expectations of child and child's ability
- Rented accommodation with shared kitchen and bathroom facilities causing tension with other tenants
- Conflict of advice given by friend and that given to her by social worker
- Found it difficult to judge what to do and who to ask for help
- Difficulty to assess who it is safe to babysit her child
- Feels depressed, lonely and powerless and wants to go back to work
- Knows people think she is unable to look after her child and thinks she is not able to as well (self-fulfilling prophecy)

Local authority Child and Family Team

- Approach and methods of assessments dictated by limited period of time (statutory time scale 35 days)
- No time to engage with Kate and establish relationship
- Lack of knowledge and experience of learning difficulty
- Lack of partnership approach with Kate/family/community support team and other agencies
- Commissioning for crisis intervention
- Assessment of problems but no provision for long-term intervention of practical support, training, preventative work
- Intention to remove child

Local authority Community Learning Disability Support Team (CLDT)

- Kate referred late to CLDT in child protection order
- Shared belief that the welfare of the child is of paramount consideration; however, unable to develop partnership working with Family Team
- Late assessment of Kate's abilities in legal process
- Deals with the emotional aspects for Kate during and after child protection order
- Recognition of need to establish/provide support networks

trust from parents and hesitancy to ask for assistance (Booth & Booth 2000). The processes of provision becomes crisis driven with tensions arising between the statutory role of professionals in child protection and an enabling role towards support for developing parenting skills (Harris 2000). There is a limitation on prevention and support to develop parenting skills including the safety and welfare of the child resulting in crisis intervention. Provision of support often results in increasing dependency behaviour and, as in Kate's situation, ultimately removal of the child rather than development of effective parenting skills. Partnership working is also limited between agencies due to lack of resources, often resulting in confusion about eligibility criteria and inadequate assessments for both child and parents.

Identifying the needs – assessment of risk

The importance of inter-agency planning has been advocated by McGaw (2000 p. 4) who advises that '"Assessments should be carried out by identifying who is best suited to assess the family," thus avoiding repetition, saving professional time and reducing wear and tear on the family'. However, in terms of parents with learning disabilities the evidence suggests that, as previously mentioned, both the process and focus of assessment and intervention are on lack of ability and inadequacies, rather than identifying strengths towards building appropriate skills (Booth & Booth 2005). Acknowledgement of the risk factors and having a 'clear understanding of the precise nature of these risks provides a good foundation for the assessment of specific risk in individual cases' (James 2004).

For occupational therapists and other members of the CLDT, inter-agency collaboration is essential, when gaining relevant information about a family before an initial assessment. It is necessary to consider and map the family's strengths and needs, which may not necessitate all members of the family being assessed (e.g. where one child or one parent is having difficulties a single assessment may be indicated). Equally, the assessments should ideally include the father or male member of the family. Both diagnostic and functional assessments to suit specific needs of the parent and family are required through joint working of the occupational therapist, psychologist, social workers, health visitors and community nurses.

A model to identify and assess the predictors of inadequate parenting skills for adults with learning disability was developed by McGaw & Sturmey (1994). The model recognizes the importance of assessing not only child care and developmental needs of the child within the home situation but also the parent's life skills, the family history, the support and resources surrounding the parents or parent. These four factors are applied to Kate in Figure 10.1. Using the model the occupational therapists can establish the areas of need for Kate and assess her abilities, including occupational areas of activities of daily living (ADL). A recent development of this model by McGaw is the Parent Multi-Dimensional Skills Model (McGaw 2006), which details the intellectual functioning and independent living skills of

Parent's life skills
Poor reading and writing skills
Poor memory and concentration on tasks
Aggressive in stress situations

Family history
Fostered from six years of age and separated from brother
No longer in contact with mother
Emotional and physical abuse in family home

Support and resources
Single mother
Isolated socially with no close friends
Keeps in contact with one of her foster parents by phone
Has boyfriends but abusive relationship
Poor financial management

Child care and development
Poor hygiene and safety awareness within flat
Child has lack of toys and play opportunity
Unrealistic expectations of 18-month-old child's ability
Poor routines for meals, sleep patterns
Poor diet

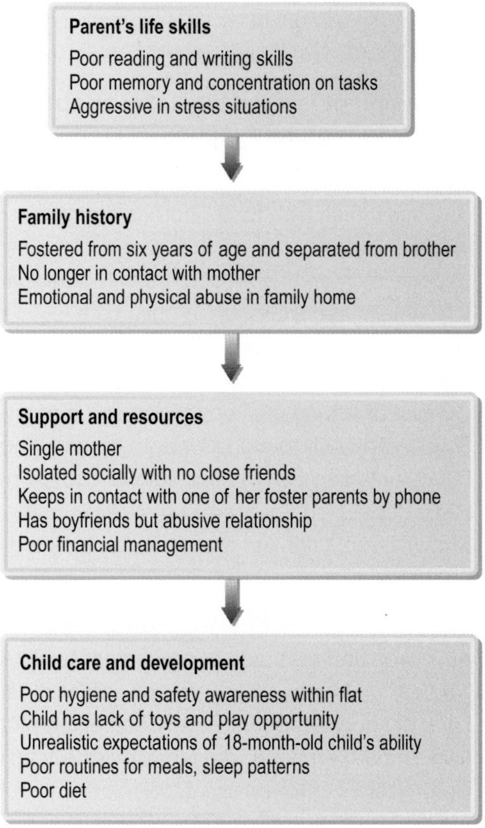

Figure 10.1 • Kate: Parenting skills model.
Adapted from McGaw & Sturmey (1994).

the parents in relation to support and resources such as employment, transport and housing. Any assessment also needs to consider those areas in which support can compensate for residual disability and recognition of 24-hour support by members of the extended family (McGaw 2000).

The occupational therapy role

The role of the occupational therapist may not initially be perceptible within a multidisciplinary context when first considering intervention with parents with a learning disability. Often, referrals received by the occupational therapist are for a joint assessment as part of a multidisciplinary team, in either a CLDT, social services team, or primary health care team. The occupational therapist has a specialist role and is well placed to be involved in a holistic approach to functional assessment. Utilizing a model of occupational practice such as Model of Human Occupation (MOHO) (Keilhofner 2002) or the Canadian Model of Occupational Performance (CAOT 1997) will help to ensure a client-centred, holistic approach for both child and parents. Using occupational therapy standardized and non-standardized assessments will more importantly highlight the abilities of the individual within the context of environmental factors, social stressors and the support available.

Assessment and planning

The mandatory process, in relation to child protection, dictates the planning, timing and frequency of the occupational therapy assessment. Within a child protection referral, all core assessments must be completed within 35 working days. The types of assessments, the planning and choice of interventions will depend on the specific situation and the need for collaborative assessments with other agencies and other professionals, such as health visitors, psychologist, social workers or community nurse. The assessments in Figure 10.2 illustrate the parenting assessment model by McGaw & Sturmey (1994) to assess skills and areas of support for Kate. Occupational therapists must also consider the important ethical issue of consent, which can be emotive and challenging. The referral for assessment must acknowledge consent unless mandatory by a court or child protection process. Informed consent is essential and information collected should be only that which is required for the intended task. For further clarification guidelines of professional practice refer to (COT 2003).

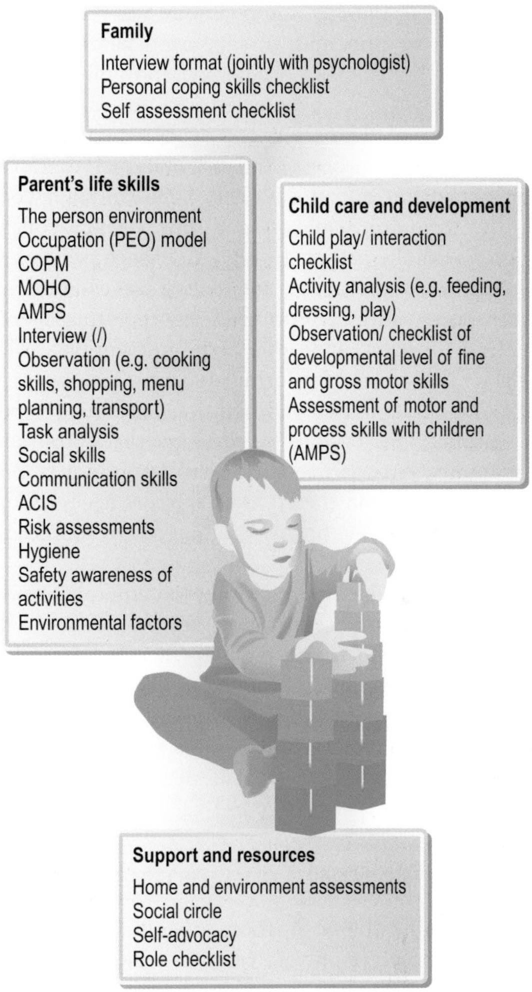

Intervention

Without experience, opportunity and choice as described by Wolfensberger (1972) people with learning disabilities are devalued and fail to learn. Applied to the parenting context this intimates that, if parenting skills are viewed as 'new skills', by questioning attitudes and providing opportunity of choice and environmental adaptations, change can be introduced to ensure better opportunity for learning and developing effective parenting skills. Booth & Booth (1996) have challenged the 'deficit model' of supporting parents and have proposed a more responsive and perceptive approach of service delivery. This is

Family
Interview format (jointly with psychologist)
Personal coping skills checklist
Self assessment checklist

Parent's life skills
The person environment
Occupation (PEO) model
COPM
MOHO
AMPS
Interview (/)
Observation (e.g. cooking skills, shopping, menu planning, transport)
Task analysis
Social skills
Communication skills
ACIS
Risk assessments
Hygiene
Safety awareness of activities
Environmental factors

Child care and development
Child play/ interaction checklist
Activity analysis (e.g. feeding, dressing, play)
Observation/ checklist of developmental level of fine and gross motor skills
Assessment of motor and process skills with children (AMPS)

Support and resources
Home and environment assessments
Social circle
Self-advocacy
Role checklist

Figure 10.2 • Occupational therapy functional assessments.
Adapted from McGaw & Sturmey (1994).

a supported parenting approach based on core principles of:

- respect for parents and the emotional context of family and child
- viewing parents as a resource not a problem
- valuing parents as people too
- support directed to the family context
- enabling parental control
- interventions based on building on strengths rather than weaknesses
- recognizing importance of the extended family, neighbourhoods and communities context
- viewing parents as active partners.

Occupational therapy interventions can contribute greatly to the principles of supported parenting and fall within the ethos of occupation and holistic practice. Whilst always acknowledging the importance of the issues of child safety and development through the assessment process, the occupational therapist can obtain critical information. This can then contribute to multidisciplinary and multi-agency collaboration with the parents to apply the above principles. Occupational therapists are skilled at establishing both short- and long-term goals incorporating client-centred, specific, individualized interventions. The intervention should be formulated on those positive behaviours, attributes and abilities combining types of learning and training centred on the home and community environments. It is also important to differentiate between the types of support needed during learning and the provision of ongoing resources to support the parents.

It is not possible in this chapter to comprehensively address all of the occupational therapy interventions for parents with a learning disability but the case of Jan Box 10.5 below, illustrates some of the specific areas of skill development and joint working. These include assessments and interventions that are based on home management, child care and skills development.

Skill development and joint working

A core skill of the occupational therapist is to identify and apply specific activities in a graded way to enable the individual to maintain or develop skills. It is, however, important not to apply generalized assumptions to each individual case as there are many risk variables that can be balanced against support from within the family and externally.

Using client-centred assessments to identify needs and strengths, the occupational therapist can use methods of intervention based on skills and experiential learning appropriate for a particular family. By grading interventions in relation to child care and safety, parenting skills and life skills of ADL, Jan can work towards optimizing learning to achieve her goals. Whilst establishing individual goals the occupational therapist will also acknowledge the ability of the parent or family to develop problem-solving skills. For Jan this included acquiring knowledge and applying it appropriately to the child's development and associated risk factors that will change as the

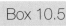

Box 10.5

Case illustration: Jan

Jan has a mild learning disability and recently moved back into the area following a split from her partner and father of her child, aged 3 years. She is 5 months pregnant and was referred to the CLDT, by the local CFT, following reported concerns about the 'neglected' appearance of her son. No notes or information had been received from the previous area but were being requested by the CFT. The case manager requested assessments from the CLDT psychologist and occupational therapist. Jan and her son lived in a first floor, council-owned one-bedroom flat. During the initial home visit, issues for Jan were discussed with the occupational therapist and she was also able to observe Jan's interaction with her son in a familiar and informal environment. The occupational therapist identified a number of risk areas including the stairs, the kitchen and bathroom in relation to her son's ability and behaviours. By establishing rapport, it was agreed to carry out further assessments on a second visit. These included a risk assessment, parenting skills assessment and the Occupational Self-Assessment (OSA) (Kielhofner 2002, pp. 179–189). These helped Jan identify her own abilities including basic literacy and numeracy skills, and her goals. The occupational therapist identified that Jan had insight into her situation and the reasons why she was finding it difficult to manage her son and a home since her partner had left her. She also had support from a close friend who lived a bus journey away. Jan's priority was to look after her 3-year-old who 'is a handful all the time'. She found it hard to get things done as 'he is always naughty'. She was fearful that once she had her baby both of her children would be taken away from her.

child grows. The intervention, therefore, facilitates opportunities for learning to achieve short- and long-term goals. The occupational therapist will also need to consider appropriate approaches to be used for the intervention (as outlined in Chapter 3). In this case the compensatory approach may be used to adapt Jan's environment and to underpin the educational or cognitive behavioural approaches used to develop parenting skills. It should also be reiterated that the occupational therapist will be working with families in a multidisciplinary context and consistency and continuity of approach is paramount when working jointly with other professions.

Interventions that address specific issues of risk will provide short-term tangible positive feedback to build on, to optimize acquisition of more complex skills. Interventions can include the provision of appropriate equipment, teaching its use or reorganizing the environment to reduce risks such as removing dangerous items from a child's level. For Jan, the occupational therapist organized immediate provision of safety equipment. This involved acquiring funding from charities for a stair gate, providing cupboard locks in the kitchen and bathroom and a safety harness for walking and use with the buggy. Funding was also provided to buy a small single bed for her son.

Once the safety equipment is in place the intervention can then focus on specific teaching programmes based on task analysis (e.g. use of safety harness for a road safety programme or getting on/off a bus). Parents with learning disabilities respond well to individual teaching programmes which, if not carried out in the home, should be in a home-like environment (McGaw 2000). There is evidence of the difficulty for parents to generalize skills programmes and they therefore need practice in the actual environments where skills are used. The occupational therapy intervention in this way identifies and builds on parental abilities that promote resilience in their home and community environments. Utilizing task analysis to develop specific teaching programmes for skills in housework can be effective if implemented within a daily routine and with ongoing support to adjust over time.

One main issue for Jan was tiredness due to going to bed late and sharing the same bed with her son. Provision of a small single bed enabled her to establish and practise bedtime routines with support. By identifying bedtime for her son, making a timetable and placing visual prompt cards in the kitchen, Jan effectively established, over a period of 6 months, timekeeping for bedtime, meal times and dressing and bathing her son. Introducing an afternoon nap for her son as a daily routine provided her with an opportunity to also rest or manage some of the household chores such as washing and ironing. A support worker continued to provide support to practise home management skills, including hygiene, nutritional shopping

and cooking. To maintain the teaching programme over a longer period will involve training others such as a home support worker or members of the family to implement the programme. In this way support networks can be established.

The long-term goals for interventions encompass addressing issues of risk as a child develops by supporting training in parental challenges related to the stage of child development and can include individualized programmes on child development, child care, identifying risk, and play. Interventions need also to address issues towards diminishing social exclusion of the child, parents and families. These may include personal skill development, including communication (i.e. using the telephone effectively), social skills, transport, accessing primary health care, etc.

The length and intensity of training for parents, either through individual programmes or through group programmes, can equate to improvement or failure in the long term. Very often, attending a large mainstream group will be too high a challenge or not meet the specific needs of a parent with a learning disability. Access to mainstream groups will also depend on availability, transport and on local resources. Small groups specifically timed and implemented with practical activities are more effective as the teaching methods can be flexible to meet the needs of parents with a learning disability (McGaw et al 2002). For Jan, individualized parenting skills interventions were incorporated into support to attend antenatal health appointments and bus training. Jan started to attend a women's group jointly run by the psychologist and occupational therapist to improve self-confidence (e.g. preparing questions to ask about her baby at the antenatal clinic), self-esteem and assertiveness. Liaison was also made to enable Jan to contact the Sure Start programme for parents and children to meet with other mothers and continue improving her literacy and numeracy.

Summary

The complexity of parenting in modern times is compounded further for a parent with a learning disability. Current ongoing changes in both service provision and legislation all have an impact on how parents with a learning disability can be supported towards developing effective parenting skills. Parenting skills models (McGaw 2006, Woodhouse et al 2001) focus on family-centred interventions to address parenting skills and personal development for parents with a learning disability. Working within the process of the child protection system is paramount, however. Parenting models offer a framework in which to identify through assessment the strengths of the parents and families and interventions to develop and learn parenting skills. Occupational therapists can use their core skills to take a role within the multidisciplinary context to enable disadvantaged mothers and fathers to develop appropriate child care skills.

with her partner (John) with whom she has two children aged 5 and 7. John is often away from home as he is a lorry driver. Both children attend a local primary school and teachers have reported that they appear sleepy and are not thriving in the classroom. They also report frequent absences from school. Although the children appeared unkempt they interact well with their mother. The case manager requested assessments by the CLDT psychologist and occupational therapist on the parenting ability of Laura when left on her own whilst John is working away from home.

Box 10.6

Case illustration: Laura and John

Laura and John have been referred by the CFT to the CLDT following a reported recent abusive situation involving Laura and her brother. As a result there is concern about risks to her children. The brother has now been arrested and is under a restraining order. Laura has a long-term relationship

Reader activity

1. Define the child protection issues in this case scenario.

2. In what way could the occupational therapist establish consent in relation to this referral?

3. How would you identify the occupational therapy assessments for Laura's and John's situation?

Further reading

McGaw S, Beckley K, Connolly N, Ball K 2000 Parent assessment manual. Cornwall Partnership (NHS) Trust

National Association of Occupational Therapists Working with People with Learning Disabilities

(OTPLD) 2003 Occupational therapy services for adults with learning disabilities. London, College of Occupational Therapists

Oakes P 2003 Sexual and personal relationships. In: Gates B (ed.) Learning disability: towards

inclusion, 4th edn. London, Elsevier Science

Sheerin F 1997 Parents with learning disabilities: a review of the literature. Advanced Nursing 28(1):126–133

Useful resources

http://www.legislation.hmso.gov. uk/acts/acts2001/20010015.htm (accessed 7 March 2008)

http://www.direct.gov. uk/en/DisabledPeople/

RightsAndObligations/ DisabilityRights/DG_4001068 (accessed 7 March 2008)

http://www.barnardos.org.uk (accessed 7 March 2008)

http://www.learningdisabilities.co.uk (accessed 7 March 2008)

http://www.afdsrc.org/parents/ completed/wellbeing.php (accessed 7 March 2008)

References

Booth T, Booth W 1996 supported parenting for people with learning difficulties: lessons from Wisconsin. Representing children 9(2):99–107 Online. Available http://www.supported-

parenting.com/publications/ art_less-wisconsin.html (accessed 7 March 2008)

Booth T, Booth W 2000 Parents with learning difficulties, child protection and the courts. Online.

Available http://www.supported-parenting.com/publications/ art_parents-courts.html (accessed 7 March 2008)

Booth T, Booth W 2005 Parents with learning difficulties in the child protection system. Experiences and perspectives. Journal of Intellectual Disabilities, 9(2):109–129

Booth T, McConnell D, Booth W 2006 Temporal discrimination and parents with learning difficulties in the child protection system. British Journal of Social Work 36:997–1015

Canadian Association of Occupational Therapy 1997 Enabling occupation: an occupational therapy perspective. Ottawa, Canadian Association of Occupational Therapy

College of Occupational Therapy 2003 Standard of practice – occupational therapy services for adults with learning disabilities. London, College of Occupational Therapists

Coren E, Barlow J 2001 Individual and group-based programmes for improving psychosocial outcomes for teenage parents and their children (Review) Cochrane Database of Systematic Reviews 2001, Issue 3 Art. No.; CD002964. DOI:10 1002/14651858 cd002964

Department of Health 1989 Children's Act. London, HMSO

Department of Health 2001a Framework for the assessment of children in need and their families. London, HMSO

Department of Health 2001b Valuing People: a new strategy for learning disability for the 21st century. London, HMSO

Department of Health 2001c National service framework for children, young people and maternity services. London, HMSO

Gender N 1998 The role of the community nurse (learning disability). People with learning disabilities. London, The Maternity Alliance

Guinea S 2001 Parents with a learning disability and their views on support received: a preliminary study. Journal of Learning Disabilities 5(1):43–56

Harris R 2000 A matter of balance: power and resistance in child protection. Journal of Social Welfare 5:332–339

James H 2004 Promoting effective working with parents with learning disabilities. Child Abuse Review 13(3) Issue 1:31–41 Online. Available: Wiley InterScience http://www.interscience.wiley.com DOI: 10.1002/CAR.823 (accessed 7 March 2008)

Keilhofner G 2002 Model of human occupation, 3rd edn. Philadelphia, Lippincott Williams & Wilkins

McConnell D, Llewellyn G, Mayes R, Russo D, Honey A 2003 Developmental profiles of children born to mothers with intellectual disability. Journal of Intellectual and Development Disability 28(2):1–14

McGaw S 1996 Service for parents with learning disabilities. Tizard Learning Disability Review 1:21–28

McGaw S 1997 Practical support for parents with learning disabilities.

In: O'Hara J, Sperlinger A (eds) Adults with learning disabilities. Chichester, John Wiley, pp 123–138

McGaw S 2000 What works for parents with learning disabilities? London, Barnardos Online. Available: http//www.barnardos. org.uk/resources (accessed 7 March 2008)

McGaw S 2006 The Parent Multi-Dimensional Skills Model. Online. Available: www.bristol.ac.uk/ norahfry/right-support (accessed 7 March 2008)

McGaw S, Ball K, Clark A 2002 The effect of group intervention on the relationships of parents with intellectual disabilities. Journal of Applied Research in Intellectual Disabilities 15(4):354–366

McGaw S, Sturmey P 1994 Assessing parents with learning disabilities: The Parental Skills Model. Child Abuse Review 3:36–51

National Assembly for Wales 2000 Working together to safeguard children: A guide to inter-agency working to safeguard and promote the welfare of children. Cardiff, National Assembly for Wales

Woodhouse AE, Green G, Davies S 2001 Parents with learning disabilities: Service audit and development. British Journal of Learning Disabilities 29:128–132

Wolfensberger W 1972 The principles of normalization in human services. Toronto, NIMR

Appendix 10.1 Case illustration: Laura, possible answers

1. Define the child protection issues in this case scenario.

   - Risk of abuse. Abuse as actions that hurt from children's uncle and family situation and legal remit under the Children Act 1989
   - Risk of neglect, i.e. Laura's lack of knowledge of child development, poor understanding and support for emotional needs for the child to develop safely.

2. In what way could the occupational therapist establish consent in this multidisciplinary working in relation to this referral?

To establish informed consent the case manager arranged for Laura to meet with the psychologist and occupational therapist. Although Laura presented as withdrawn, unkempt, with low mood and uncooperative, she did agree for the occupational therapist to do a home visit to 'help me sort out the housework'. Through the home visit the occupational therapist established informed consent by clarifying the reasons for involvement and who would be involved (i.e. John her partner, a support worker and the psychologist).

3. How would you identify the occupational therapy assessments for Laura's and John's situation?

Apply the parenting skills model – you would consider assessing the issues by identifying strengths and needs in relation to:

Parents' life skills

Use a model framework (i.e. MOHO or COPM) to assess all areas including the environment.

Home visit: This is the initial assessment and starts forming a relationship built on getting to know what are the issues for Laura. As Laura was very often left alone whilst John was away working, the occupational therapist needed to explore Laura's ability to maintain routines for the children whilst managing areas of self-care and productivity (i.e. housework).

Observation: During the subsequent home visit the occupational therapist discussed the areas that were causing her difficulty including getting the children up in time for school, especially when John was working.

Occupational analysis: The occupational therapist observed that in each room there were piles of clothes which Laura said "… needed to be sorted". This was something she repeated often and also that the cooker was broken. Both these were of concern for Laura which she wanted to sort out.

Parents' lifeskills

Information was gained from the case manager and a joint meeting with the whole family, in conjunction with the case manager and psychologist helped to identify issues.

Support and resources

Role or interest checklist: Identify who was around to offer support within the family and neighbourhood.

Child care and development

- Observation/checklists of developmental level, fine/gross motor skills
- Social skills
- Communication skills
- Risk assessments in the home and getting to and from school.

Chapter Eleven

11

Loss and bereavement

Jenni Hurst

Overview

This chapter will focus on the loss and bereavement that can occur across the lifespan when someone close to you dies. This can be very painful if the death involves the loss of a valued carer or the death of a loved relative. Due to developmental delay a person with a learning disability will sometimes not reach the level of maturity attained by their peers of a similar chronological age and may have difficulties in understanding the concepts of loss and bereavement. In Chapter 9 you have looked at the importance of attachment and how that helps people cope with transitions through the lifespan. Bowlby (1988) suggests that the strength and type of attachment formed through bonding with the parent will affect the way an individual approaches the loss experience throughout their lives. Summers (2003) examines the conflicts that can arise for someone with a learning disability when attachment difficulties are present when a parent dies. Research into the emotional lives of people with a learning disability and an understanding of how they interpret loss and bereavement is limited but authors do reach similar conclusions (Arthur 2003, Oswin 1991). Oswin (1991)

identifies some of the difficulties that people with a learning disability and their family or carers experience when they lose someone close to them. For a health or social care practitioner working in this area it is essential to have an understanding of the grieving process. Although an understanding of death as a process may not be fully understood by some people with a learning disability, the assumption that they may just need 'cheering up' and 'will soon forget it' should be avoided.

Equally, there is a lack of support and understanding for relatives and carers who need to deal with the complexities of communicating with a person with a learning disability about these emotional events (Bloom 2005, Oswin 1991). People with a learning disability will also need understanding and support as they face their own death, and some of these issues are addressed in Chapter 12. While they can be told about what is involved through the use of different media, for example how a funeral is arranged, this abstract learning opportunity is very different to the actual experience of coping with the death of a relative. This chapter will assist you to understand these complex situations and suggest some approaches that will enable you to support

clients, relatives and carers and each other as members of a specialist learning disability team.

Learning Outcomes

By the end of the chapter you will be able to:

- Understand the importance of acknowledging loss especially during the grieving process
- Understand the role of occupation in contributing to the individual's ability to cope at this time
- Identify resources which can be used to support someone with a learning disability to understand the grieving process
- Be able to apply this knowledge when working with people with learning disability and the networks that support them.

Overview of key concepts

Two things are certain in life, birth and death, and the way in which these events are managed will have cultural and ethnic rituals of importance to all concerned in the process. The recent increase in genealogical research indicates that people like to know how they fit into the family, although changes in the UK population have resulted in an increasingly secular society so some funerals have less structure and ritual. Births and deaths are no longer recorded in the family Bible and fewer families keep detailed records. It can therefore be difficult for a person with a learning disability to see how they fit into family relationships and structure.

When someone dies there can be tensions because those working with a person with learning disability may want to include them in the rituals associated with a death. This may be very difficult for the family and some family members may think it is in their best interests to exclude the individual. There may also be difficulties when a person with a learning disability has a terminal illness and you can explore this in Chapter 12. Raji & Hollins (2003) found that there was a lack of awareness from both religious groups and funeral directors regarding the role of a person with learning disability in funeral proceedings. It is important to acknowledge that some people with a learning disability may be able to differentiate between loss and death especially if they understand the concept of death and dying. As with all other aspects of communication, they need to be able to understand and make sense of the rituals that surround death. They also need acknowledgement of their feelings and the emotional turmoil that can engulf the individual when dealing with the death of someone they love.

Unruh et al (2004) suggest that meaningful occupations may help people cope with a life crisis. It is therefore important to ensure that the person with a learning disability receives support to continue with meaningful occupations. Staff in a residential setting can fail to appreciate how much a move that occurs because of the death of a relative disrupts a service users' occupational form. This can easily occur if they have not had any training in bereavement and can lead to them not making allowances for the impact of the grieving process on occupational performance. In this situation an occupational performance analysis completed before the loss can help illustrate the impact of the loss to both the service user and the support staff. Worden (2003) suggests that during the normal grieving process the psychological changes that occur may leave an individual unable to focus on embedded occupational tasks. This is frustrating for any individual and it is important to view this as part of the grieving process and to remember that people with learning disability may find it difficult to communicate how they are feeling. At this time it is also important to consider the cultural and ethnic implications of the way loss and death are viewed within the family unit and community as this will be of significance to the grieving process. Evidence exists that supporting someone through this period is influenced by a cultural approach to loss. Dodd et al (2005) compared the attitudes of carers in Ireland to findings from a previous project in the UK completed by Murray et al (2000). While both of these staff groups would have benefited from more information and training, they found cultural differences in the way staff supported service users. They found that the staff group in the study that they completed in Ireland had more understanding and that culturally loss was acknowledged in a more positive way. While this was just the result from one study it does indicate the cultural differences that need to be explored as carers want to be able to support those they work with (Bennett 2003).

Loss and bereavement are not always formally acknowledged within the United Kingdom and after the funeral and what is deemed a suitable period any further mention of the loss is often avoided. One consequence of this is the emergence of voluntary counselling organizations, such as CRUSE Bereavement Care UK, that offer both professional training and support to those who need it during the grieving process. It is important to realize that these attitudes do not only apply to people with learning disability and can be found in the general population. A woman recently widowed described how people crossed the road rather than speaking to her (Parkes 1998). The rationale often given is that talking about the loss can upset the individual, but those missing the person who has died do need to talk about the death as part of the grieving pro-cess (Worden 2003). In particular, holidays, anniversaries and birthdays will often remind the person of the loss they have experienced.

Death of a loved friend or relative is one of the most difficult times in any person's life, having to try and make sense of the events happening around you while experiencing a range of emotions (Worden 2003). Each individual will have at some time in their lives the experience of grieving the death of someone close to them. It can be argued that the closer the person and the more integrated they are into your daily routine the greater the sense of loss. For a person with a learning disability this time can be even more confusing as they may not even recognize the concept of dying and the fact that someone will not appear again. Although their need to be included has been identified, those closest to them, who wish to protect them, may still exclude them from the funeral (Dodd et al 2005, Bennett 2003, Oswin 1991). Occupational therapists can contribute, with other professionals, to ensure that both the people with learning disability and those who support them understand the implications of loss and bereavement.

When a sudden transition occurs, it is usually due to the death of a parent and the need to find suitable accommodation for a suddenly homeless person. People do not always understand the sense of unreality following a sudden death, especially if this is their first experience of having someone close to them die. McEvoy et al (2002) found that people with learning disability can have difficulty understanding the phrases used to describe what happens when

Box 11.1

Case illustration: Joe

Joe has Down's syndrome and when he was 10 and away on holiday his elder sister was killed in a road traffic accident. His parents left him staying with his relatives until after the funeral as they felt that he would not understand what was happening. Joe could understand that his aunt and uncle were upset, especially as this meant that they did not go to the funeral and this worried him. He then returned home to find his beloved sister had 'gone away to heaven'. It was many years before he was told the truth and could start to grieve for his sister. His parents reflected that this had also made it very difficult for them to cope with their grief. He would get upset because they would not let him go and see his sister in heaven and because of lack of comprehension would frequently ask to be taken to see her.

someone dies. There are some useful resources and books available; for example, Read (2006) has produced a series of small books which can be useful to service users, their families and professionals. It is important to consider your response; if, for example, you have religious beliefs, you may tell a recently bereaved person with a learning disability that you know the person who has died has 'gone to heaven'. Reflect on the confusion when they get to the funeral and you tell them that the person who has died is in the coffin. They are now not sure if heaven is in the coffin or that the coffin is going to heaven. Additional difficulties can arise when the coffin is either interred or cremated. Being clear and open can also cause difficulties for parents and there will usually be an element of protection from distress. This is illustrated by what happened to Joe (refer to Box 11.1.)

Understanding the grieving process

This section of the chapter will consider the components of normal grief as described by Worden (2003) and consider how this process may influence the feelings and behaviours of the people who have experienced the death of someone close to them. Worden (2003) suggests that people in the general population who do not handle grief well can be identified as those who have been overly dependent on the loved one who has died. It must be remembered that while clinical depression can be the result of unresolved grief, normal grieving is a painful process. The grieving process is complex and fluctuating and will affect the individual's feelings, physical health, cognition and behaviour (Worden 2003). Once the shock starts to wear off, feelings experienced will include sadness, anxiety and loneliness but they may feel guilty and worry that the death was their fault. This can contrast with labile mood swings, which alternate between anger and a sense of being abandoned; crying and pining are also experienced. If the roles have changed and the person with a learning disability has been involved in caring for the parent, the sense of guilt may be because there is a sense of emancipation and relief that the person they have been caring for has died. Physically, breathlessness can occur due to anxiety, and insomnia or appetite disturbance are also common. Someone with learning disability will not necessarily associate physical pain and fatigue with grief. Cognitively, poor concentration and regression resulting in the loss of ability to perform familiar tasks can add to the sense of insecurity. Confusion and hallucinations may occur so seeing or hearing the person who has died is not uncommon and can be very frightening. Behavioural changes often result in low vitality, with the person staying in bed, while hyperactivity and sleepless nights are also common. Lack of interest in normal activities should be expected and sadness should not be confused with clinical depression in the early stages of grief (Read 2006, Worden 2003).

If the person with a learning disability is still living with a parent then the death of that parent will be of great significance. While increasing numbers of people with a mild learning disability live alone, they usually are still in contact with services. They may not view themselves as dependent on a care worker but this can change if this person leaves or retires. However, one skill they may have learnt is to cope with frequent staff changes by not becoming attached to staff so the significance of this type of event is reduced. For people with profound and multiple disabilities the loss of a carer may have greater significance. Sheehy & Nind (2005) highlight the importance of understanding the emotional needs of people with profound and multiple disability. Expressing concerns about how difficult this area is to research they suggest that reaction to loss may only be apparent in changes to behaviour. The loss of someone who understands how to communicate with you and gives assistance for activities of daily living such as dressing, bathing and feeding could be viewed by that individual as a major trauma, which they are unable to communicate. Having to adapt to new people who do not fully understand how you are used to having these tasks performed must be very difficult. Hewitt & Nind (1994, 1998) have explored how interaction occurs for people who have communication difficulties, providing approaches for professionals and support workers. Even if only limited evidence exists that people with profound and multiple disability form relationships, they can certainly exhibit behaviours that indicate upset if an important person no longer appears in their daily routine. The discussion that occurs regarding at which developmental age an individual has a concept of death is not relevant in this instance. Adverse reaction to new support workers should therefore be viewed in the context of someone coping with loss.

Reader activity

- Have you ever been in the situation where as an adult you have had to receive personal care? What were or might be the issues for you if you suddenly found yourself needing support for all your self-care tasks?
- As an adult how do you feel about your parents caring for you?

While this chapter cannot explore the components of the grieving process in depth, health and social care professionals working with people with a learning disability should seek training on this topic. Occupational therapists who understand the grieving process will therefore have insight into the implications of death on occupational performance and be able to factor this into their assessment process (Hurst 1998).

Coping with grief

Parents also have to cope with grief if their child dies before them; a parent once discussed her grief and feelings of guilt saying that she had 'lost her daughter twice'. This had happened for the first time in the hospital when she was told that her new baby daughter had been diagnosed with Down's syndrome and now when she had just died from the complications arising because of Alzheimer's disease. The relief that she was experiencing as part of the grief related to the fact that she would not have to die worrying about how her daughter would cope without her and who would care for her. She was able to discuss this with a professional who had been involved with her daughter and who was not shocked by these feelings. While it did not diminish her loss it helped her to acknowledge that this was a normal component of grief. It can be seen from this example that grief is very complex and should always be viewed in the widest context.

Support workers who work in health and social care day and residential settings may have to cope with the death of the people that they have worked with for years. In residential homes, they face the challenge of having to explain this to the other people living there in a way that they understand and be able to support their grieving (Bennett 2003). Often not acknowledged is the fact that staff will also need to grieve, therefore offering training can help them as well as the people they support. Staff may not have been given the opportunity to explore their own understanding about death and dying and if they have worked with someone closely over a period of years will have to address their own grief as well as support others (Bennett 2003). McEvoy et al (2002) found that it can be difficult to ascertain how emotionally aware a person with learning disability is, but coping with grief is unique to the individual and the circumstances surrounding the death. It is therefore wise to assume some sense of loss and explore if any changes in behaviour are a way of expressing the loss even if the concept of death is incomplete.

The feelings that the person may be experiencing are confusing for anyone trying to cope with both the sadness of the loss and being angry with the person who has died and left them. In the situation when the death was unexpected, the shock will last some time, and equally those who have expected someone to die are often shocked when it actually happens. Following the death of a parent, the individual may be moved into residential care, and although surrounded by people, will feel very lonely and anxious. Memories are important and photographs can give some reassurance if they can be shared with new people. As mentioned previously, insomnia can often occur and resulting fatigue may mean that the person cannot cope with occupational tasks, especially if they have

moved and are expected to adapt to the expectations of the new environment. Sometimes emancipation is experienced, which can occur when a person with a mild learning disability gradually changes roles with a parent and becomes their carer. Maggie, who was 45 when her mother died, is an example of the emancipation process that can occur (Box 11.2).

The above experience illustrates that not all people with a learning disability are bereft when someone dies and some do have ideas about what they would like to do with their future. Maggie saw herself as free and able to choose for the first time in her life. The occupational therapist quickly realized that she had a range of occupational performance that would allow her to live independently with minimum support. This resulted in Maggie eventually moving to a small flat in her own town and although she grieved for and missed her mother she enjoyed the freedom that not having to care for her gave her. She also joined some local clubs and developed her own independent social life.

It can also be difficult to explain to someone with a learning disability the physical changes associated with anxiety that can occur at this time, such as breathlessness or lack of energy, so that they do not want to engage in daily routines. In fact, expecting a bereaved person to want to do this is unrealistic because people need time to rest and to think about

Box 11.2

Case illustration: Maggie

Maggie had lived at home with her mother all her life and was viewed by her siblings, as 'the burden mother had to bear'. In recent years, as her mother had aged, she relied on Maggie to do the chores. Maggie had gradually acquired the skills from her mother that she needed to run the home and pay the bills at the post office from their allowances. Living in a small town helped Maggie as she and her mother used the same shops and kept to the same routines. Maggie first came in contact with the specialist learning disability services when her mother died and her siblings wanted to sell the house. Maggie was therefore homeless and bereft; her siblings had no clear idea about the level of her occupational performance and asked for her to be cared for in supported accommodation.

the loss. Oswin (1991) gives examples of staff trying to 'keep them occupied' when this is the last thing that is required. Cognitively, the individual is trying to cope with disbelief, confusion and may be preoccupied with thoughts about the death.

Worden (2003) suggests that mourning is concerned with a series of tasks and that the reality of the loss has to be accepted before the individual can move on to a life following the loss of the loved person. He also points out that grieving is not a continuous and smooth process but will vary from day to day. Even if the person with a learning disability is able to accept the death of someone close, they may still be preoccupied with thoughts about the death and not understand what has happened. Accepting the reality of the loss is a difficult task and will not be possible if confusion exists. An additional burden for a person with a learning disability is if they are not told if someone important to them is ill. Preparation means that they are more likely to cope with the loss and/or to be involved with the funeral arrangements at a level appropriate to them.

By understanding the grieving process staff can provide reassurance to the service user who does understand the concept of death that it is acceptable to be able to express their emotions and will provide support when they need to do this. They will also need to be reassured, as will the rest of the population, that feeling deskilled and unable to remember simple tasks or appointments is normal and to recognize this temporary confusion is part of the grieving process. Another difficult aspect of coping with grief can be the physical manifestation of the person who has died. People often report seeing the loved one sitting in a chair or hearing them walking around the house. This is often not shared, as 'seeing and hearing things' has mental health implications and should not be dismissed if a service user starts to talk about mum or dad talking to them.

Engaging in occupation

In an ideal world the occupational therapist working in a specialist team will already know the individual concerned and have completed an intervention with them; this will give insight into any changes in their occupational performance. If this is not the case, then understanding the cultural and ethnic implications of occupational meanings is always important when completing an assessment. This is of significance if

adherence to rituals is expected during a period of mourning. As discussed throughout this book, the occupational therapist needs to complete an assessment with the client and work with other members of the multidisciplinary team and support staff. Families may have strong beliefs and opinions about the occupational performance of their family member who has a learning disability. This happened with Maggie who had little support from her family when caring for her mother. Being aware of the way grief will affect even habitual tasks is an important factors when assessing a new client. Through contact with the service users' previous support network, you can gain as much information as possible. Finding out the nature of the relationship with the person who has died and listening to the narrative of the experience will all help establish a therapeutic relationship. The circumstances of the death are also important, especially as a person with a learning disability may have been 'protected' by the family, who did not want to upset them (Oswin 1991). This should be viewed as a time to support and encourage existing meaningful occupations rather than trying to teach new skills. Other aspects, also relevant, are the individual's personality, their other experiences of loss and the cultural implications of loss within their family.

Helping people with a learning disability understand the process of death and dying

This last section of the chapter focuses on how people with a learning disability can be given the opportunity to find out about what happens when someone is terminally ill and what happens to their body when they die. Whilst certain rituals apply after death that are culturally specific, similarities are found in how families deal with death. By acknowledging these contexts, one method of helping them prepare is to understand why people die. Depending on the needs of the individual, this opportunity can be facilitated through working with an individual or with a small group. Whilst research has been completed on groups that were established to identify how to contribute to individuals' understanding of emotion or bereavement (Mckenzie et al 2000, Stoddart et al 2002, Mappin & Hanlon 2005), there is little evidence of the application of a more occupationally focused approach. Most individuals, including those who do not have a learning disability, have a hazy idea of what actually happens when someone dies until they find themselves dealing with a personal loss. A practical approach worked with a group of four individuals to explore what they wanted to know about the process of coping with a funeral and what happened when someone dies. The group visited the funeral director, the registrar, the crematorium and cemetery to find out what happens at each stage (A Jones, personal communication 2006). This approach promotes autonomy and empowerment as the individual can make sense of what happens when someone dies within the context of his or her own occupational form. Understanding what will happen can help someone when they have to cope with a loss and enable them to behave appropriately in these settings. As this was part of a funded project, it also gave an opportunity for the service users' to present their knowledge to others. Weeks et al (2006) found that some people with a learning disability valued the opportunity to learn how to train each other and that role play was a powerful tool. Information produced from this project will also have the advantage of being produced from professionals and service users working together. Ward & Townsley (2005) suggest that consultation at every stage is the way to produce accessible information that is meaningful and therefore useful for service users. Raji & Hollins (2003) found that other professionals, such as clergy and funeral directors, also need more information on helping people with a learning disability cope with bereavement. While books, videos and DVDs provide opportunities to see others dealing with grief, and to see if the people concerned recognize the emotions, they do not replace the opportunity to see the physical environment that they might have to visit later. To reflect on how much you know about what happens when someone dies please complete the reader activity:

Reader activity

How much knowledge do you have about what needs to be done when someone dies? Make a list of what you think needs to happen and compare it with the list of questions given for possible group visits.

The following approach is one that an occupational therapist could contribute to as part of a multidisciplinary team as it selects occupations that will help the group understand the complicated process.

A group approach

What happens when people die? Through using a group the individuals participate in the occupation by actually physically engaging with the environments involved and by seeing what happens from an occupational perspective. There is also opportunity to ask questions of the people who provide the service when a death occurs. This allows them to advocate for themselves by giving the service providers the opportunity to ask questions about preferences which can contribute to their learning and insight (Raji & Hollins 2003). Some of the tasks that could be explored through the group approach are listed below:

- Does the group want to know where people die; is a visit to the local hospital or hospice appropriate?
- Where can you get information about a funeral?
- Was the death expected? If so, then a death certificate will be issued; who signs this depends on whether it is a burial or a cremation. An unexpected or traumatic death may have additional bureaucratic complications. How do you register a death?
- What are the implications of the culture/faith/beliefs for the funeral service?
- Who deals with the body? The role of the funeral director needs to be understood and where the body is kept until the funeral. Some cultures pay respects to the person who has died by viewing the body.
- What happens at the funeral? This will involve several scenarios, as it may be a church ceremony followed by interment or crematorium.
- What happens after the funeral? Is there any ceremony that involves a celebration of the life of the person who has died?

Exploring the issues raised by the above list can identify that when someone dies the rituals will vary in importance depending on a range of factors. The coping skills needed at this time will vary but an understanding of the process beforehand can help the person with a learning disability make sense of what is happening. Members of the group will also be able to support each other in the future if one of them experiences a death in the family, as they will have some concept of the process, which will enable them to discuss this. Service users need consideration at a time of loss and bereavement and occupational therapists need to have an awareness of the process to contribute to the service provided.

Summary

This chapter has highlighted the importance of acknowledging loss and bereavement for people with a learning disability. It has emphasized the need for all concerned to understand how they can support both service users and themselves through the grieving process. It has established that maintaining meaningful occupation is significant to the grieving process. Finally, it has suggested ways that service users can find out for themselves what happens when someone becomes ill and dies. Now look at the next reader activity, which involves Joe at a later stage in his lifespan (Box 11.3). A discussion about these questions can be found in Appendix 11.1.

Box 11.3

Case illustration: Joe (continued)

Joe remained happily at home with his parents and attended a local day centre for many years. He enjoyed his lifestyle with the family, going on holidays and other social events and his glass of wine with his evening meal. He had remained fit and healthy because he walked regularly and his bedroom was decorated to his taste with his own television and stereo system so he had privacy if he needed it. His social ability and friendly personality ensured that he was integrated into the voluntary learning disability services of the small town that they lived in and regularly attended social activities. When his father became terminally ill his parents discussed this with him and the general practitioner contacted the local specialist team to ask for help for Joe to leave home.

Reader activity

1. What are the implications for Joe of leaving home at this time?

2. How may moving to other accommodation change Joe's occupational form?

3. How can you assess Joe's current occupational performance levels?

4. What does Joe need to enable him to communicate the happy and fulfilling life he has enjoyed with his parents to others in the future?

Further reading

Oswin M 1991 Am I allowed to cry? A study of bereavement amongst people who have learning difficulties. London, Souvenir Press

Worden JW 2003 Grief counselling and grief therapy: a handbook for the mental health practitioner, 3rd edn. Hove, Routledge

Useful resources

Assessment of Motor and Process Skills: http//www.ampsintl.com/ (accessed 7 March 2008)

British Institute for Learning Disabilities has a range of publications: http://www.bild.org.uk/ (accessed 7 March 2008)

Cruse Bereavement Care has helpful advice and links to local groups: http://www.crusebereavementcare.org.uk (accessed 7 March 2008)

MENCAP has useful publications: http://www.mencap.org.uk/ (accessed 7 March 2008)

St George's University of London has a range of resources available online: http://www.intellectualdisability.info/home/authors.htm (accessed 7 March 2008)

The Valuing People support team has produced a useful site with a wide range of resources you can download: http://valuingpeople.gov.uk/index.jsp (accessed 7 March 2008)

References

Arthur AR 2003 The emotional lives of people with learning disability. British Journal of Learning Disabilities 31:25–30

Bennett D 2003 Death and people with learning disabilities: empowering carers. British Journal of Learning Disabilities 31: 118–122

Bloom J 2005 Breaking bad news. In: Grant G, Goward P, Richardson M, Ramcharan P (eds) Learning disability: a life cycle approach to valuing people. Maidenhead, Open University Press

Bowlby J 1988 A secure base. London, Routledge

Dodd P, McEvoy J, Guerin S et al 2005 Attitudes to bereavement and intellectual disabilities in an Irish context. Journal of Applied Research in Intellectual Disabilities 18:237–243

Hewitt D, Nind M 1994 Access to communication. London, David Fulton

Hewitt D, Nind M 1998 Interaction in action: reflections on the use of intensive interaction. London, David Fulton

Hurst J 1998 Loss and bereavement in people with learning disabilities. British Journal of Therapy and Rehabilitation 5(9):468–471

Mappin R, Hanlon D 2005 Description and evaluation of a bereavement group for people with learning disabilities. British

Journal of Learning Disabilities 33:106–112

McKenzie K, Matheson E, McKaskie K et al 2000 Impact of group training on emotion recognition in individuals with a learning disability. British Journal of Learning Disabilities 23:143–147

McEvoy J, Reid Y, Guerin S 2002 Emotion recognition and concept of death in people with learning disabilities. British Journal of Developmental Disabilities 48(95):83–89

Murray G, Mckenzie K, Quigley A 2000 An examination of the knowledge and understanding of health and social care staff about the grieving process in individuals with a learning disability. Journal of Learning Disabilities 4(1):77–90

Oswin M 1991 Am I allowed to cry? A study of bereavement amongst people who have learning difficulties. London, Souvenir Press

Parkes CM 1998 Bereavement: studies of grief in adult life, 3rd edn. London, Penguin

Raji O, Hollins S 2003 How far are people with learning disabilities involved in funeral rites? British Journal of Learning Disabilities 31:42–45

Read S 2006 Bereavement counselling for people with learning disabilities. London, Quay Books

Sheehy K, Nind M 2005 Emotional well-being for all: mental health

and people with profound and multiple learning disabilities. British Journal of Learning Disabilities 33:34–38

Stoddart P, Burke L, Temple V 2002 Outcome evaluation of bereavement groups for adults with intellectual disabilities. Journal of Applied Research in Intellectual Disabilities 15:28–35

Summers SJ 2003 Psychological intervention for people with learning disabilities who have experienced bereavement: a case study illustration. British Journal of Learning Disabilities 31:37–41

Unruh M, Versnel J, Kerr N 2004 Spirituality in the context of occupation: A theory to practice application. In: Molineux M (ed.) Occupation for occupational therapists. Oxford, Blackwell

Ward L, Townsley R 2005 'It's all about a dialogue…' working with people with learning difficulties to develop accessible information. British Journal of Learning Disabilities 33:59–64

Weeks L, Shane C, MacDonald F et al 2006 Learning from the experts: people with learning difficulties training and learning from each other. British Journal of Learning Disabilities 39:49–55

Worden JW 2003 Grief counselling and grief therapy: a handbook for the mental health practitioner, 3rd edn. Hove, Routledge

Appendix 11.1 Case illustration: Joe, possible answers

1. What are the implications of Joe leaving home at this time?

Joe's mother is still at home so he is not able to help her if he leaves. This will not be a problem if he moves somewhere close to home so he can visit when he wants to. Living locally will also help him keep in contact with his friends and provide some continuity to the move. He will also be able to attend his existing daytime occupations and this will provide structure to his daytime productivity.

2. How may moving to other accommodation change Joe's occupational form?

Moving somewhere new will mean that Joe has to adapt to the routines of a new home. This can be difficult, especially as he will be living in residential care or someone else's home. The occupational therapist can assist Joe with any negotiations that affect valued occupations.

3. How can you assess Joe's current occupational performance levels?

A full observational assessment of relevant occupational performance areas, using Assessment of Motor and Process Skills (AMPS) if the occupational therapist is trained, will provide a baseline for the future. An interests checklist will indicate what he values and allow staff to explore possible opportunities.

4. What does Joe need to enable him to communicate the happy and fulfilling life he has enjoyed with his parents to others in the future?

Life books are always useful; Joe was keen to compile one and he was fully involved in directing this, even chose the colour of the book cover. He came from a large family and they all had to have a place. Life books are an excellent aid to communication and help explain the narrative of a life; they have an added advantage over photograph albums as they can have text and other mementos added. Joe also had a speech defect and could have captions underneath the photographs that gave enough information for someone new in his life to understand significant people and events. This provided a valued occupation for Joe and supported him through his time of change.

The older adult and life changes

Jenni Hurst

Overview

This chapter will consider the implications of becoming an older person with a learning disability. Improvements in public health have resulted not only in people living longer but also delaying, in some instances, the health problems that used to be attributed to ageing. The expectation in both the Valuing People White Paper (DoH 2001a) and the National Service Framework (NSF) for Older People (DoH 2001b) is that people with a learning disability will continue to live in the community and have access to and support from primary care as they age. It is envisaged that the needs and therefore the support required for people with a learning disability will increase in old age in line with the rest of the population. For people with learning disability and their families this is a relatively new experience. Until recently people with a learning disability and their families did not usually consider the implications of living longer. The change in medical expertise and the social care offered to people with a learning disability mean that they now have a higher profile in the community. The changes in policy in the last twenty years and the expectations of the Valuing People White Paper mean that they now should

have access to community services. As people with a learning disability live longer evidence is emerging that some of them may age prematurely. In particular, Down's syndrome in early onset Alzheimer's disease, or the rarer Seckel's syndrome, will result in premature old age including dementia. Managing these conditions provides a challenge to current service provision.

Learning Outcomes

By the end of the chapter you will be able to:
- Understand the implications of government policy and its effect on the occupational choices of older people with a learning disability
- Be able to support older people with a learning disability to choose supportive environments and meaningful occupations for their retirement
- Be able to contribute to the screening and support for people with Down's syndrome due to their increased risk of Alzheimer's disease.

The implications of growing older with a learning disability

When people with learning disabilities reach this stage of the lifespan the balance of their needs may change, so it is important that any intervention considers how the relevant policy documents influence the intervention. The needs of older people with a learning disability are addressed in Chapter 8, Quality Services, Valuing People (DoH 2001a) and links to the NSF for Older People (DoH 2002b). The NSF for older people clarifies the service provision required for those working in these services. Both documents acknowledge that a change in service provision is required because of people with learning disability living longer. As you will be aware from reading about the historical perspective of service provision in Chapter 2, many factors contribute to people with a learning disability having a lower than average life expectancy (Gates 2005). While people with profound and multiple disability may still die younger, a significant number of people are now living to retirement age. Some of the generation that was sent to long-stay hospitals for a variety of reasons had relatively mild learning disabilities and they are now becoming older. Bigby (2005) suggests that they are the survivors of the system and this means they are remaining fit and healthy as they age. Having had the opportunity to live in the community they will also have learnt new competencies and will be able to relate to other older people if they do move to a residential setting. While the closure of the long-stay hospitals in the UK is almost complete, there are still older people being discharged who have spent a part of their lives in forensic settings because they became part of the criminal system. They still have to overcome years of institutionalization and can find it difficult to adapt to living in a community home.

Older people with a learning disability should have their needs assessed within the framework of the NSF for Older People, which categorizes people as those entering old age, those in transition and frail older people. It is clear that older people, including those with a learning disability, need to have an assessment that recognizes their age as well as other aspects of their life. This may be difficult for professionals working in specialist learning disability teams who have supported people living successfully in the community in their own accommodation. A move to residential care may be difficult to accept even though the majority of services for frail older people are in residential or nursing settings. During this time it can be difficult to identify an advocate to support the service users with proposed changes

and by now most of them will have a reduced social network.

It is important to be aware of the definitions given in the NSF for Older People. These are listed as:

- People with a learning disability over the age of seventy-five who meet the criteria for high dependency needs that are predominantly those of an older person, and need their person centred plan linked to services for older people.
- Older people with a learning disability who are both mentally alert and mobile should be able to have packages of occupational and recreational activities that meet their needs.
- People with a learning disability who develop the signs and symptoms of Alzheimer's disease will need specialist support (DoH 2001b).

One of the challenges for people working with service users is to establish and maintain social networks. Grant (2005) highlights how important involvement in the wider community rather than just paid support is for people with a learning disability especially as they are living longer. As people age their social networks change and may disproportionally diminish for people with a learning disability (Bigby 2005). In addition to limited social networks, few are married and may be dependent on siblings and their children to keep up family relationships. Bigby (2005) highlights the importance of a key person to support the service user who may be a sibling or a long-term family friend who can assume the support role as an advocate. Care managers need to be able to identify and include that person to assist the service user in completing the person-centred plan if this is to include their needs as well as the service implications.

Maintaining occupation through physical changes

The changes that occur as people age will vary for people with a learning disability, as they will in the rest of the population. Increasingly, evidence is emerging of the effect of the individual's lifestyle as well as genetic predisposition. For example, all individuals who spend little or no time weightbearing will have an increased risk if osteoporosis; this is true whether you spend your spare time on sedentary pursuits after a day sitting at a desk or are dependent for your mobility on a wheelchair. The need to prevent falls is clearly identified within the NSF for Older People as poor balance has been identified as a major factor that influences occupational performance. People with a learning disability also need support to help them improve their balance and need to be able to access groups run by primary care allied health professionals.

The role of the occupational therapist, if someone is moving from a group home into a residential setting, is to ensure that the staff group has a clear understanding of the service users' occupational performance. Moving into residential care is a major transition for anyone and maintaining occupational performance during this time will help maintain independence. Being able to engage in familiar occupations will provide a sense of continuity and affirmation of the individual's abilities.

Schkade & Schultz (2003) discuss the importance of occupational adaptation and how the framework of productivity, play/leisure and activities of daily living (self-care) used by occupational therapist can influence an individual's occupational environment. Establishing a routine and eating a healthy diet with moderate exercise will all contribute to a healthy old age (Bigby 2005). Older people have an increased chance of hospital admission and those returning to their own home after an admission to hospital can be assessed by an occupational therapist working in an acute setting. If this occurs then the role of the occupational therapist in the specialist team will be one of liaison with a colleague in acute or community setting as required. This will enable specialist advice, if available, on the service users' occupational performance prior to the illness that caused the occupational disruption and to contribute to the assessment prior to rehabilitation. At this point it is essential that the predominant need be recognized, as the occupational therapist working in the specialist team will not always have been involved with a service user. As with any older person who is remaining fit and healthy, any opportunities for health promotion in older age should have come from the primary care team. To illustrate this, please read about what happened to Mary (Box 12.1).

Life changes for Mary

The consequences of a stroke will result in occupational disruption and consequently occupational

---

Box 12.1

Case illustration: Mary

Mary had a mild learning disability and lived in a group home that she shared with two other people. Mary got on well with the support staff and the people she lived with and was happy and contented with her life. As she was well and healthy she had not recently visited her GP. Staff knew that Mary did not like doctors as she had lived for some of her life in a long-stay hospital. Staff had found that she became upset if she had to take what she described as 'doctor's pills'. She was the most independent of the three people in the home, being able to take care of her self-care needs and enjoyed keeping her own bedroom clean and tidy. She had recently celebrated her 65th birthday and had started going to a local centre run by Age Concern. Mary really enjoyed looking after others and was helping as a volunteer assisting in the serving of refreshments. One morning she did not get up at her usual time so staff knocked and went into her room. They found that she was unable to tell them what was wrong and she could not get out of bed, as she was not able to move her right arm and leg. The doctor was called and diagnosed a cerebrovascular event (CVE). Mary suddenly found herself in an ambulance and taken to the ward of an acute hospital which was an unknown setting for her. Despite this Mary recovered some of her cognitive functioning and speech but was still only able to transfer to a chair/wheelchair with assistance when the hospital was ready to discharge her. As Mary had a learning disability they had already contacted the care manager at the specialist learning disability team.

---

dysfunction for a signification number of people who experience a cerebrovascular event (CVE) and it is the third leading cause of death and a major cause of adult disability (Morgans & Gething 2002). Mary had not visited her doctor recently, which indicates the importance of a health action plan as she could have had hypertension without anyone being aware of it. Support staff could have sought advice from the specialist team as Mary had a fear of seeing the doctor. Liaison with the primary care team is very important in these circumstances, as Mary should have been offered health checks. The specialist nurse became involved to ensure that Mary had a health action plan when she returned home. This included advice for Mary and her keyworker on how to prevent further strokes. Because of the occupational dysfunction followed the CVE the fact that Mary has a learning disability ceased to be of major significance. The main impact on Mary's ability to perform tasks was because of the CVE, as it was this that had altered her occupational performance and impacted on her occupational form with such dramatic impact. As Mary was an active person, she still had a work role with her voluntary work that also provided her with social contacts. Although the specialist team occupational therapist had not previously met Mary she was able to gain a useful narrative from the support staff about her previous occupational performance and pass this information to the occupational therapist responsible for Mary's rehabilitation (Morgans & Gething 2002). It then became clear that the multidisciplinary team were dealing primarily with the motor, perceptual, sensory, cognitive and communication difficulties that she was experiencing as a consequence of the stroke rather than her learning disability. It is important to reduce the stigma due to lack of understanding in hospital settings that can be attached to people with a learning disability. In some Foundation Hospitals a specialist learning disability liaison nurse has been appointed to ensure this does not happen. This was vital for Mary as she was unable to communicate on admission but she still needed an explanation of what was happening to reduce her fear.

In Mary's case this illustrated that her needs reflected the consequences of her CVE rather than her learning disability. As Mary shared a bungalow, suitable equipment and staff training resulted in her returning home. The care manager ensured that funding was available as it was still cost-effective for Mary to stay in the bungalow and she was happy with the staff and other residents. Further rehabilitation from the intermediate care team and support from the specialist team nurse, occupational therapist, speech and language therapist and physiotherapist resulted in a successful discharge. Mary's CVE also affected the other residents and the support staff. Appropriate and timely support and resources from all the teams contributed to Mary's return home.

The specialist occupational therapist helped Mary to look for opportunities to expand her social interaction outside her home and she joined the local stroke club and enjoyed her monthly visits and the friends that she made.

The physical changes that can occur as the body ages may also require support from members of the specialist team. People with a learning disability and associated physical disability may find that their mobility is affected due to physical changes occurring as part of the ageing process. The reader can further apply what has been learnt from reading about Mary to the changing needs of Arthur, at the end of this chapter (refer to Appendix 12.1, End of chapter case illustration: Arthur).

Down's syndrome and dementia

The incidence of dementia

The second part of this chapter discusses one of the possible consequences of living longer for people with Down's syndrome which is the increased risk of developing Alzheimer's disease. While people with a learning disability, along with the rest of the population, may develop dementia as part of getting older, evidence is emerging of an increased incidence of early onset dementia in people with Down's syndrome (Hogg et al 2000, DoH 2006). To put this into perspective it has been suggested that people over 50 with Down's syndrome are six times more likely to develop dementia than a person in the general population (Turk et al 2001). Watchman (2003), whilst advocating routine health screening should be available to all adult's with Down's syndrome, highlights the importance of multidisciplinary screening for dementia. Raising concerns about service provision, she identifies the following areas as all needing consideration by service planners: diagnosis, accommodation, training and experience of staff and the role of the family. Forbat (2006) describes a research project that focused on the needs of older adults with a learning disability, noting the lack of research into this area. This project is of interest because the interviews were conducted with individuals who were all in a position to influence learning disability policy. One of the themes that emerged was the need for more training for staff both at support and general practitioner level, with an emphasis on communication skills. The influence of the Mental Capacity Bill (UK Government 2006) has yet to be established, as it is still being fully implemented, but it will have some impact on people with a learning disability. Another area of concern will be the rights of carers to challenge decisions made for their relatives who have a learning disability and dementia with regard to the medication available following the National Institute for Health and Clinical Excellence guidelines (NICE 2005). Other issues raised included daytime activities, family respite, flexible finance and housing. Supported housing models that meet the needs of people with dementia are of real relevance to people with a learning disability. Having to move from a familiar physical environment and known carers will increase the stress and add to confusion.

Occupational therapists' contribution to health screening for people with Down's syndrome

Screening of people with Down's syndrome to provide a baseline assessment, will enable comparisons to be made if concerns arise and is now being offered in some health trusts. Care pathways have been produced to deal specifically with this although it is essential that all other causes are eliminated, such as medical conditions or the consequences of a reaction to bereavement. These care pathways for assessment will have been established involving members of the specialist team. Occupational therapists will usually work with the care manager, nurses, psychologists, physiotherapists and speech and language therapists, who may all be involved at different stages of the dementia pathway.

Huxley et al (2005) suggest that behavioural changes that occur when people with Down's syndrome experience dementia mirror those of the non-learning disabled population; they reflect that it is an area which has 'largely been ignored by research' (p. 189). They conclude that people with Down's syndrome who also show evidence of signs of dementia are more likely to have an increased frequency and severity of behaviours that challenge than those who do not. By focusing on behaviour it is easy to ignore the occupational perspective: an individual who is experiencing difficulties in functioning in their familiar occupational form can become

frustrated and lack the communication skills needed to express this. Lynggaard & Alexander (2004) report on the work they completed with a group of people with learning disabilities who lived with two people who were in the early stages of dementia. The difficulties in comprehension that they addressed with this group illustrate how difficult it is for anyone to understand why someone is losing their ability to perform familiar occupational tasks. One of the exercises they used involved making a cup of tea, which effectively illustrated what happens when sequencing is disrupted. It also needs to be remembered how confusing this is for the person in the early stages of dementia, especially if they do not have the concept of memory. Informed consent and the ethical issues that arise when obtaining this are complex when working with people with a learning disability. This issue needs to be acknowledged and addressed by service providers who seek to offer a screening service to people with Down's syndrome. Occupational therapists will want to discuss this as part of the specialist team approach. As has been noted, it can be difficult to identify if changes in occupational performance and social behaviour are occurring because the person is experiencing the early stages of Alzheimer's disease. However, the Down's syndrome Association, as a means of ensuring that there is adequate service provision when it is needed, supports screening as an option.

Occupational therapists are able to use a range of functional assessments including observational assessments to contribute to the screening process. These can then be repeated if concerns arise and families or staff identify behavioural or functional change. The Assessment of Motor and Process Skills (AMPS) is an established and validated assessment that allows the therapist to identify strengths and weaknesses in a service users' motor and processing skills (Fisher 1999, Kielhofner 2002). This is a task-based assessment used by an occupational therapist trained in the use of AMPS to work with people who wish to improve their motor and processing skills. However, this assessment can equally be used to provide a baseline that can be repeated in the future on the selected tasks if concerns are noted. For occupational therapists who have not yet been able to complete the AMPS training, a functional assessment of occupation performance in selected familiar tasks will also provide a useful baseline assessment Kielhofner (2002) paper 94 demonstrates.

AMPS will assess motor skills:

- posture
- mobility
- coordination
- strength and effort
- energy.

AMPS will also assess process skills:

- energy
- using knowledge
- temporal organization
- space and object
- adaptation.

As one of the first signs of Alzheimer's disease may be behavioural change, completion of the Assessment of Communication and Interaction Skills (ACIS) as part of the screening process will again provide a baseline for future use (Forsyth et al 1998). ACIS collects assessment data from three domains: physicality, information exchange and relations. This assessment is designed to inform an occupational therapy intervention but can be equally useful in providing information for staff working with the service user. A copy of these assessments included in the service users' health action plan will give the information needed to identify changes in occupational performance or communication and interaction that cannot otherwise be attributed to changes in health or in the occupational form.

Continuing occupation through the stages in the dementia process

The early stage

Early changes in the behaviour and occupational performance of a person with Down's syndrome may be observed, especially if they still live with their family or in a small group home where people may notice subtle changes. However, if they are in a residential setting with frequent changes of support worker these may not be noticed. Unlike dementia in the general population, it appears changes in behaviour are often one of the first indicators that the signs of dementia are present in that individual. Loss of temper and irritability as well as difficulty in short-term memory may lead to arguments, especially if the individual cannot remember eating lunch or thinks that they have mislaid a coat (Lynggaard & Alexander 2004). This may also be because the service users are unable to find strategies to cover up the memory difficulties that they are experiencing, unlike the general population who are more skilled in dissembling.

The importance of context

At this stage, the person is living in a familiar environment and dealing with a structure that is familiar, if increasingly confusing, to them. The value of an AMPS assessment is that it can contribute to the risk assessment that needs to be completed for at-risk tasks such as using public transport or cooking. Difficulties in retaining short-term memory and learning new tasks mean that there is a need to find methods of structuring occupational performance to retain embedded skills and memory aids can be useful during this stage. These may include:

- ensuring that there is a clear routine for each day for self-care tasks
- using a wall chart as a calendar; this can incorporate photographs of people or places
- encouraging and supporting previously valued occupations
- ensuring the physical environment does not provide any obstacles to mobility, especially on stairs or steps
- if acceptable to others who may be sharing the house, using visual symbols to indicate the contents of cupboards or keeping kitchen equipment on open shelves
- using the life book to remind them of the significant people in their life or making a life book if one does not already exist.

Middle stage

In the middle stages of dementia, people are unable to remember names of familiar people or objects and may not recognize the familiar home environment. This can be a stressful time for those living with them, as behavioural disturbances occur that may involve sleep disruption and agitation and changes in social behaviour (Lynggaard & Alexander 2004). During this difficult stage it is important to provide the person with a safe and supportive environment to help reduce stress. Unfortunately, this is often the time that staff will be unable to cope and the person with Down's syndrome is moved to a residential setting over which they and those close to them do not always have control and choice. The occupational therapist, along with the rest of the team, can provide support and continuity. Staff working in dementia services should already understand how important preserving occupation is, but information about how someone new entering the home is functioning should be offered. Occupational therapists can contribute by:

- ensuring the physical environment mirrors the one that the person is moving from, including position of furniture and fittings in the bedroom and bathroom
- attention to meeting the spiritual needs of the person
- attention to sensory input, including textures of clothing and food, adapting food presented to meet changes in ability to drink and chew
- transferring intact occupational routines including self-care and bedtime routines.

End of life issues

At this stage the end of life issues for people with Down's syndrome and dementia mirror those of anyone with end-stage dementia. Occupational therapists should be aware that the National Network for Palliative Care of People with Learning Disabilities (NNPCPLD) aims to provide support and share good practice. One issue they seek to highlight is pain management and access to hospice support. They also provide support for people with a learning disability who are terminally ill with cancer. While they need access to the oncology services which serve the rest of the population, some specialist services are being developed to disseminate expertise.

In the final stages of dementia the fact that the person has a learning disability is no longer their primary difficulty. This is a difficult stage for all concerned as the service user will often be unresponsive even to those closest to them have little mobility and difficulty eating and drinking. They will also have an assortment of health problems and will now require 24-hour care. For people at this stage the influence of pain should be of prime consideration. Reynard

et al (2003) completed a study looking at how the experience of pain was communicated by people with severe communication problems and Kerr et al (2006) completed a study, part of which explored how those working with people who have a learning disability recognized pain. The role of the specialist nurse as a health facilitator can help reduce pain but the use of correct equipment and position is also essential for people who are terminally ill.

The role of the occupational therapist, although limited at this time, can still contribute by ensuring that equipment is available to support those caring for the person and seeking opportunities for meaningful occupation by:

- ensuring the right equipment is in place and staff understand how to use it
- supporting the spiritual needs by exploring any sensory input that still calms or engages the person when they are in distress
- liaising with specialist palliative care services.

It is also important after the death that all concerned have a chance to mourn the death and to support each other through the grieving process. While this is important for the person's family, others who have been close to them will also need support. This includes other people with a learning disability who they may have lived with for years, prior to the illness, staff members and those working in the specialist team (see Chapter 11, Loss and bereavement).

Summary

This chapter has enabled you to look at how current health policy applies to older people with a learning disability and to reflect on how becoming an older person with a learning disability can in some instances lead to a restriction of occupations available. This is especially so if people have to move into residential or nursing care offered to the general population. Finally, it looked at the increased risk of developing dementia for a person who has Down's syndrome and the way that occupational therapists can encourage them to preserve elements of their occupational performance for as long as possible. To consolidate your learning complete the final reader activity and answer the questions about Arthur.

Box 12.2

Case illustration: Arthur

Arthur, aged 64, has been referred by his general practitioner to the specialist learning disability team for assessment following a recent fall in his home. Arthur, who has a moderate learning disability, has lived in a shared home with two other gentlemen of similar age since all three of them were resettled in the community 10 years ago. Arthur has epilepsy, which is controlled by medication, and in the last 5 years he has developed Type 2 diabetes. As a consequence of this condition he has recently developed peripheral neuropathy in both feet. He is finding that he frequently stumbles and knocks his lower legs on furniture or steps. As a result he has an unhealed ulcer on his lower shin. In addition, his osteoarthritis has deteriorated and both knees have, over the last few months, become more painful and stiff.

Arthur lives in a Victorian three-storey terraced house on the side of a hill in an old mining town. There are three railed steps up to the front door that enters onto the middle floor of the house. The house is owned and run by an independent organization and provides Arthur and his friends with day care and sleep-in cover at night. Arthur's bedroom and the sleep-in room are on the middle floor but the kitchen/diner and bathroom/toilet are downstairs in the basement. There is also a bathroom on the top floor shared by the other two tenants. Support workers are concerned that he is finding it increasingly difficult to manage the stairs and is sometimes unable to access the toilet in time, leading to continence difficulties for him. They also note that an increase in frequency of falls is reducing his confidence walking unaided and leaving the house to access outside services.

This is clearly a complex situation and it is recommended that Arthur's needs be considered in relation to the recommendations of both Valuing People and the NSF for Older People. On completion of the reader activity, possible answers to the questions can be found in Appendix 12.1.

Reader activity

1. Is this a referral for the specialist team and if so who should be involved?

2. How can an occupational therapist contribute to the team assessment of Arthur's needs?

3. What short-term solutions could be offered by an occupational therapist?

4. What are the long-term solutions that should be considered and by whom?

Further reading

Kerr D, Cunningham C, Wilson H 2006 Responding to the pain experience of people with learning disabilities and dementia. York, Joseph Rowntree Foundation

Reynard C, Matthew D, Gibson L et al 2003 Identifying distress and its causes in people with severe communication problems. Journal of Palliative Nursing 9(4):173–176

Useful resources

Down's Syndrome Association 2007 The dementia workbook (authors: Dodd, Kerr and Fern)
The Down's Syndrome Association, Langdon Down Centre, 2 A Langdon Park, Teddington, Middlesex TW11 9PS. Email info@downs-syndrome.org.uk

British Institute of Learning Disabilities has produced three booklets: About dementia, About my friend and The journey of life (authors: Dodd, Turk and Christmas). Available from orders@booksource.net

The National Network for Palliative Care of People with Learning Disabilities (NNPCPLD). Website http://www.helpthehospices.org.uk/NPA/learningdisabilities

References

Bigby 2005 Growing old. In: Grant G, Goward P, Richardson M et al (eds) Learning disability: a life cycle approach to valuing people. Maidenhead, Open University Press

Department of Health 2001a Valuing People: a strategy for the 21st century. London, HSMO

Department of Health 2001b The National Service Framework for Older People. London, DoH

Fisher AG 1999 Uniting practice and theory in an occupational framework. American Journal of Occupational Therapy 532(7):509–520

Forbat L 2006 Valuing people: hopes and dreams for the future. British Journal of Learning Disabilities 34:20–47

Forsyth K, Salamy M, Simon S et al 1998 A users guide to the assessment of communication and interaction skills (ACIS). Chicago, Model of Human Occupation Clearinghouse, Department of Occupational Therapy, College of Applied Health Sciences. University of Illinois at Chicago

Gates B (ed.) 2005 Learning disabilities: towards inclusion, 5th edn. London, Churchill Livingstone

Grant G 2005 Healthy and successful ageing. In: Grant G, Goward P, Richardson M et al (eds) Learning disability: a life cycle approach to valuing people. Maidenhead, Open University Press

Hogg J, Lucchino R, Wang K et al 2000 Healthy ageing – adults with intellectual disabilities: ageing and social policy. Geneva, World Health Organization

Huxley A, Van-Schalk P, Witts P 2005 A comparison of challenging behaviour in an adult group with Down's syndrome and dementia compared with an adult Down's syndrome group without dementia. British Journal of Learning Disabilities 33:188–193

Kerr D, Cunningham C, Wilson H 2006 Responding to the pain experience of people with learning disabilities and dementia. York, Joseph Rowntree Foundation

Kielhofner G 2002 A model of human occupation: theory and application, 3rd edn. Philadelphia, Lippincott, Williams & Wilkins

Lynggaard H, Alexander N 2004 'Why are my friends changing?' explaining dementia to people with learning disabilities. British Journal of Learning Disabilities 32:30–34

Morgans L, Gething S 2002 Cerebrovascular accident. In: Turner A, Foster M, Hopson S (eds) Occupational therapy and physical dysfunction: principles skills and practice. Edinburgh, Churchill Livingstone

National Institute for Health and Clinical Excellence 2005 Final Appraisal Determination: donepezil, rivastigmine, galantamine (review) and memantine for the treatment of Alzheimer's disease. Online. Available http://www.nice.org.uk (accessed 12 March 2008)

Reynard C, Matthew D, Gibson L et al 2003 Identifying distress and its causes in people with severe communication problems. Journal of Palliative Nursing 9(4):173–176

Schkade JK, Schultz S 2003 Occupational adaptation. In: Kramer P, Hinojosa J, Roveen CB (eds) Perspectives in human occupation: participation in life. Philadelphia, Lippincott Williams & Wilkins

Turk V, Dodd L, Christmas M 2001 Down's syndrome and dementia: briefing for commissioners. Foundation for People with Learning Disabilities. Online. Available http://www.learningdisabilities.org.uk (accessed 11 March 2008)

United Kingdom Government 2006 Mental Capacity Act. London, HMSO

Watchman K 2003 Critical issues for service planners and providers of care for people with Down's syndrome and dementia. British Journal of Learning Disabilities 31:81–84

Appendix 12.1 Case illustration: Arthur, possible answers

1. Is this referral appropriate for the specialist team and if so who should be involved?

As Arthur lives in funded accommodation, he already has a care manager who is co-coordinating care and has referred him to appropriate health professionals on the team. It is appropriate that the GP referral should go to the care manager, who has overall responsibility for Arthur's service provision. In this case, although Arthur was accessing primary and secondary care services, his learning disability meant that he needed support in understanding the consequences of the change in his physical condition. The care manager is responsible for completing a yearly review that notes any changes in Arthur's person-centred plan. As Arthur's health status has been changing in the last few years the community nurses from both the specialist team and the primary care team were involved and addressed the following issues. The specialist team nurse has already assisted him in writing his health action plan and supporting him with accessing appropriate services, with assistance from the community nurse; this included:

- Diabetes – support at diabetic services/clinic regarding medication/wound healing/chiropody
- Vision – support with attending eye clinic/ophthalmologist (with diagnosed diabetes he should already be known to a clinic) Deteriorating sight may be a factor in increased trauma and falls
- Epilepsy – support to review profile and medication with clinic appointments as necessary as poor control of epilepsy could be another factor in increasing falls. Nurse could ask care staff to monitor any seizure activity
- Continence assessment – refer if necessary to continence advisor to rule out any underlying reason for occasional inability to control bladder/bowel, or is this purely due to poor access or mobility.

As the situation had deteriorated in recent weeks the care manager discussed the situation with Arthur and a care review was held.

2. What can an occupational therapist contribute to the team assessment of Arthur's needs?

At this stage there would need to be some discussion about who would be the most relevant occupational therapist to be involved. Assessment of and funding for an adaptation in the home is usually part of the social services occupational therapist's remit. Arthur, however, lives in provider accommodation and not his own home, so different funding arrangements may apply. An occupational therapist will need to complete the following assessments:

- An assessment of Arthur's current occupational performance relating to his self-care skills and ascertain any difficulties in washing, toileting and dressing due to decreased sensation in his legs, care of the ulcer, and restricted lower limb mobility due to his osteoarthritis
- A joint assessment with the physiotherapist to focus on mobility inside the house, especially on stairs, and the need for any stabilizing rails both inside and at the entrance to the house. As Arthur is in provider accommodation this was in the form of joint risk assessment
- Assessment of the physical environment in relation to the height/design of seating, bed, toilet, shower used by Arthur
- An assessment of Arthur's occupations outside the home, in this case visits to a local dinner club twice a week and a walk to the corner shop several times a week
- Attendance to a falls group to improve his mobility. While this would have been in line with current guidelines, Arthur was not willing to do this and in view of his deteriorating condition this was not pursued.

The physiotherapist also needed to complete an assessment, which was part of a joint assessment visit with the occupational therapist, and the following additional aspects were assessed:

- Assessment of knee joint pain and range of movement to ascertain problematic activity. Liaison with nurse or GP regarding prescribing of, or effectiveness of, existing pain relief medication

- Assess gait and refer to an orthotist for special footwear to improve stability, support and protection of feet from knocks
- Assess overall current levels of general activity to ascertain if current situation is due to long periods of inactivity, poor sitting position or overdependence on staff?
- Assess support workers' input into assisting Arthur when necessary
- Assess for possible walking aid.

3. What short-term solutions could be offered by an occupational therapist?

The occupational therapist worked closely with the physiotherapist to assist Arthur with some short-term solutions which included the following aims:

- Provision of a high-back, high-seat chair and a larger television as Arthur enjoys watching the 'soaps' in the evening
- To identify all possible causes of falls and manage them appropriately
- To reduce pain and stiffness in knees by increased level of activity, possibly including new outside activities
- The provision of walking aid and/or appropriate footwear to reduce risk of skin trauma from furniture and falls
- Provision of attendant-propelled wheelchair for use outdoors, although this was dependent on provision of suitable rails so that Arthur could manage the three steps to the front door

- To increase safety in home – installation of rails on steps, stairs and in the bathroom and recommendation for the installation of a walk-in shower in the bathroom
- Provision of a commode in his bedroom to reduce need to access toilet at night or during periods when mobility is poor.

4. What are the long-term solutions that should be considered and by whom?

Arthur and his friends were faced with the consequences of the discharge process from the hospital setting. When the accommodation was initially purchased the future health of those who were moving into the accommodation was not considered. Members of the specialist team felt that it would be in Arthur's best interests if he and his friend were re-homed in purpose-built ground floor accommodation, to include level access and adapted features for future possible use with a wheelchair. In reality, due to shortage of funds and lack of availability of suitable housing in the area, Arthur was eventually moved into a nursing home. His entire medical and care needs were taken over by the nursing and support staff in the home. The specialist team, occupational therapist and physiotherapist were consulted on occasions to monitor mobility and provide advice on handling techniques and equipment as Arthur's condition deteriorated.

Section **Four**

The context of the chapters in this section is to explore the role of occupational therapists in collaborative working, be it with service users, carers or for research purposes. Occupational therapists have a role and responsibility in the development for service users of self-determination, advocacy and to carry out evidence-based practice and research activity. In Chapter 13 Rhonwen Parry and Edwin Jones will first describe how user participation has been researched, which in turn has promoted inclusive methods with service users. They continue by presenting and explaining practical examples of service user involvement in research involving service users in South Wales. A definition of participation and person-centred approaches for more severely disabled service users is discussed in relation to total communication and active support. Inclusive models of practice in learning disability services from a user perspective are discussed and the chapter outlines specific research methods and issues that can help occupational therapists to challenge their practice.

As stated in Chapter 14, the occupational therapist may select one or more of several different roles described in the Valuing People White Paper. This may involve working with the individual and their immediate network (therapeutic and/or advisory), working with organizations, teaching or becoming involved in service development. In this chapter Sally Donati identifies who may be part of the network and defines the roles of the occupational therapist as they relate to Valuing People. The complexity of issues that can arise is illustrated through case illustrations and reflective questions. The concluding chapter is a personal comment by the editors exploring the issues of change in the current services for people with learning disabilities.

Chapter Thirteen

13

More than having a say – user participation in learning disability services

Rhonwen Parry • Edwin Jones

Overview

Occupational therapists have a role and responsibility to carry out evidence-based practice and research activity (COT 2005). In practice, it is often difficult to carry out this role regardless of the field of work for reasons of time, resources and expertise. This is reflected within the field of learning disabilities where there has been a paucity of research evidence until recent years and much of this has been exclusive of people with learning disabilities.

This chapter focuses on service user involvement in both research and service development and links the role of evidence to developing services that include service users in positive ways. The chapter draws on existing research evidence, looking at service and policy development and then considers specific research methods and issues that can help occupational therapists to challenge their practice.

For occupational therapists interested in enabling occupation, it is helpful to consider inclusive ways of providing their services and research possibilities that can enhance future practice and the lives of people with learning disabilities. This chapter will firstly present and explain

some practical examples of inclusive models of practice in learning disability services, from a user perspective. It then goes on to describe how user participation has been researched, which in turn has promoted inclusive methods with service users. Structured approaches, that have been developed in support services, and place the person with a learning disability at the centre of their plan of care, are then considered.

Finally the chapter explores issues in carrying out inclusive research with people with learning disabilities and offers possible methods that occupational therapists could consider when involving service users in research studies. A case study is used to illustrate the concepts presented in the rest of the chapter.

Learning Outcomes

By the end of this chapter, the reader will be equipped to:
- Define the main principles of user participation
- Present examples of how policy has helped to set the agenda for user participation in research
- Identify how service users can be involved in research and provide feedback on services

- Explain ways in which an occupational therapist can promote user participation in daily life; such as active support and person-centred planning approaches.

User participation – definition of terms

User participation is generally understood to mean active involvement in decision-making and inclusion in all aspects of daily life. Aichison et al (2001) suggested that the fundamental building blocks to successful engagement of service users include: communication, leadership, independent advocacy and the need for recognizing and developing a 'culture' of partnership from both sides.

'User participation' as a concept is now well accepted within the field of learning disability; however, this does not mean that it is clearly defined or consistently understood. In this chapter, we define user participation as a process by which people with learning disabilities are active participants not only as subjects, but also as initiators, doers, writers and disseminators of good practice and research. Further, in line with the established value base in learning disability services, underpinned by social role valorization (SRV) principles (as described in Chapter 2), user participation must also address wider issues of social inclusion. Social inclusion involves the extent to which people, especially those with more severe learning disabilities, are supported to be included in daily life and have opportunities to participate in typical activities in their homes and communities. This is central to the role of the occupational therapist in enabling occupation and engaging people in meaningful life experiences that enhance their occupational performance (CAOT 1997).

Levels of participation

User participation is not a single event but should rather be considered as a process. Strong & Hedges (2000) provide a useful framework to conceptualize this process. In this framework, user participation can be seen as four distinct steps (Figure 13.1), similar to a ladder that has to be climbed one step at a time, each of the steps building on the one before it.

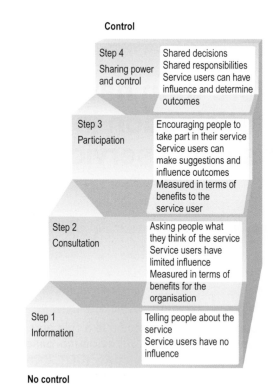

Figure 13.1 • Four steps to service users' participation.

The level of service user participation at each stage may be assessed by considering the following examples:

- Information leaflets about an occupational therapy service written in a user-friendly format would demonstrate that *Step One* has been achieved
- An occupational therapist could run a focus group, asking service users to provide feedback on the service they receive. This would demonstrate that *Step Two* has been achieved
- The occupational therapist could invite service users to design or share ideas about how things could be improved. This consultative approach would demonstrate more active involvement from service users at *Step Three*
- Achieving *Step Four* may be more of a challenge, as many service users require a considerable amount of support to actively participate in, for example, service planning meetings. Step Four also requires service managers to consider user participation at an organizational level.

In Chapter 4 inclusive methods of communication are presented and this is one way in which service users can be supported at each stage of the process. There are no shortcuts and if things are done too quickly or steps missed out there is a risk of a user involvement initiative becoming ineffective. Further, it can be perceived as tokenistic to expect service users to participate effectively at the organizational level if they are not able to participate at the individual and service levels in the places where they live, work or socialize. Occupational therapists could consider their role at each stage of the process and use ideas presented in the rest of this chapter to either implement or support strategies for inclusion within their own practice or to consider ways of influencing services to enable service users to take a more proactive role at all levels of delivery.

Reader activity

Think about your own service for a moment and consider:

- What is happening already to enable service user involvement at each of these levels?
- What could you do to increase involvement in your service at each level?
- What would be your first steps towards increased service user involvement?

Policy development

It is not possible to consider user participation without thinking about how policy has shaped the agenda in learning disability services, particularly in user involvement research. Over the past 30 years, there have been a number of philosophical influences on service development in learning disability services. This section builds upon Chapter 2, which presents the major historical influences on the development of learning disability services.

Early research in this area involved the analysis of situations that people with learning disabilities were faced with. This was heavily influenced by normalization (Aichison et al 2001, Wolfensberger 1972), later renamed SRV (Wolfensberger 1983), the social model of disability (Oliver 1996) and the growth of self-advocacy. Although normalization may have created the conditions for considering user participation, in practice much of the early work in this area

did not include people with learning disabilities views directly. More recent policy developments (for example Valuing People, DoH 2001) focusing on integrated services delivered in the communities where people with learning disabilities live, allied with a social model of disability, have raised the stakes for carers, professionals and researchers in learning disability services who aspire to work in more inclusive ways.

Research: Social Role Valorization (SRV)

To understand the context of user participation, one needs to question why it has emerged as a key theme over the past three decades. SRV had a very important influence on UK service development and more indirectly on social policy during the 1970s and 1980s and began shaping the research agenda. In the United Kingdom, the influence of SRV ideas can be clearly seen in the three principles of the All Wales Strategy (Welsh Office 1983):

1. People with a mental handicap have a right to ordinary patterns of life in the community.

2. People with a mental handicap have a right to be treated as individuals.

3. People with a mental handicap have a right to additional help from the communities in which they live in order to enable them to develop their maximum potential as individuals. (Welsh Office 1983, quoted in Felce & Grant 1998 p. xii).

This resulted in a massive closure programme of long-stay hospitals and development of alternative community services. This was probably the most sustained attempt in the UK to develop a coherent approach to service provision for people with learning disabilities.

SRV has also had an international influence, for example, in Australia, the principles of the Victorian Legislation (Intellectually Disabled Person Services Act, 1986) stated among other things:

- The needs of intellectually disabled persons are best met when the conditions of their everyday life are the same as or as close as possible to norms and patterns which are valued in the general community

- Services should promote maximum physical and social integration through the participation of intellectually disabled persons in the life of the community (Victorian Government 1986, Section v).

In research terms, Chappell (1992) argues that SRV spawned a wealth of research that attempted to evaluate the quality of services (for example, Blunden 1988, Humphreys et al 1987, Mansell et al 1987). PASS (Wolfensberger & Glenn, 1975) and PASSING (Wolfensberger & Thomas 1983) tools to evaluate service quality from a normalization perspective, were two of the most potent means of spreading normalization ideas. Much activity in the 1980s was taken up by PASS Workshops where participants experienced service provision by becoming a participant observer (service user) for a period of time and then evaluating this experience in relation to their own practice. Much research inspired by normalization has taken the service as its focus and the audience, service providers rather than users (Felce & Grant 1998). Whilst the research in this area has been greatly influential, in terms of evaluating new services, less attention has been paid to the central concepts of SRV. SRV's central concepts, stated very basically, are that if people could occupy socially valued roles then their image and social status would be enhanced, enabling them to get the good things in life that typical members of society take for granted. As Chappell (1992) writes: 'it neglects issues outside the narrow world of service provision' (pp. 35–51).

Chappell (1992) further argues that since the 1980s SRV has influenced applied research, which set out to investigate and evaluate the quality of services including areas such as participation (O'Brien & Johnson 1987) and advocacy (Nicholls & Andrew, 1990). However, there are limitations and although applying SRV principles may have helped create the conditions in which people with learning disabilities could speak up, Atkinson (2001) argues that in practice this is not always the case. Also SRV principles were not based on gathering the views of people with learning disabilities but rather on assumed knowledge of them (Chappell 1992).

One can attribute, however, to SRV a role in making inclusive research and service development possible and a continuing influence. It helped form the view that people with learning disabilities were human beings deserving ordinary patterns of living and encourages others to view them as potential and valued contributors to service development and research. Occupational therapists can play a key role in this by being aware of both the principles and tools available to support inclusion.

The more integrative policies of hospital closure, rights to school education, etc., influenced by SRV have meant that people with learning disabilities are more aware of their rights and are becoming more willing to be involved in research and take opportunities to tell their interesting stories. The opportunity to learn more about their own life histories through access to research skills and to benefit others is a significant development for people with learning disabilities (refer to Chapter 2). Certainly, the experiences of de-institutionalization and community living have been major areas where researchers have tried to get inside the experience from a user's point of view (Atkinson 1986, Potts and Fido 1991). The importance of researchers acting as advocates for people so that they can participate fully is one role that occupational therapists may consider. Inter-professional working and seeking support from other team members may also help to develop useful, inclusive research studies that have clear links between research and service development.

A possible reason why research has not addressed the issues of whether enhancing social roles results in an improved quality of life as theorized in SRV, could be that these concepts are very difficult to measure. Occupational therapists can contribute to this with use of outcome measures (i.e. Assessment of Motor Processing Skills (AMPS), Canadian Occupational Performance Measure (COPM)) and longer-term studies that seek to measure views and behaviours, before and after resettlement, for example.

Disabled people's movement

Research on the rights of people with disability has also influenced the development of policy. Ideas developed by disabled people about the importance of research being a tool for social change, about the need for disabled people to control the agenda, processes and outcomes, and about the necessity of accountability to organizations of disabled people have been taken up (Aspis 2000). However, much of the research in this area has focused on physical disabilities and less so on the issues of people with learning disabilities. This is partly due to the fact that people with learning disabilities have received little assistance in participating in, or carrying out research.

Self-advocacy has been of vital importance in enabling people to find a voice and in recognizing the value which research may have for them (Goodley 1998). People First (Open University 1996), a national self-advocacy charity, describes self-advocacy as:

- speaking up for yourself
- standing up for your rights
- being independent
- taking responsibility for yourself.

Many researchers have worked successfully with individual self-advocates and with groups to undertake participatory research and insights into the perspectives of people with learning disabilities have been gained. Some have expressed reservations about tokenism; others about the potential of relatively able self-advocates to represent issues related to people with more severe learning disabilities (Walmsley & Downer 1997). More recently, some individual self-advocates and one or two groups have begun to question the role of non-disabled allies (researchers) and their right to do research, which are seen to be the rightful property of self-advocates (Aspis 2000). This has, to some extent, created tensions in learning disability services and some dilemmas for those conducting research. The subject of research enquiry can also extend beyond the individual receiving services. One also needs to consider the contexts in which services are actually delivered.

An occupational therapist in learning disability services may be part of a community multidisciplinary team, working alongside colleagues from health and social services. Thus while the team might view themselves as one, members might well be managed and governed by two organizations, one in health and the other in social services, each one having its own set of standards and targets. Involving service users would thus include different organizational systems. The service user might only be aware of those individuals they have direct contact with. Other people within the system, such as clinical supervisors, could well influence a clinical outcome but this would not necessarily be visible to the service user. Research methods that cut across different elements of the service user's system of support need to be developed further. Occupational therapists are well placed to influence breaking down of service barriers to inclusive research because of their role in both health and social care settings.

Reader activity

Reflect on what role as an occupational therapist you might take to facilitate research across health and social care settings.

- Who would you need to liaise with to make this possible?
- Are there any barriers to this happening?
- How could you engage the service user?

Another factor that has received little attention in research is related to intellectual competency. Research should be as inclusive as possible and the challenge for researchers and service providers is to address how one can assist people with significant intellectual impairments and limited communication to participate. This also raises issues around how one might obtain informed consent from potential research participants. The Mental Capacity Act (2005), implemented in April 2007, sets out key principles in determining capacity around specific decision-making. Occupational therapists need to be aware of the provisions of the Act and seek advice from their colleagues (for example, the team speech and language therapist and/or psychologist) if it is unclear whether a person has capacity to consent to participate in research.

Person-centred planning and action

The broad definition of user participation described earlier in this chapter demands at least some discussion of person-centred planning (PCP), particularly as this is now a major component of policy, both within the UK as part of the Valuing People initiative (DoH 2001) and internationally. However, the intention is not to explain PCP in great detail here as it has been comprehensively described elsewhere (e.g. DoH 2002, Holborn & Vietze 2002, O'Brien & O'Brien 1998, 2002, Ritchie et al 2003, Sanderson et al 1997). The following section will, however, provide a basic overview and make a number of key points in relation to service user involvement.

Basic overview of PCP

There are various ways of implementing PCP and, although each one has a slightly different emphasis and format, they all share the common themes and features expressed in the definition below:

A process for continual listening and learning, focusing on what is important to someone now and in the future, and acting upon this in alliance with family and friends (DoH 2002).

The key features of PCP are described by the Department of Health (2002) as:

- The person is at the centre (and is often referred to as the 'focus person')
- PCP includes family members, friends and others as full partners or team members
- PCP reflects the person's capacities, what is important to them, and specifies the support they require to make a valued contribution to the community
- PCP builds a shared commitment to action that will uphold the person's rights
- PCP leads to continual listening, learning and action, and helps the person get what they want out of life
- PCP requires organizations to change the way they do things and adopt a person-centred approach.

The different PCP formats can be adapted or combined to meet the needs of each person, their family and staff team. Most PCP processes have the following in common:

- A committed team of significant people in the person's life, such as family members, friends and others, assist the person to plan and develop a support package to live the life they want to live
- The work is done in small groups and members facilitate decision-making and write up key points, sometimes using graphics, photos and other innovative formats, to assist the person in describing the kind of life they wish to live.

Clearly PCP has great potential to increase the involvement of individual service users in planning their own services, and the careful incremental introduction of PCP using independent facilitators is widely recommended (DoH 2002, Ritchie et al 2003). However, there are concerns about its ability to transform radically services in the strategic way envisaged in Valuing People (refer to Mansell & Beadle-Brown, 2004a, 2004b, Felce 2004). Rather, person-centred 'action' is required to promote service user participation and guard against the risk from attempts to introduce PCP alone. This will simply lead to some people having plans, but no real changes in their quality of life or in service provision (Mansell & Beadle Brown, 2004a, 2004b; Emerson & Stancliffe, 2004, Towell & Sanderson 2004, Felce 2004).

Reader activity

Occupational therapists can play an important role in facilitating PCP. Reflect on the following questions to consider how this role might be implemented in your service:

- How could you use your occupational therapy skills to enable service users to prepare for their person-centred plan?
- What specific occupational therapy skills and intervention tools are available to occupational therapists to contribute to the PCP process?
- How might you enable service users to identify their strengths and needs on which to build their plan?
- What part could an occupational therapist play in enabling service users to put their agreed plans into practice?

There are several examples of person-centred actions that can assist with this these, including the following:

- individualized funding arrangements (Beadle-Brown 2006)
- the development of positive behavioural support (Kincaid & Fox 2002) and
- the use of active support (Jones et al 1999, 2001a, b, Felce et al 2002, Mansell & Beadle Brown 2004a, 2004b, Emerson & Stancliffe 2004, Sanderson et al 2001). Also implementation of the total or inclusive communication approaches described in Chapter 4 will enable the PCP process.

Whilst the role of the occupational therapist provides opportunities to make very valued contributions to PCP in general, active support provides a set of evidence-based, person-centred procedures that constitute the type of action required to achieve person-centred aspiration in practice and are of particular relevance to occupational therapists.

Active support for inclusion and participation in learning disability services

Participation and inclusion in all levels of daily life should be a fundamental service aim in all services for people with learning disabilities. There is, however, a risk of failing to achieve breadth of user participation due to inconsistent expectations across services. For example, some services require participation in complex organizational issues such as how services are managed, policy development or research, in the absence of clear methods for assisting all service users to participate fully in daily life.

This highlights the potential for participation to become merely a gesture reserved for service users with relatively mild or borderline' learning disabilities. Indeed, there are similar concerns around the lack of any clear methodology within PCP approaches to gain the views and aspirations of people with more severe disabilities who characteristically have major problems with communication, and subsequently a very limited 'voice' to influence services.

One way of helping to guard against these risks is to take a more comprehensive view of participation by seeking to achieve active participation at all organizational levels and providing support for all service users including those with more severe disabilities.

Low levels of participation in activity by residents and inadequate staff–resident interaction were common features of traditional institutional services such as the large long-stay hospitals (Moores & Grant 1976, Burg et al 1979, Oswin 1971). Most of these have now closed and the people 'resettled' into the inherently richer environment of community-based ordinary housing. As a result, whilst research has shown a general improvement in quality of life it also shows considerable variability amongst the new services. Problems of inadequate staff support and low levels of service user participation in activities, even within 'ordinary' homelike settings with high staffing levels and contemporary service values are highlighted (Bratt & Johnston 1988, Felce & Perry 1995a, Emerson & Hatton 1994, Jones et al 1999, 2001a, b).

Although most contemporary housing services for people with learning disabilities may claim to have a value base that empowers service users and promotes inclusion in practice, many deliver a service that prevents people from participating in daily life. This has been characterized as a 'hotel' model, where staff control and run the household, undertaking all domestic activities, excluding service users and leaving them with little to do between scheduled and, in some cases, relatively infrequent external activities

(Felce & Perry 1995b). A hotel-model culture can be evident with a tendency to blame the victim (e.g. the service users' lack of ability, behavioural problems or health and safety issues, etc.) rather than recognize that the service is failing to take full advantage of the improved environment an ordinary house provides. Despite modern services often having higher staff to service user ratios, with a wider range of typical activities that are much more readily accessible than they were in institutions, the new environment can still be deficient. This may be due to staff skills, attitudes and organizational culture functioning as a disabling barrier, preventing service users from participating in daily life, being included as valued members of their own household and communities, and developing their own skills. The research cited earlier suggests that this problem is widespread and that elements of 'hotel' culture can easily creep even into otherwise well-designed services, resulting in a 'vicious circle of disempowerment' as shown in Figure 13.2 (Jones & Lowe 2005).

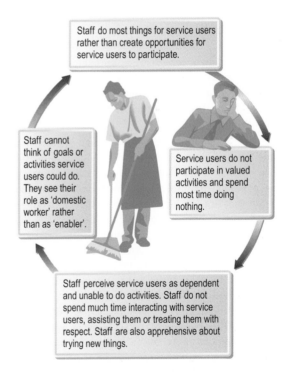

Figure 13.2 • A vicious circle of disempowerment in hotel models.
From Jones and Lowe (2005).

Whilst the risk of having one's life wasted in a hotel model is often greater for people with higher support needs, individuals that are more able can also be bored and excluded from daily life. People with a mild learning disability may, alternatively, be given too much participation in their own environment without the necessary guidance or support to make this a satisfying experience. These problems are a key concern for occupational and other therapists and difficult if not impossible to solve without a concerted multidisciplinary working approach. It also involves residential and other services directly addressing the issue of staff skills and organizational culture and a clearer view about 'whose job' it is to resolve some of these problems.

Reader activity

As an occupational therapist working, with a service user in a supported living environment, consider the actions necessary to support the:

- individual service users to participate in their home environment; for example skills training, advocacy
- staff in the home; for example training, advice, consultancy, implementing skills programmes
- client family or other carers; for example advice, advocacy, training
- members of the wider team; for example the occupational therapist involved in joint working and training.

The key factors associated with high quality outcomes in terms of this aspect of service user participation are how staff interact with service users, and the planning, monitoring and management arrangements that are in place to support this. Indeed, the first demonstration projects in the early 1980s such as NIMROD (Lowe & de Paiva 1989, 1991a, b, Lowe et al 1993) and Andover (Felce 1989) developed these factors as core components, and these have more recently come to be known as active support (Mansell & Beasley 1993, McGill et al 1994, Felce 1991, McGill & Toogood 1994, Jones et al 1999, 2001a, b). These projects were established to test the feasibility of radical, community-based alternatives to traditional institutional provision, and were informed by behavioural psychology research, combined with a value base derived from normalization (Wolfensberger 1972).

Both the Andover and NIMROD projects did not simply set out to discover whether people with learning disabilities could exist outside institutions, but to what extent they could be involved in daily life, develop skills and have an improved quality of life. The focus was on staff interaction and service user participation on a micro level, emphasizing service user 'engagement in activity' as a key outcome. Consequently, carefully selected ordinary house environments were designed to promote developmental progress by providing structured opportunities to learn and participate. Of crucial significance was the concentrated management attention on practical training for support staff to interact positively with service users to promote engagement, backed up by positive monitoring and feedback to staff. The longitudinal evaluations of these projects showed impressively positive results, including gains in service user's participation levels, skills and use of community facilities being sustained over time.

The current deficiencies in service provision represent a dilemma of particular relevance to human services. The usual expectation in other sectors, such as information technology or car manufacture, is that successful prototypes lead to better and better outcomes over time as they are replicated on a wider scale and further improved. However, in the field of learning disabilities national policy and service development initiatives focused only on partial elements of the model projects, emphasizing the need for small groupings in ordinary housing, but ignoring active support and associated practical staff training (Felce & Perry, 1995b). A number of factors may account for this: policy was developed prior to the publication and dissemination of the comprehensive research findings from the pilot projects; the physical structures such as the 'bricks and mortar' of the settings were more obvious than the more subtle, but crucially important operational procedures. Whilst normalization and its more recent reformulated version SRV (Wolfensberger 1983) has been essential in clarifying the value base, or what services should achieve, it has been criticized for its lack of clarity on how these values can be achieved in practice and failure to provide enough practical guidance. Contemporary housing services may have aims and mission statements which seek to enable service users to participate and live as independently as possible, but many would appear to lack the technology to achieve such laudable objectives. Importantly, however, there is evidence that active support, although by no means 'rocket science', can provide part of a multifaceted solution to such a complex problem and be successfully introduced to services to improve levels of service user participation (Jones et al 1999, 2001a, b, Bradshaw et al 2004).

What is active support?

Active support comprises two basic elements: positive interaction and a set of organizational systems for planning and monitoring. Although many of the principles (refer to Box 13.1) will be very familiar to occupational therapists, they are still not widely applied by staff in supported housing services.

Positive interaction

Positive interaction has been adapted to the context of ordinary housing and led by contemporary values of inclusion, rights and choice to enable support staff to make full use of the opportunities available to involve service users in daily life. Based on evidence from earlier experimental evaluations of an applied behavioural approach (Porterfield & Blunden 1979; Porterfield et al 1980, Mansell et al 1982) the process of positive staff interaction, shown in Figure 13.3 (Jones & Lowe 2005), consists of the following three main elements:

1. Different levels of assistance
2. Thinking in steps
3. Reinforcing participation.

The first element of 'different levels of assistance' guides staff in providing the right level of help according to each service user's ability. This is presented as a graduated hierarchy of assistance that progresses from 'ask' (1); the lowest level, through verbal instruction (2); to the non-verbal levels of physical prompting (3); and demonstration (4); with physical guidance (5) as the highest level. The basic approach is to give each person the right level of help to participate successfully. Whilst 'ask' and 'instruct' depend on the ability of the individual to understand language, if someone has only limited comprehension then reducing the number and complexity of words is a useful strategy. A range of non-verbal forms of assistance may then be used to enable more disabled service users. These include physical prompts e.g. pointing and other gestures, repositioning materials

Box 13.1

Learning points: Principles of active support

- Active Support is a technology about supporting people with learning disabilities to participate and being included in daily life
- As stated earlier, many of the components of active support will be familiar territory to occupational therapists; the aim of this section has been to explain what active support should be about and how to ensure quality
- A key issue concerns the advantages of training support staff in basic approaches, and incorporating these into the cultures of organizations and teams. Providing active support should be within the purview of mainstream providers. Creating a more conducive environment allows occupational therapists to provide specialist input that fulfils their specialist role rather than trying to deal with basic service deficiencies
- This specialist role is clearly up to occupational therapists to define but supporting and extending the model by providing specialist advice on diagnostic issues, specialist equipment and other complementary approaches and in producing structured teaching plans seem obvious areas. Indeed, the involvement of occupational therapists as external specialists could make a great contribution in ensuring the quality of active support
- Active support has parallels with the total or inclusive communication approach described in Chapter 4, but with a different focus on support to participate in activity. It is important to stress that both approaches are required, as key elements of the technological mix required in high quality services for people with learning disabilities.

and equipment, using 'objects of reference' (Park 2002) showing or demonstrating what needs to be done, and then prompting the person to do the same thing immediately afterwards. Providing hand-on-hand guidance is often the right level for some people when undertaking an unfamiliar and relatively complex activity for the first time. Once the person

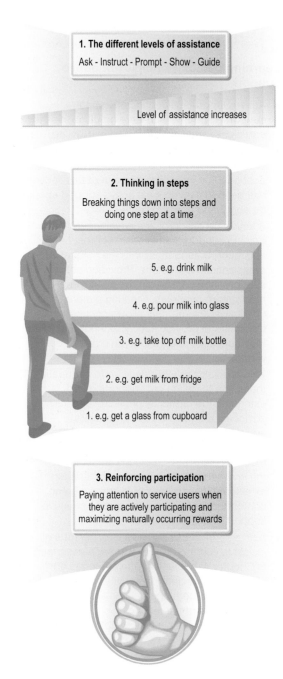

Figure 13.3 • The model of positive staff interaction.

make unfamiliar or complex activities easier to do by breaking them down into a series of steps (Gold 1980). This combines with the first element to provide the most appropriate level of assistance at each component step depending on the service user's ability and experience. Steps are broken down further and higher levels of assistance provided where a service user has difficulty, and component steps are combined and assistance faded as the service user becomes more proficient through regular practice.

The third element shown in Figure 13.3 'positive reinforcement', ensures that the person gets something pleasant or enjoyable (a reward) immediately after they have participated in the activity, increasing the likelihood that they will behave in the same way in the future. Not all people find the same things rewarding, therefore a variety of strategies are required. However, praise and attention should always be incorporated, as they are effective, easily adaptable and require no additional resources. Naturally occurring rewards are also used and can be maximized by starting at a step near to getting a reward, such as stirring a cup of tea before drinking it, and then introducing the other component steps by 'backward chaining', e.g. adding sugar, then stirring the tea before drinking it, and so on. Using the 'Premack' principle (refer to glossary) of linking a less preferred activity to a more preferred activity is also a useful reinforcement strategy, e.g. sweeping the floor and then having a cup of tea as a reward.

As well as these three elements, another crucial aspect is the style of staff interaction. To ensure both ethical and practical perspectives to promote participation and avoid challenging behaviour, the tone of voice and body language must be supportive and encouraging rather than demanding or domineering. Effective communication skills also involve verbal economy such as avoiding the use of overly complex words and phrases, not repeating verbal instructions so they become 'nagging', or distracting people by talking too much.

Planning and routines

Planning is part of an ordinary life; typically people constantly plan a wide range of things, from daily activities such as what to wear, eat and do, to more occasional activities such as holidays. Many people also rely on some form of written plan, such as lists, wall calendars, appointment diaries, for at least some

is able to participate successfully, assistance can be gradually faded to promote independence.

The second element in Figure 13.3, 'task analysis' is a tried and tested behavioural approach used to of the time. The more people that are involved and the more complicated their arrangements, the greater the need for structure in planning and one of the consequences of having a learning disability is that people need more help with planning.

Residential services for people with learning disabilities are complex environments, often with several service users who have different needs and interests, supported by numerous staff on rota systems, which means that only a limited number of staff are available at any one time. As limited planning of service users' activities occurs in 'hotel' models, service users are often left with too little to do. More sophisticated planning is, therefore, a central part of the active support model. Making plans for personal routines, domestic tasks, leisure pursuits, daily, regular and occasional activities, as well as the necessary staff support, helps to ensure that residents have full and busy lives, and the opportunity to experience the range of activities that represent a typical lifestyle. Two basic components address the issue of participation by morning routines and daily participation plans, with two further components of opportunity plans and teaching plans to address the issue of skill development.

In the hotel model it appears that the more disabled a person is the more likely they are to get 'processed' by staff during personal care activities or in other words have things done to them without their active involvement. Further, particularly when working on a one-to-one basis, staff, quite understandably, are unlikely to be consistent, because they cannot observe exactly what their colleague does. Ten staff members are, therefore, likely to provide personal care in 10 slightly different ways. Written routines are designed to address these key problems for people who need help with personal care. Staff can promote involvement and provide consistent support and the service user is more likely to be able to predict what will happen next, increasing their control. Each step of the task is listed in detail, with the level of help given in parentheses, e.g.:

- Jane gets out of bed (ask)
- Jane fills the bath (instruct) – staff check temperature
- Jane gets in the bath (hand on hand)
- Jane washes her hair (prompt), and so on.

Involving the staff team in producing personal care routines with this level of precision has several benefits. First, it sets the scene for the person to participate and learn. Second, it highlights areas where support can be decreased systematically to encourage independence. Third, it helps new staff to know exactly what support to give, and it helps in the management of transition.

Shown in Figure 13.4 is an extract for a Monday morning from a set of daily participation plans that covers the whole week. There are two columns for each service user, one for activities, with any regular planned activities already included and one for support staff initials. The 'household' column lists a menu of daily domestic and other activities required to run the house, and an 'options' column lists a menu of other optional activities that can be offered including leisure, social, etc. Daily participation plans are written following a person-centred approach, as they must reflect individual service user's personal preferences and activity patterns. Several times over the course of each day, staff, together with the service users wherever possible, meet briefly using the plan to agree which service users will do what activities and the staff who will support them. Because the activities are in half-hour slots, gaps in service users' schedules quickly become apparent, and the menu of activities in the household and option columns is used to fill these gaps. Staff deploy themselves to support the service users' activities and write their initials in the relevant columns. Planning in this way allows flexibility to respond to changing circumstances, gives service users and staff structure and ownership, and helps to ensure that service users are supported to be constructively engaged in living a typically full life, involved in daily decision-making and more likely to know what will happen next. Versions of the plans using pictures and symbols can also be developed to promote greater involvement of service users. Care should, however, be taken within the planning process to ensure that people do have time to do nothing as well and not fall into the trap of making people fill every waking moment or miss their need for time alone or just being.

In addition to these basic planning tools, 'opportunity plans' (Toogood et al 1983) and more formal skill teaching plans can be introduced to help people develop specific skills through regular practice. In both methods, goals are written in clear performance terms (i.e. who will do what, where, when, how often and with what level of help) (Houts & Scott 1975), but the degree of precision varies. Introducing skill

Monitoring progress is an important part of the process. Each time a person participates in an activity, this is recorded very simply on an individualized participation grid. These are summarized weekly and used as part of a positive monitoring approach that provides general performance feedback to staff. Ideally this is by the first-line manager through regular staff team meetings, with a particular emphasis on what has worked well and agreeing remedial action to address areas where improvement is required.

The key to implementing active support is the skills and motivation of the staff team. The literature on staff training in services for people with learning disabilities recommends that combinations of different training techniques, reinforced by ongoing management attention, are most effective in changing staff behaviour and maintaining improved ways of working. Wherever possible the key 'mediators' or those people who spend most time in contact with service users are trained in key skills (e.g. Anderson 1987, Jones et al 1987). These recommendations have been incorporated into the design of the active support training with a particular emphasis on a practice-based 'interactive training' session of around 2 hours with each individual member of staff working with service users in their own home (Toogood 1995). This form of training is often referred to as 'in vivo' or 'in situ' training in the literature and is widely recommended as essential in translating theory into practice (Anderson 1987). It is important to train all members of a staff team and involving managers in the training is essential if they are to have the operational expertise to implement and maintain the model, by specifying clear goals, monitoring progress, removing obstacles, helping staff to solve problems and providing performance feedback to motivate and reward staff in the long term. Managers also need to work in a multidisciplinary way with therapists (occupational, speech and language, physiotherapists), psychologists, community nurses, to ensure greater accessibility, such as in kitchens and providing more equipment that is suitable, more creative management of risks, and more targeted interventions etc.

The benefits of active support

There is a good evidence base for active support dating back to the early model projects, and the effect of introducing active support into well-established

17 Morgan Street   Monday Morning

Staff names and shift times:

1...............from........to....... 2...................from.........to........
3...............from........to....... 4...................from.........to........

Time	Ann	S	Mark	S	Janet	S	Household	Options
6.30					Gets up Cup of tea			
7.00	Gets up Cup of tea		Gets up Breakfast		Shower		Put bins out	
7.30	Back to bed		Cup of tea Shower		Dress Hair		N.B. all prepare own breakfast	Sort mail
8.00	Gets up Cup of tea		Shave		Breakfast		Change bed	
8.30	Shower Dress						Clear up Load dishwasher	Go for walk
9.00	Hair						Clean bathroom	Water plants
9.30	Breakfast Medication						Make coffee/tea Wipe surfaces Mop floor	Ironing
10.00			Clean bedroom		Go to bank Collect £		Local shop Break and milk	Swimming and sauna
10.30	Exercise video		Hoover, dust and polish		Photography class		Load and start washing machine	Mow the lawn
11.00					at			Gardening
11.30					Valley college		Prepare lunch	Hang washing out
12.00								Golf
12.30			Lunch		Lunch			Lunch out
1.00	Lunch						Load and start dishwasher	

Figure 13.4 • Daily participation plan.

teaching in the general context of promoting participation that follows the introduction of active support appears to be much more effective than attempting to teach service users skills in a hotel-model setting.

staffed community houses has been formally evaluated twice (Jones et al 1999, 2001a, b). Both these studies showed positive results, with significant gains in the amount of time service users participated in activities and in the level of positive interaction they received from staff. The pattern of staff contact also changed to more closely match service user needs. Prior to introducing active support the more able service users received the greatest amount of attention; afterwards this became more equitable and there was a slight tendency for the less able people to receive more assistance. Indeed, the amount of assistance given to the less able people increased by up to five times and the quality of assistance provided by staff was enhanced, becoming more effective at enabling service users to participate. There was no reduction in the amount of social contact, so an informal and friendly atmosphere was maintained in the houses.

Service users have been very positive about active support, and their views were independently surveyed by People First groups (Jones et al 2001a). Whilst this survey only canvassed the views of more able people, most were overwhelmingly positive about the change in their lives, stating that doing things for themselves, learning new skills and being involved in their homes were positive and enjoyable experiences. Indeed, service users made a number of insightful comments both about themselves and the role of staff such as : '...it was boring before, now I do lots of things in the house'; 'We do so much more now we've got plans'; 'It's important we know when things are going to happen' and '...it's good to see men doing the housework in our house!'; 'it gives staff an idea of what they are meant to be doing'...'I didn't know staff could teach me so well! They are good teachers'.

Although staff views have not been formally surveyed, direct and indirect feedback has been readily available both during the studies and in subsequent years of delivering the training. Staff often express mixed views during the workshops, with some staff clearly resistant and sceptical as to its efficacy or applicability to service users they work with (particularly if they have more severe disabilities or challenging behaviours) whilst others are enthused and eager to try working in the way described. The interactive training component makes a great difference in promoting staff acceptability and commitment to active support. Most staff are not only surprised at what they can help service users to achieve by translating the theory into practice, but even the most initially resistant staff find this extremely rewarding. They report increased job satisfaction and a closer match between their original reason for working with people with learning disabilities and work following active support training. Key qualitative outcomes, repeatedly borne out when this model is fully implemented, are that service users (including the most severely disabled who have great difficulty expressing opinions) enjoy participating and staff enthusiasm and satisfaction can increase as they become more skilled and experienced in the interactive approach. We have described this as a virtuous circle, as shown in Figure 13.5 (Jones & Lowe 2005).

It seems entirely appropriate for a service user who said 'We've got too much to do now' to have one of the last words on active support. This comment can be interpreted as a negative one, but we would argue that it shows that the person is more included in daily life as experienced by most typical active members of society. The most appropriate response is therefore 'welcome to the real world'.

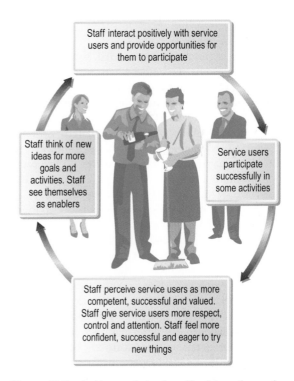

Figure 13.5 • A virtuous circle of positive interaction and empowerment.
From Jones and Lowe (2005).

209

User participation in research

Research involving people with learning disabilities has had a relatively short history dating from the late 1980s. Richards (1984) could only find five studies in the previous 20 years which had featured people with learning disabilities even as respondents. Research in learning disability was, and to some extent still is, heavily influenced by a medical model of learning disabilities that sees learning disabilities as an unalterable condition. The researchers' task in this instance is to describe and analyse the behaviour or characteristics of the people so-labelled. Kiernan (1999) characterizes traditional research as being very much on method rather than with people and states:

> In the traditional model, participation 'of subjects' is strictly limited. The researcher decides on the research question, develops and employs what are felt to be suitable measures, analyses the ensuing data and interprets the results in terms of the original hypothesis. The subjects of research studies are therefore almost entirely passive in the research process (pp. 43–47).

This type of research has tended towards quantitative research methods whereas more inclusive research may lend itself better to qualitative approaches. Being able to focus on the actual lived experiences of research participants would be the aim of inclusive methodologies. Qualitative methods have developed significantly over the past decade, which has made research involving service users more possible.

As an occupational therapist embarking on a research study involving service users it is important to choose methods that are appropriate for the questions being explored and quantitative and qualitative methodologies may each play a part in involving service users, depending on the aims of the study. For example, if you wish to seek the views of service users on the service they received you could choose to use a structured questionnaire scored against quantitative criteria or you may use an individual interview of a qualitative nature – both methods would elicit their views. However, the way in which the service user was involved in the research may be different, so in the first case the person may be a research participant, consultant or advisor about the type of questions to ask. In the second case, they may be participants or facilitators.

As services for people with learning disabilities have moved away from institutions to community care, this has made the capacity of families to care for people with learning disabilities a significant policy issue. A large number of studies have therefore focused on how they view their disabled offspring. Walmsley and Johnson (2003) argue that researchers in this area have failed to represent the perspectives of people with learning disabilities in their research.

Early research focused on carers rather than the 'cared' for. This is not to argue that families and carers do not deserve consideration – they do. However, current thinking recognizes that the views of people with learning disabilities must be central rather than considered as an after-thought. Walmsley and Johnson (2003) suggest that for research to be inclusive, the research problem should be owned by service users, it should be collaborative, it should be in the interests of people with learning disabilities and the process and outcome reports made accessible to people with learning disabilities. Occupational therapists should, therefore, consider how to put research and inclusive methodologies into place in their practice. Being involved in research activity may represent a meaningful occupation for some service users and the occupational therapists may become involved in supporting a service user to fully contribute to this role or to learn new skills in order to participate.

Managing inclusive research

A range of research methodologies have been promoted over recent years, giving people with learning disabilities an active role in the research process. Regardless of whether you choose qualitative or quantitative methods for your research study or a combination of the two, there are specific roles that people with learning disabilities have played in research. Some of these are presented below with their pros and cons.

Advisory or focus groups

Advisory or focus groups have continued to be a popular and often a successful way of ensuring that people with learning disabilities have ongoing investment in a research project. Ward & Simons (1998) cite the practical benefits of having input from advisors on, for example, designing letters to participants, and pictorial questionnaires. Rodgers (1999) highlights the need for one to consider the expectations of the degree to which people with learning disabilities should be included. She stresses the benefits of people contributing to such a process. However, one must consider the capabilities of people with learning disabilities to understand and influence the research process. Advisory or focus groups are therefore just one method and for people to fully participate and have their views represented, this must be combined with other methods. Researchers in this area have highlighted their own experiences of focus groups feeling tokenistic, to the extent that individuals that are more able tend to participate, excluding those who lack either the capability or confidence to present their views in such a forum. The skills of the facilitator in enabling participation would also play an important part in this process.

However limited advisory or focus groups may be in giving real power, they do have many advantages in a practical sense. Researchers can and do benefit from advice from people with learning disabilities, on understanding the issues they encounter as people with learning disabilities and on putting things in a way that the respondents are likely to understand. In one service in Wales, a follow up project on people who had been resettled from institutions 'A Better Life' (Parry R, Potter R 2006 'A Better Life' Bro Morganwg Service Development Report, unpublished paper) ran a series of focus groups. The 'Better Life' focus groups enabled the researcher to understand which issues had real meaning for those in the group and helped the researchers consider how to interpret the findings such that they related to people's 'real' experiences (see Box 13.2: A Better Life).

Co-researching

Co-researching implies an equal partnership where researchers work with people with learning disabilities to pool expertise. Usually it involves researchers bringing their knowledge and skills and people with learning disabilities bringing their unique perspective. Of all the forms of research in which people with

Box 13.2

'A Better Life'

A study of the effects of institutional closure on two cohorts of participants resettled from long-stay learning disability hospitals.

Research questions

- What was the impact of institutional closure on the people resettled to their local communities?
- To what extent were people engaged in the process of receiving and obtaining information about their resettlement?
- Had their lives truly changed once they had left the hospital?

Participants – two cohorts of participants resettled from two long-stay institutions with an additional small sample of individuals who were residing in hospital at the outset of the study. The smaller cohort was followed up over a nine-month period. The remaining participants had been established in their local communities (a range of 3 months to a maximum of 9 years).

The method

Stage One – In order to address the broad research questions, the researcher was involved in a number of different research activities over a twenty-four month period. The initial stage involved qualitative interviews with a cross-section of managers who had been involved in planning the hospital closures. The researchers used a grounded theory approach to analyse the content of the responses. The responses shaped the development of the research questions.

(Continued)

Box 13.2 (Continued)

Stage Two – The researcher designed and conducted a semi-structured qualitative interview. This involved the use of symbols and photographs to supplement the questions. Consent was considered at this stage and a pictorial consent booklet was designed for the purpose of the research. Careful consideration was made of inclusion criteria for participation in the research. The key criterion was the ability of individuals to engage in an interview on a one-to-one basis. All interviewees were given the option of having a carer or an advocate or a member of their family to be present in the interview.

Stage Three – Follow up interviews were conducted and the researcher ensured that participants were still consenting to participate in the project. The content of the qualitative follow up interviews was compared with the preliminary interviews and a summary report was produced.

Stage Four – Facilitation of focus groups. Given the small sample size, the researchers were concerned about the extent to which the narrative generated by participants could be generalized. The main findings were presented to a number of 'People First' self-advocacy groups across the geographical regions in which the research was conducted. Feedback from these groups was then used to reflect on the themes generated by the main participants.

Results

The study provided a description of the experiences of participants being resettled out of two long-stay hospitals. Themes generated were consistent with the issues identified by service managers and the focus groups. Experiences were mixed. Whilst resettlement was viewed generally as a positive experience, participants highlighted the negative aspects of being resettled into the community. Themes around social isolation, being devalued in their local society and realizing lost opportunities were produced by some. This highlighted the failure of some services to address these issues on an individual basis, particularly in the transition period between moving out of hospital and into their new homes. The study revealed how the resettlement process was influenced by two different ways of thinking: the rights of individuals to move to their local community; and the management of the process. The study identified those aspects of the resettlement process that could have been managed better in order to enable individuals to lead more integrated lives in their local community (Parry R, Potter R 2006 'A Better Life'. Bro Morganwg Service Development Report. Unpublished briefing paper for Bro Morannwg NHS Trust, Directorate of Learning Disabilities. Bro Morgannwg NHS, Cardiff).

---

learning disabilities have been major participants, the *autobiography* probably holds the greatest potential for full and equal partnership since the person who tells is unambiguously the 'expert'. The telling and recording of one's own story as an autobiography is an important way in which people may choose how they are portrayed, how their identity is presented and claimed by the person rather than constructed by 'powerful others' as case notes or biographical fragments (Atkinson & Walmsley 1999). This gives more of a balance in the research process, with the storyteller, and the researcher guiding the process, having an equal part to play in presenting information about the service user's experiences and/or accounts of themselves.

Occupational therapists will be familiar with the role that story telling and narrative can play within interventions. The importance of recognizing people's history and the path they have taken before they meet the therapist is central to occupational therapy practice. Using this knowledge to support people involved in autobiographical research is one contribution that the occupational therapist can make to inclusive research in this field.

Service evaluation

Another area where people with learning disabilities have been engaged to carry out research is in evaluation of services. Again this is an area where there is considerable value in user participation, not least because it presents a direct account. As Whittaker (1997) puts it:

> *User evaluators see services from a different angle, which gives a more complete picture. People with learning disabilities may well give*

more honest answers and may know better what questions to ask because they have experience of being on the receiving end (p. 28).

Inevitably, involvement in service evaluation adds value to positive imagery both for people in the service being evaluated who see people like themselves in valued roles, and for people who do the work, who learn new skills, get out and about and get paid for their efforts.

Users as 'consultants'

Involving people as co-researchers in more complex research projects is much more challenging. Mitchell (1997) explored the impact of self-advocacy on families. Three members of a Self-Advocacy Group for Learning Disability 'People First' participated in the study. Mitchell aimed to involve people with learning disabilities in the whole research process. The title 'consultants' was adopted and Mitchell made it her business to summarize the research on families with sons and daughters with learning disabilities for the benefit of the co-researchers. The co-researchers also assisted Mitchell in drawing up a list of factors they thought should feature in home life in which self-advocacy was recognized and encouraged. However, there was a limitation in how the co-researchers were able to participate and they were not able to actually carry out the interviews or analyse the data. This was largely their decision because of matters of confidentiality. The very fact that people with learning disabilities might not have the experience or skills to analyse data should not prevent them from being involved in the process. For example, Rolph (2000) ran a memories group, which invited people to present stories about their experience of life in their hostels. They contributed to the group reminiscence exercises and became involved in analysing the data. Aspects of data analysis began to take place from early stages of the group. Members began to prioritize the most important aspects of their lives in the hostels, highlighting themes for further discussion. Comments from some members contested the evidence representing the official voice challenging the known history (pp. 125–126). The contribution of Rolph (2000) was to produce a summary of relevant data and historical information to inform the memories group discussions and of course to act as facilitator, recorder and scribe and ultimately to write this up as a PhD project.

Action methods

Action methods cover a range of approaches that aim to involve participants directly in the research process. This ensures that participants are fully engaged through their own experiences (refer to glossary). One of the earliest ways in which people with learning disabilities have been directly engaged in major research projects has been participation in advisory or reference groups. Ward & Simons (1998) cite a number of practical benefits of having input from advisors on, for example, designing letters to participants and pictorial questionnaires. Rolph (2000) also used advisors in the Memories Group study. They met throughout the period of the research project, assisted in shaping the direction and content and were specifically able to agree on recording method, duration and reporting of outcome. An advantage of action methods, directly involving service users, is that one can engage a number of people in the research at the same time. This also gives participants an opportunity to interact with each other (whether they are service users, therapists or managers), giving an added richness to the narratives that service users provide.

Occupational therapists have a role alongside others to consider how they can actively involve service users in aspects of their service, including research. This may seem a daunting task so it is important to start small. Considering some of the information in this chapter in relation to your own service may act as a starting point. The reader activity below is intended to get you thinking about how you might start this process.

Reader activity

- What aspects of service delivery and user participation could be the subject of a research study or audit evaluation?
- What research methods could best be applied to this research study?
- What active role could service users play in the research process?
- How would service users be identified to become involved?
- How would service users be engaged and supported to play an active role throughout the process (consider the ethical issues)?

- Who would be able to support service users and the researcher throughout the process (e.g. organization, manager, colleagues, service user groups)?
- What are the first steps to start the research?

Ethical issues in participatory research

Working ethically raises a number of issues that cut across all types of inclusive service evaluation and research. All researchers are now required to find ethical approval for their studies and this can be a lengthy and difficult process, particularly if service users from any field are directly involved in the study. The process is rigorous and involves ethics committees, parents or others (such as advocates). Thomas & Woods (2004) state that at the planning stage ethical criteria have to ensure not only informed consent, but confidentiality, absence of harm and that the contribution is a positive one (p. 253). In the field of learning disabilities the researcher has the added issue of how to engage research participants with these dilemmas so that as participants they are fully aware of the implications of being involved in the study and as researchers they are enabled to implement any procedures that protect participants in the study.

Some of the additional areas that may need addressing in learning disability research are explored further below. Occupational therapists and others have a key responsibility when engaging service users in research to be aware of these factors and put mechanisms in place to address them. Using existing support from ethical committees and research groups within your setting and from your professional body should ensure that ethical practices are adhered to. This includes being aware of different requirements in different agencies and seeking advice from those who have implemented similar work before.

The context of care

A significant proportion of health provision is provided in social care settings and service users may find it difficult to separate aspects of the care they receive from different agencies, such as health-specific services, supported accommodation, local authority day centres, and support from the voluntary sector. Experiences in one setting may for many individuals with learning disabilities be transferred to other settings, making accurate appraisal of their experience difficult. Any research or service evaluation would need to consider the context in which a person receives care and support and where people are receiving services across agencies to find ways of cross referencing experience. The views of others in a particular context may be one way of checking research data or evaluating service policies and written records. This would help the researcher separate those elements that are relevant to the particular research question.

Levels of intervention

Many people with learning disabilities receive direct and indirect interventions from a range of professionals in the services which support them. This might include indirect interventions such as staff training as well as direct clinical intervention. In carrying out any type of service evaluation, occupational therapists would have to make it clear at the outset which element of the service they are evaluating and on whom it impacts.

Research participants should be provided with clear information that clearly states what the study is about, what their role in it would be, how they will be supported to participate and what the expected outcomes will be. An important consideration is how the ethical dilemmas will be dealt with, such as confidentiality within the study and how any products of the research will be shared. As stated earlier in this chapter, good information presented in a user-friendly format is more likely to lead to active participation in making decisions about treatment options and feedback on what service users receive.

Population

In conducting research in learning disability services, objective research methods such as randomized controlled trials are harder to achieve given the small population and the fact that a great proportion of service users present with severe communicative difficulties and significant intellectual impairments. This would make it difficult to match control groups for utilizing quantitative research methodologies.

Qualitative methods lend themselves to exploring and understanding by interpreting the life experience of others. Qualitative methods also ensure that the subject being explored or investigated is set within the context of an individual's experience, life circumstances or indeed any other information that is pertinent to the issue in hand. Occupational therapists can be in a good position to evaluate these areas in their direct work with people with learning disabilities. Very often therapists work with individuals on an individual basis to explore issues relevant to occupational balance and by using a method such as single subject case study can objectively measure and analyse changes in occupations which also can demonstrate an individual's progress (Wilson 2000). Other methods include the use of narrative (Wicks & Whitefield 2003) or establishing a focus group (Bloor et al 2001) to explore common issues around service delivery. Useful further reading can be found in social research based books such as Bloor et al (2001), Denzin & Lincoln (2000).

Finding participants

Occupational therapists wishing to conduct inclusive research with people with learning disabilities need to consider that for many individuals this will be a new experience. It may also be a new experience for the therapist. Walmsley (1993) speculated on the viability of approaching people with learning disabilities who are relative strangers to the researcher, with an invitation to participate in research. For the person with a learning disability, research is a somewhat esoteric activity beyond their usual experience. The problem is exacerbated by the stigma associated with learning disabilities and researchers may avoid telling people this is why they are of interest as it could lead to individuals refusing to take part.

Self-advocacy groups are another avenue to explore for research participants. The support afforded for individuals or groups belonging to a self-advocacy organization is one reason for their use as a source of participants. The problem with self-advocacy is that it may also restrict the number of people who participate in research, as some people participate time after time and others remain excluded.

To summarize the above issues, the key to any success in inclusive research is to ensure that individuals are clear about their participation, that there are opportunities for accountability and that user participation as discussed at the beginning of this chapter is meaningful rather than tokenistic (refer to Box 13.3).

Informed consent

Informed consent must be seen as more than a single 'signing off' of a single event. Consent must be viewed as a decision process in which an individual is

Box 13.3

Learning points: user participation

- User participation should be understood in its broadest sense as a key issue concerning the social inclusion of people with learning disabilities. It includes how people are involved in decisions about their own services and the extent to which they are supported to be part of society
- Normalization or SRV has set basic principles in learning disability services, which have included the views of people with learning disabilities
- Normalization has meant that people with learning disabilities are more available to provide feedback on their experiences
- Normalization has ensured that people with learning disabilities are valued and need to be central to service planning, evaluation and design
- Although the principles of normalization are well established in learning disability services, service planning and research involving people with learning disabilities is limited
- Service planning and research initiatives need to consider making service users more widely represented (to escape tokenism) and relevant to people's actual experiences
- Service users need to be more supported to take part in planning and providing feedback on services
- Person-centred planning (PCP) has been adopted in recent policy initiatives and provides potential for service users' views to be very influential in service planning and delivery. It also provides a means to begin to address the issues of social inclusion. However, these are not inevitable outcomes of simply introducing PCP but are dependent on services changing and promoting person-centred action.

presented with information and gives assent or provides acceptance of something done or planned by another. Gaining informed consent is not something that can be captured by even the most sophisticated of inclusive research methodologies. McCarthy (1998) argues that:

It is one thing to consent to the face-to-face aspects of the research i.e. consent to talking to an individual researcher and it is quite another thing to consent to the hidden or behind the scenes aspects of research i.e. the researcher going away with your answers, analysing them, coming to conclusions about you and your situation and then informing other people what they have discovered about you and people like you (p. 143).

The issue of informed consent presents one with a dilemma in learning disability services. Confining research only to those who can truly give informed consent may well exclude a larger number of people with learning disabilities from being involved at all. One way to overcome this is to use reference or advisory groups such as a People First campaigning self-advocacy group or local MENCAP group to assist and explore ways to make sure that consultations with participants about informed consent are as open and accessible as possible. The use of advocates or guardians who can give informed consent on behalf of another is one way to ensure that exploitation is minimized. However, this presents with the additional problem that once a third person is involved in this way, there may be issues related to confidentiality and privacy. A good balance needs to be struck, therefore, by the researcher in consultation with the reference group, in exploring the ethics of this particular issue. However, the use of third parties to resolve this issue can only be to address broader issues. Specific issues related to the person, which may be sensitive ones, would need to be addressed at an individual level with the person and/or another who can advocate for them.

Payment

Some research has gone to great lengths to ensure that people are paid and recognized for their work. However, much inclusive research operates outside normal funding processes so often there is no funding to pay people the going rate for a particular job. In reality, a good proportion of research relies on the goodwill of participants and those supporting them, with limited funding of expenses incurred for participating such as transport. This illustrates the difficulties of introducing the principles of inclusive research without fully planning or acknowledging implications or provision for research participation. A practical way of addressing this is to air the issues and concerns and allow those taking part to make informed decisions on how they can be rewarded for their contribution and time.

Power

Reference has already been made to the extent to which researchers determine the research process and outcome. Considering the questions below can help the researcher to address the power imbalance between researchers and participants. Addressing these questions jointly with research participants, advisors, and co-researchers may be one way of working.

Reader activity

- What are the problems that any participants may encounter in their involvement? For example, confidentiality, not being able to speak for themselves, the use of advocates, etc.
- Is this research going to make a positive contribution to people's lives?
- Do the advantages of this research outweigh any disadvantages?
- Would I be willing to participate in this research in its current form?
- Does this research focus matter to people with learning disabilities?

Exploring and answering these questions creates a grounded approach, addressing the key issue of whether the research is relevant to a person's life and will make a difference to them or the service they receive in the long run. It also enables the researcher to make any changes and adjust research plans prior to ethical approval being sought.

Skills

One issue that has not been addressed fully in participatory service evaluation and research relates to individuals with learning disabilities acquiring skills. Most professionals and researchers would have received some training to learn about specific methods and how to use research. People with learning disabilities may wish to develop such skills themselves. A challenge for professionals within services is to cascade such skills to the people for whom they offer a service. In the absence of this, professionals and researchers have a duty to consider the relevance of research and the impact on particular individual service users. Walmsley et al (2003) suggest that user participation could be increased in user controlled organizations, for example, 'People First'. The user organization might well hold funds and employ researchers providing the necessary training and support. In the UK, the number of leading self-advocacy groups is very limited and confined to a few service vanguards. The four step model of user participation presented in this chapter needs to underpin every aspect of service delivery. Any inclusive research or service evaluative approach needs to be considered with a staged model in mind.

Summary

User participation is a broad area and an important issue, but there is no right way to enable service users to participate. There is a need to explore different strategies and possibilities depending on the needs of the individual or group and the objective of the particular task.

In this chapter, we have endeavoured to identify areas that are relevant to user participation. We have identified some of the dilemmas in attempting to be totally inclusive in learning disability practice and in research. Whilst researchers in the field of learning disabilities have looked for more inventive ways to enable people with learning disabilities to do research one must recognize that a good proportion of the population would not demonstrate the necessary skills or understanding to do so. However, this does not mean that the issue of participation is not relevant for them. Given our wider definition of participation, person-centred approaches using total communication and especially active support can enable even the more severely disabled service users to participate in daily life. Indeed, it should be noted that it is unlikely that every person with learning disabilities may want to get involved in research or service evaluation. It is more likely that most people would like to enjoy some of the good things in life such as having interesting things to do, and rewarding relationships with other people who interact positively and communicate effectively with them.

We have presented a consistent argument that participation is about enabling people with learning disabilities to get a better quality of life by helping to make services more responsive and relevant to their needs. With this in mind, occupational therapists have a duty to consider all aspects of their practice and to take responsibility for making user participation possible at a level by which they can influence. The failure of health professionals to explain not only what we do, but also how and why we do it has often led to the mystification of health service delivery and further marginalization rather than inclusion of service users. Occupational therapists have key philosophies and principles that embrace service user participation and are therefore well placed to introduce and advocate for people with learning disabilities within their role and to make inclusive service provision a central role.

Box 13.4

Case illustration: service users' participation

This case illustration explores the underpinning philosophy discussed in this chapter and the processes involving facilitating service users' participation towards supporting an individual in accessing community facilities. From this, the reader is encouraged to reflect on evaluation and consider how this process might be taken forward to involving service users in research.

Daniel has a diagnosis of Fragile-X syndrome. Most boys with Fragile-X syndrome are described as having moderate or severe learning disability with difficulties adapting to the environment, problems with thinking, problem solving, concept understanding, information processing and overall intelligence. Daniel has a moderate learning disability with cognition problems associated with short attention span and difficulty staying on task. He also presents with sensory motor problems including clumsiness, difficulties with walking and balance and sensitivity to light or sound.

He demonstrates anxiety when there are changes in routine, upcoming stressful events, difficulty coping with crowds or new situations, which can lead to distractibility and impulsive behavioural problems. Daniel finds conversation difficult, with perseveration of speech and has poor eye contact.

Daniel appears very interested in activities such as cooking, but has not had any opportunities to get involved and wants to participate in a range of activities in the community such as shopping,

(Continued)

Box 13.4 (Continued)

swimming etc. He needs to have the appropriate support to participate in any of these activities. Currently, there is a change in the support staff to do this and recruitment of new staff is being planned to support Daniel in accessing community facilities.

Reader activity

1. How would the occupational therapist ensure participation and Person-centred planning for Daniel in the first phase of the assessment process?

2. By applying the four steps to user involvement (refer to Figure 13.1) describe how Daniel's involvement illustrates the processes of the active support model.

3. How does Daniel's situation illustrate the principles of SRV and present day service provision?

4. Reflect on facilitating service user involvement in service development or research.

Further reading

Bloor M, Frankland J, Thomas M, Robson K 2001 Focus group in social research. London, SAGE

Denzin NK, Lincoln YS (eds) 2000 Handbook of qualitative research. Thousand Oaks, CA, Sage

Hollis V, Openhsaw S, Goble R 2002 Conducting focus groups: purpose and practicalities. British Journal of Occupational Therapy 65(1):2–8

Laver Fawcett A 2007 Principles of assessment and outcome measurements for occupational therapists and physiotherapists: theory, skills and application. Chichester, Wiley

Miles BM, Huberman MA 1994 An expanded sourcebook: qualitative data analysis, 2nd edn. Thousand Oaks, CA, Sage Publications

Thomas D, Woods H 2004 Working with people with learning disabilities. Theory and practice. London, Jessica Kinglsey Publishers, pp 246–257

Useful resources

http://www.dh.gov.uk/en/SocialCare/Deliveringadultsocialcare/Learningdisabilities/index.htm

References

Aichison J, Greig R, Hersov E et al 2001 Deciding together: working with people with learning disabilities to plan services and support. London, CCDC, Kings College London

Anderson SR 1987 The management of staff behaviour in residential treatment facilities: a review of training techniques. In: Hogg J, Mittler P (eds) Staff training in mental handicap. London, Croom Helm, pp 343–367

Aspis S 2000 Researching our history: Who is in charge? In: Brigham L, Atkinson D, Jackson M et al (eds) Crossing boundaries: Change and continuity in the history of learning disabilities. Kidderminister, BILD

Atkinson D 1986 Engaging competent others: A study of the support networks of people with mental handicap. British Journal of Social Work 16:83–101

Atkinson D 2001 Researching the history of learning disability using oral and life history methods. Unpublished PhD thesis. Milton Keynes, Open University

Atkinson D, Walmsley J 1999 Using autobiographical approaches with people with learning difficulties. Disability and Society 14:203–216

Beadle-Brown J 2006 Person-centred approaches and quality of life. Tizard Learning Disability Review 11(3):4–13

Bloor M, Frankland J, Thomas M, Robson K 2001 Focus group in social research. London, SAGE

Blunden R 1988 Quality of life in persons with disabilities: issues in the development of services. In: Brown R (ed.) Quality of life for handicapped people. London, Croom Helm

Canadian Association of Occupational Therapists 1997 Enabling occupation: an occupational therapy perspective. Ottawa ON, CAOT Publications ACE

Chappell A 1992 Towards a sociological critique of the normalisation principle. Disability, Handicap and Society 7(1): 35–51

College of Occupational Therapists 2005 Code of ethics and professional conduct. London, COT

Denzin NK, Lincoln Y (eds) 2005 The sage handbook of qualitative research, 3rd edn. London, Sage Publications

Department of Health 2001 Valuing people. London, HMSO

Department of Health 2002 Valuing people: guidance for implementation groups towards person centred approaches. London, HMSO

Department of Health 2005 The Mental Capacity Act. London, HMSO

Emerson E, Hatton C 1994 Moving out: relocation from hospital to community. London, HMSO

Emerson E, Stancliffe RJ 2004 Planning and action. Comments on Mansell and Beadle-Brown. Journal of Applied Research in Intellectual Disabilities 17(1):23–27

1989 Staffed housing for with severe and profound handicaps: The Andover t. Kidderminster, BIMH ations

991 Using behavioural les in the development ctive housing services for with severe or profound handicap. In: Remington) The challenge of severe handicap. London, John pp 285–316

004 Can person-centred g fulfil a strategic planning omments on Mansell and -Brown. Journal of Applied ch in Intellectual Disabilities 27–30

Felce D, Grant G (eds) 1998 Towards a full life: researching policy innovations for people with learning disabilities. London, Butterworth Heinemann

Felce D, Perry J 1995a The extent of support for ordinary living in staffed housing: the relationship between staffing levels, resident dependency, staff/resident interactions and resident activity patterns. Social Science and Medicine 40:799–810

Felce D, Perry J 1995b Living under the strategy: do outcomes for users of Welsh community residential services live up to the All Wales Strategy underlying principles? British Journal of Learning Disabilities 23: 102–105

Felce D, Jones E, Lowe K 2002 Active support: planning daily activities and support for people with severe mental retardation. In: Holburn S, Vietze PM (eds) Person-centred planning; research, practice, and future directions. Baltimore, Paul H Brookes

Gold MW 1980 Try Another Way Training Manual. Illinois, Research Press

Goodley D 1998 Appraising self-advocacy in the lives of people with learning difficulties. Unpublished PhD Thesis. University of Sheffield

Holburn S, Vietze PM (eds) 2002 Person-centred planning; research, practice, and future directions. Baltimore, Paul H Brookes

Houts PS, Scott RA 1975 Goal planning with developmentally disabled people. The Pennsylvania State University College of Medicine. Pennsylvania, The Milton S. Hershey Medical Centre

Humphreys S, Evans G, Todd S 1987 Lifelines: an account of life experiences of seven people with a mental handicap who use the NIMROD service. London, King's Fund

Jones AA, Blunden R, Coles E, Evans G, Porterfield J 1987 Evaluating the impact of training, supervisor feedback, self monitoring and collaborative goal setting on staff and client behaviour. In: Hogg J, Mittler P (eds) Staff training in mental handicap. London, Croom Helm, pp 213–300

Jones E, Lowe K 2005 Empowering service users through active support. In: O'Brien P, Sullivan M (eds) Allies in emancipation: shifting from providing service to being of support. South Melbourne, Thomson/Dunmore Press

Jones E, Perry J, Lowe K et al 1999 Opportunity and the promotion of activity among adults with severe intellectual disability living in community residences: the impact of training staff in active support. Journal of Intellectual Disability Research 43(3):164–178

Jones E, Felce D, Lowe K et al 2001a Evaluation of the dissemination of active support training in staffed community residences. American Journal of Mental Retardation 106(4):344–358

Jones E, Felce D, Lowe K et al 2001b Evaluation of the dissemination of active support training and training trainers. Journal of Applied Research in Intellectual Disabilities 14:79–99

Kiernan C 1999 Participation in research by people with learning disability: origins and issues. British

Journal of Learning Disabilities 27(2):43–47

Kincaid D, Fox L 2002 Person-centered planning and positive behaviour support. In: Holburn S, Vietze PM (eds) Person-centred planning; research, practice, and future directions. Baltimore, Paul H. Brookes

Lowe K, de Paiva S 1989. The evaluation of NIMROD a community-based service for people with a mental handicap. The service, staff and clients. Cardiff, Mental Handicap in Wales Applied Research Unit

Lowe K, de Paiva S 1991a NIMROD: An overview. a summary report of a 5 year research study of community based service provision for people with learning disabilities. London, HMSO

Lowe K, de Paiva S 1991b Clients' community and social contacts: results of a 5 year longitudinal study. Journal of Mental Deficiency Research 35:308–323

Lowe K, de Paiva S, Felce D 1993 Effects of a community-based service on adaptive and maladaptive behaviours: a longitudinal study. Journal of Intellectual Disability Research 37(1):3–22

Mansell J, Beadle-Brown J 2004a Person-centred planning or person centred action? Policy and practice in intellectual disability services. Journal of Applied Research in Intellectual Disabilities 17:11–19

Mansell J, Beadle–Brown J 2004b Person-centred planning or person centred action? A response to the commentaries. Journal of Applied Research in Intellectual Disabilities 17(1):31–35

Mansell J, Beasley F 1993 Small staffed houses for people with a severe learning disability and challenging behaviour. British Journal of Social Work 23:329–344

Mansell J, Felce D, de Kock U, Jenkins J (1982) Increasing purposeful activity of severely and profoundly mentally handicapped adults, Behaviour Research and Therapy 20: 593–604

Mansell J, Felce D, Jenkins J, de Kock U, Toogood S 1987 Developing staffed housing for people with mental handicap. Tunbridge Wells, Costello

McCarthy M 1998 Interviewing people with learning disabilities about sensitive topics: a discussion of ethical issues. British Journal of Learning Disabilties 26(4):140–145

McGill P, Toogood S 1994 Organizing community placements. In: Emerson E, McGill P, Mansell J (eds) Severe learning disabilities and challenging behaviour; designing high quality services. London, Chapman & Hall, pp 232–258

McGill P, Emerson E, Mansell J 1994 Individually designed residential provision for people with seriously challenging behaviours. In: Emerson E, McGill P, Mansell J (eds) Severe learning disabilities and challenging behaviour; designing high quality services. London, Chapman & Hall, pp 119–157

Mitchell P 1997 The impact of self-advocacy on families. Disability and Society 12(1):43–56

Moores B, Grant GWB 1976 On the nature and incidence of staff interactions in hospitals for the mentally handicapped. International Journal of Nursing Studies 13:69–81

Nicholls R, Andrew R 1990 A stand for advocacy: Report of the Advocacy Project. Melbourne, The Office of the Public Advocacy

O'Brien J, O'Brien CL (eds) 1998 A little book about person centred planning. Toronto, Inclusion Press

O'Brien J, O'Brien CL 2002 The origins of person-centred planning: a community of practice perspective. In: Holburn S, Vietze PM (eds) Person-centred planning; research, practice, and future directions. Baltimore, Paul H. Brookes

O'Brien S, Johnson K 1987 Improving Consumer Participation. Community Quarterly 13:4–14

Oliver M 1996 Defining disability and impairment: issues at stake. In: Barnes C, Mercer G (eds) Exploring the divide. Leeds, The Disability Press

Open University 1996 Learning disability: working as equal people. Milton Keynes, Open University

Oswin M 1971 The empty hours. Harmondsworth, Penguin

Park K 2002 Objects of reference in practice and theory. London, Sense

Parry R, Potter R 2006 A better life. Bro Morganwg Service Development Report. Unpublished briefing paper for Bro Morgannwg NHS Trust, Directorate of Learning Disabilities. Cardiff, Bro Morgannwg NHS

Porterfield J, Blunden R 1979 Establishing activity periods in special needs within adult training centres. A replication study. Cardiff, Mental Handicap in Wales Applied Research Unit.

Porterfield J, Blunden R, Blenitt E 1980 Improving environments for profoundly handicapped adults: Using prompts and social attention to maintain high group engagement. Behaviour Modification 4: 225–241.

Potts M, Fido R 1991 A fit person to be removed. Plymouth, Northcote House

Richards S 1984 Community care of the handicapped: Consumer perspectives. Birmingham, University of Birmingham

Ritchie P, Sanderson H, Routledge M, Kilbane J 2003 People, plans and practicalities, achieving change through person centred planning. Edinburgh, SHS Ltd

Rodgers J 1999 Trying to get it right: undertaking research involving people with learning difficulties. Disability and Society 14(4): 421–433

Rolph S 2000 The history of community care for people with learning difficulties in Norfolk 1930–1980. In: Walmsley J, Johnson K (eds) Inclusive research with people with learning disabilities: past present and

future. London, Jessica Kingsley
Publishers, p 152

Sanderson H, Kennedy J, Ritchie P,
Goodwin G 1997 People, plans
and possibilities, exploring person
centred planning. Edinburgh,
SHS Ltd

Sanderson H, Jones E, Brown K 2001
Active support and person centred
planning: strange bedfellows or
ideal partners? Tizard Learning
Disability Review 7:31–38

Strong G, Hedges Y 2000 Too
many pages. SCOVOS guide
to involving service users to
make services better. Cardiff,
Standing conference of voluntary
organisations for people with a
leaning disability in Wales

Thomas D, Woods H 2004 Working
with people with learning
disabilities. Theory and practice.
London, Jessica Kingsley
Publishers, pp 246–257

Toogood S 1995 Interactive training
materials. Clwyd Health Authority

Toogood S, Jenkins, J, Felce D,
de Kock U 1983 Opportunity
plans. University of Southampton:
Health Care Evaluation Research
Team. Southampton, University of
Southampton

Towell D, Sanderson H 2004 Person-
centred planning in its strategic

context: reframing the Mansell/
Beadle-Brown critique. Journal of
Applied Research in Intellectual
Disabilities 17(1):17–22

Victorian Government 1986 The
Intellectually Disabled Persons
Services Act, Section V. Mental
Illness. Melbourne, Victoria,
Awareness Council

Walmsley J 1993 Women first: lessons
in participation. Critical Social
Policy 38:86–99

Walmsley J, Downer J 1997 Shouting
the loudest: self advocacy, power
and diversity. In: Ramcharan P
(ed.) Empowerment in everyday
life. London, Jessica Kingsley
Publishers

Walmsley J, Johnson K 2003 Inclusive
research with people with learning
disabilities. Past, present and
future. London, Jessica Kingsley
Publishers

Ward L, Simons K 1998 Practising
partnership: Funding people with
learning difficulties in research.
British Journal of Learning
Disabilities 26(4):128–131

Welsh Office 1983 The All Wales
Strategy for the Development of
Services for Mentally Handicapped
People. Cardiff, Welsh Office

Whittaker A 1997 Looking at our
services: service evaluation by

people with learning difficulties.
London, King's Fund Centre

Wicks A, Whitefield G 2003 Value
of life stories in occupation-based
research. Australian Occupational
Therapy Journal 50:86–91

Wilson SL 2000 Single case
experimental designs. In:
Breakwell GM, Hammond S, Fife-
Schaw C (eds) Research methods in
psychology, 2nd edn. London, Sage,
pp 59–74

Wolfensberger W 1972 The principle
of normalisation in human services.
Toronto, National Institute on
Mental Retardation

Wolfensberger W 1983 Social role
valorization: a proposed new term
for the principle of normalisation.
Mental Retardation 21:234–239

Wolfensberger W, Glenn L 1975
Program analysis of service
systems: handbook and manual,
3rd edn. Toronto, National
Institute on Mental Retardation

Wolfensberger W, Thomas S 1983
Passing (Program Analysis of
Service System's Implementation
Of Normalisation Goals):
Normalization criteria and ratings
manual. Toronto, National Institute
on Mental Retardation

Appendix 13.1 Case illustration: service users' participation, possible answers

1. How would the occupational therapist ensure participation and person-centred planning for Daniel in the first phase of the assessment process? How could the active support model be used to help Daniel?

The occupational therapist's primary role is to ensure Daniel has control of his own life by helping him to make his own lifestyle choices and ensuring his wishes are supported by the carers. This will involve the occupational therapist working with Daniel through the occupational therapy process to identify his perception of needs and supporting his involvement in training carers to give Daniel appropriate support.

By establishing a working relationship and taking time to get to know Daniel the occupational therapist can start to assess his skill abilities to access community facilities. This involves non-standardized assessments using observation, self assessment checklist and risk assessment to ensure safety issues are taken into account. Using a standardized observational assessment such as AMPS enables the occupational therapist to develop a profile of that person's ADL motor and process raw scores. In this way the therapist is able to identify which of the individuals skill's/actions are effective and which are not. This information explains why the person experiences a difficulty. The benefits of using a standardized tool are:

- It predicts what level of task challenge Daniel can manage
- It gives an indication of Daniel's capacity to benefit from restorative interventions or compensatory interventions. Individuals with lower ADL ability may be less responsive to restorative occupation, but possibly able to benefit from adaptive occupation
- It gives an objective measurement of any performance improvement that occurs following interventions and aids ongoing quality assurance measurements and evaluation.

2. By applying the Four Steps to User Involvement (Figure 13.1) describe how Daniel's involvement illustrates the processes of the active support model.

Step 1: Assessment – getting and giving information

To identify how Daniel's problems were affecting his capacity to cross roads to access community facilities, the occupational therapists used non-standardized assessments (e.g. self-assessment checklist) as well as a standardized test (e.g. AMPS) to gain a better understanding of his cognition, visual spatial skills, attention to task and motor processing skills. This helps to ensure a person-centred approach by identifying the individual's occupational capacities and to coherently explain to his carers the probable reasons for his difficulties.

Step 2: Planning and consultation

The therapist collaborates with Daniel to identify and agree what support is needed and what the potential risks are. After gaining consent Daniel was videoed using pavements and crossing roads. Afterwards, together they reviewed the video, which was paused at key stages. Daniel, using a pictorial self-assessment, circled the skill areas where he needed further learning and/or additional carer support. During the video analysis Daniel recognized that:

- He was unable to filter sound and visual stimuli effectively, which gave him difficulty focusing on the task
- His cognition and safety awareness were faulty e.g. he did not consistently stop at busy entrances and look for cars that were exiting/entering
- He did not have the visual–spatial ability to judge the speed and direction of the vehicles and make a judgement about when to cross
- His ataxic gait and lack of task focus (looking around rather than ahead) led to him weaving across the pavement with a risk of inadvertently stepping into the path of oncoming traffic
- He also had difficulty passing pedestrians walking in the opposite direction.

Step 3: Interventions and participation

Daniel identified with the occupational therapist the need to create a tool to train carers (family, paid, voluntary and friends) to show them how to give him appropriate support for crossing roads to access community facilities.

He had enjoyed the videoing and it was agreed that a training video could be produced to demonstrate best practice. This was achieved through a graded process of task analysis to formulate:

- Cue cards designed with digital photos of Daniel explaining his wishes inside speech bubbles
- Performance assessments were created (with photos and text) so that Daniel, or someone nominated by him, could assess and sign off carer competence.

Step 4: Outcome and evaluation

To enable Daniel to establish both autonomy and control of his goals a process of shared decision-making with his support manager and occupational therapist identified that the video could form the basis of a pilot for video-based training for staff. In this way Daniel was taking responsibility in the process of staff recruitment for himself. With support Daniel piloted the video on 18 job candidates, many of whom had no previous experience as carers. He showed each candidate his video and gave them his cue cards to study. They then did a job test, supporting him on a community presence outing. Every candidate, even those who, following interviews, were not considered suitable for employment, accurately followed the guidelines. The only change needed to the video was to add a more robust explanation of how to help Daniel appropriately to stop and check for traffic at entrances.

3. How does Daniel's situation illustrate the principles of SRV and present day service provision?

Services should treat people with respect and dignity and support them in overcoming barriers to inclusion.

The vision for adults is that everyone has a contribution to make and the right to control their lives.

Services should be person-centred, seamless and proactive. They should support independence, not dependence and allow everyone to enjoy a good quality of life, including the ability to contribute fully to our communities.

Service providers should focus on positive outcomes and well-being, and work proactively to include the most disadvantaged groups by ensuring they have more control, giving them more choices and helping them decide how their needs can best be met. This involves giving them the chance to do the things that other people take for granted and giving the best quality of support and protection to those with the highest levels of need.

Through current legislation and policies this will be achieved by changing the ways social care services are designed. Individuals will be given more control through self-assessment and through planning and management of their own services; this will be achieved by developing new and innovative ways of supporting individuals. Since April 2002 all social care organizations registered with the National Care Standards Commission have to comply with National Minimum Standards. Formulating person-centred planning and staff training will assist carers to understand the principles of care, understand their role and understand the particular needs of the individual while maintaining safety.

4. Reflect on facilitating service user involvement in service development or research.

Benchmarking

The video training package, put together collaboratively by Daniel and local health care professionals, is a vital component of providing safe care and establishing a competent work force. It is an effective and sustainable way to improve carer performance.

The video is a benchmark of the care requested by Daniel and enables him to influence and provide carers with the necessary learning support. It can also form the basis on which Daniel can establish effective outcome and service evaluation. The benefit of training carers in this way enables Daniel to be involved in all decisions taken about his care. It allows him to take the lead role in training carers who work with him and ensures consistency of practice and staff performance.

Service user participation and research

Daniel's situation identifies the advantage of directly involving service users in their goals. By employing similar methods to those used by Daniel to ensure clear information, the potential of involving action research methods with service users can be established. Establishing clear criteria and taking into account ethical considerations there is potential for the service user to participate, to inform and change current practice. Equally, the use of qualitative research methods such as single case study, narrative or focus groups can form the basis of establishing appropriate skills towards involvement in research.

14

Working with people with learning disabilities and their networks

Sally Donati

Overview

One of the privileges of working with people with learning disabilities is meeting and joining the complex networks that are often part of their lives. The challenge for the occupational therapist is to clarify the focus of involvement in order to be as effective as possible. It is therefore important at the outset to establish what is being asked for and how to work collaboratively with the network in the best interests of the person with learning disabilities.

This chapter describes the range of people who may be part of the network. It clarifies the roles of the occupational therapist as a member of specialist health care services and relates these to Valuing People (DoH 2001) and associated documents. It then goes on to outline a collaborative approach that recognizes and builds on the strengths and resources of the network. This approach is then described in detail from the point of referral to closure.

Learning Outcomes

By the end of this chapter you will be able to:
- Identify some of the people who may be part of the network of a person with learning disabilities
- Identify the range of different roles the occupational therapist may adopt when working with the network
- Apply the processes for clarifying referral, assessment and intervention
- Discuss collaborative working practices
- Identify approaches to risk management
- Describe closure processes when working with networks.

People who may be part of the network of a person with learning disabilities

Some people with learning disabilities live in their own homes and access their local community with little or no additional support. They may only become known to specialist services if circumstances change, for instance because of concerns from another agency about their coping skills, a change in their health, or in their informal support networks.

The majority of people with learning disabilities, however, will have lived in complex systems of support for much of their lives. Valuing People (DoH 2001) acknowledges this when it emphasizes the role of specialist health services in enhancing the competencies of paid staff in both specialist and mainstream services as well as working therapeutically with families and people with learning disabilities. The term 'network' covers a range of different people. Many people with learning disabilities live in their local community with, or close to, their families (Williams & Robinson, 2001). Apart from family members, the informal network may comprise neighbours, friends, shopkeepers or people in the local pub. Formal support is usually provided by professionals and support workers from specialist respite, day, domiciliary and employment services. Individuals not living with family increasingly live in supported living where they have their own tenancy and support arranged according to need. Although the number of people with their own tenancy is increasing, a much larger number of people still live in residential homes (Emerson & Hatton 2000) or in long-stay hospitals, residential campuses or private institutions (Mansell 2005).

The terms informal and formal support are used throughout this chapter rather than 'carer', which is only used when referred to in the literature. Many so called 'carers' dislike the term, as it fails to acknowledge the range of possible roles and relationships they may have, many of which are reciprocal (DoH 2001; Williams & Robinson, 2001). Table 14.1 summarizes

the range of accommodation and resources people with learning disabilities may access in different settings.

Apart from families, a wide range of people might consult the specialist health care service. These include paid staff, health care professionals and people working in community resources (e.g. occupational therapists in other services such as social services or wheelchair clinics, college tutors, employers, care managers, people working in leisure centres, employment schemes). As people with learning disabilities increasingly use local non-segregated community resources, occupational therapists will find themselves relating to a wider group of people.

Occupational therapy roles in working with the support network

This next section outlines the roles of the Specialist Healthcare Team as described in Valuing People

Table 14.1 Summary of resources that people with learning disabilities may use in different settings

	Institutional	Moving out	Community living
Where the person lives	NHS Institution/residential campus/forensic service/large registered care home	Registered care home Hostel Group home Adult placement	Own tenancy in a general needs housing or supported living project. Separate support arranged as and when required
How the person spends their time	In house daycare/sheltered workshops or horticultural opportunities or college usually in segregated groups or settings	Day centre/sheltered employment/training scheme Segregated youth and clubs (e.g. Gateway clubs) Holidays with other residents	Range of opportunities from college classes, mainstream community leisure and recreational activities, supported and open employment, selected and accessed independently
How health care needs are met	In house and/or local health care provision. Where NHS funded, Continuing Care review and advice from specialist health care service from NHS Trust in place of origin	In house and local health care provision. Referrals to specialist learning disabilities service from provider staff on behalf of service user	Local primary and secondary health care provision independently accessed or facilitated by specialist learning disabilities service where necessary

(DoH 2001) and explores the occupational therapy contribution in particular.

Valuing People describes the roles of the Specialist Healthcare team as follows:

1. Clinical and therapeutic

2. Health promotion

3. Health facilitation–linking with primary and secondary health care teams

4. Teaching

5. Service development.

In broad terms these describe the individual clinical, therapeutic as well as advisory, teaching and service development roles. Occupational therapists engage in these both in a profession-specific capacity and as members of the specialist team. The term 'non-profession specific' is different from the term 'generic'. The term non-profession specific describes a specialist role in learning disabilities services that contributes to the shared tasks of the service e.g. representing the team at a school transition meeting, but is not occupational therapy specific. A generic role could describe a task unrelated to learning disabilities such as teaching assessment of wheelchairs. It is important for the occupational therapist to be aware of balancing the different roles taken on.

The report New Ways of Working in Health Services for People with Learning Disabilities (Valuing People Support Team 2004a) emphasizes the need for specialist health care teams to focus less on individual clinical and therapeutic interventions and instead to work with staff in specialist and mainstream resources. The request to the team from a network might be described as an invitation to be a resource to the network in order that they can continue in their supporting role. Jones (1995) highlights the fact that the occupational therapy interventions in adult learning disability services assist the social and physical environment to accommodate the needs of individuals and provide opportunities for development. This is different from the developmental approach, which often underpins adolescent and children's services, where the focus is on developing the skills of the child or young person.

The following case in Box 14.1 illustrates how the occupational therapist may take on all five of the above roles when working with one client.

The clinical and therapeutic role describes work with individuals, families and members of the network in relation to specific issues. People with learning disabilities seldom refer themselves, and requests for support or advice are usually made by someone in the network. Clinical intervention may then involve the referrer and/or the person with learning disabilities in various combinations described in more detail later in the chapter.

Requests for involvement from the occupational therapist are often made in relation to the following issues.

- Transition from children's to adult services. Guidance recommends that health, education and social services work together to involve as many family members as possible in planning for transition (DoH 2001, Tarleton & Ward 2005). Occupational therapists are most likely to become involved when the young person has complex needs, e.g. physical, behavioural or emotional. The focus of involvement will often be to assess and contribute to the planning of the support and environmental needs. Placements that demand unrealistic levels of independence can result in distress for the person with learning disabilities and disappointment for the staff (Clegg & King, 2006).

- Planning for the future is a concern for older parents, 40% of whom are aged 60 and over (Morgan & Thomson 2000). It is important for services to be proactive in identifying and planning for the future needs of these families (DoH 2001). Many older parents have low expectations as a result of unhelpful responses from services in the past and limited alternatives to institutional care (Swain & Thirlaway 1999). Issues that have been identified as important for services to consider when planning for the future with these families are:
  - Proactive planning processes to include information about services
  - Review of the appropriateness of activities for the older person with learning disabilities
  - Consideration of the effect of any change on ageing parents
  - Development of leisure activities and friendships outside the home for the person

| Box 14.1 |

Case illustration: how an occupational therapist may use the full range of interventions described in Valuing People in one referral

Sandra is a young woman in her early 30s who has profound learning disabilities and epilepsy. She lives in her own flat with a new team of paid support workers. The care manager has referred Sandra and her team of workers as they are concerned that the combined effect of her profound learning disabilities and her seizures makes it difficult for her to engage in activities and she therefore sleeps a lot during the day.

- *Therapeutic* – as the occupational therapist does not know much about Sandra, she decides to spend a couple of sessions with her and the key-worker getting to know more about Sandra's interests, methods of communicating likes and dislikes, how she engages when she is feeling lively and alert and how she is after seizures.

- *Health promotion and health facilitation* – the occupational therapist recommends to the staff that they make an appointment for Sandra to see the neurologist and together they make a list of concerns to be taken to the appointment. As a result, Sandra starts a new drug regime, with the effect that she is less sleepy. The occupational therapist works with the staff team to identify the times she is most alert, the sorts of things she likes and could be involved in, aspects of the environment and the type of support that enables optimal engagement. The occupational therapist does this with the whole staff team, organizing their ideas on a piece of flipchart paper using the above headings. She then takes this away and develops some guidelines on behalf of the staff. Subsequently, it emerges that although the staff have ideas about outings with Sandra they are finding it difficult to identify meaningful ways of involving Sandra in the everyday running of the house.

- *Teaching* – the occupational therapist and staff team agree that a workshop on 'active support' would be very helpful.

- *Service development* – the occupational therapist has experienced a number of people like Sandra who do not have many opportunities to meet and do things with others. She, together with the speech therapist and physiotherapist on the team, decide to set up a social group at a local community centre with a focus on fun, communication and physical activity. They develop a structured programme, which they document. The running of the group is then handed over to a development worker at the community centre.

with learning disabilities to include transport where needed

- Short breaks to include preparation for moving away from home
- Trained and reliable staff who can inspire confidence (Morgan & Thompson 2000).
- Change in health, behaviour or circumstances of the person or their support. Changes in health may or may not be directly related to the person's learning disabilities. However, any change in health status will have an impact on the person and their network which may result in a referral to the Specialist Healthcare Team for re-assessment of their needs.
- Conflict sometimes occurs within the network due to a number of factors. Expectations of family members and staff are often different. Like most people, the person with learning disabilities may behave differently in different settings.

Resentments and conflict can arise if the person is more or less independent or has more opportunities to socialize and develop relationships in one setting than another. Methods of communication will often be different between family members and staff (this is developed further in Chapter 4). For example, some families are more directive with the person with learning disabilities, whereas staff are more likely to focus on development of opportunity, choice, rights and responsibilities.

The occupational therapist may be asked to act as 'expert' by providing an assessment of skills to establish a person's abilities. In such a situation where an assessment might be used to arbitrate between the two parties it may be more helpful for the therapist to facilitate discussion about a way forward in the best interests of the person with learning disabilities. Recognition of different rather than right or wrong approaches promotes an exchange of ideas and experiences that will identify areas where consistency might be helpful but also recognize and value difference. Rikberg Smyly (2006) describes some approaches to these situations. However, an independent assessment may be helpful and these options need to be weighed up to achieve the most constructive outcome.

Health facilitation and promotion

This relates to work with individuals, members of the network, specific work with primary and secondary health care teams as well as teaching and service development. All occupational therapy interventions have the ultimate goal of promoting healthy lifestyles within a given context (Molineux 2004) but the following examples focus on interventions where the link is most obvious.

Occupational therapists often become involved in liaising with primary and secondary health in the course of their clinical and therapeutic role and GPs are informed of involvement (see Chapter 5). For example, functional changes sometimes occur as a result of medical interventions such as in-patient treatment, changes in medication or surgery. The occupational therapist's role in these instances might involve identification of support needs on discharge reflecting the person's change in function or possibly to advise a period of rehabilitation based on their knowledge of the community setting of the person. If the occupational therapist has been the only professional from the team involved, they may need to refer to other team members and take on a coordinating role until the others become fully engaged. Another coordinating role that the occupational therapist may adopt is described under the Care Programme Approach when clients have additional mental health needs.

Other areas of work that promote health include:

- advice on adapting environments and providing equipment
- in leisure facilities such as swimming pools, computer resources, etc.
- promoting out-of-wheelchair activities
- development of groups to promote physical exercise and self-care or strategies to manage stress and anxiety
- service developments that address the specific needs of people with learning disabilities who also have autism, dementia, mental health needs, complex physical and sensory needs
- teaching and training.

Teaching

Teaching may take place with individuals, families or groups. An example of an individual teaching role may be helping a day centre worker structure a group to engage a person with particular difficulties, or advising a social worker to structure a parenting assessment to take account of the effects of learning disabilities.

Specialist health care services often become involved in teaching groups of staff or professionals in order to help them to work most effectively with people with learning disabilities. Sometimes these become formalized training or workshop sessions. Ideally, service users and their families and carers are involved in some way, e.g. through video recordings or in the development or evaluation of training. Some examples of training topics that the occupational

Table 14.2 Range of teaching topics that may involve the occupational therapist and the multidisciplinary team

Session topic	Professions that might join the occupational therapist
Multisensory training	Speech and language therapist
Epilepsy and effects on everyday life	Learning disability nurse
Difficulties with eating and drinking	Speech and language therapist and physiotherapist
Supporting people with additional mental health needs	Psychologist/psychiatrist/ community mental health nurse
Supporting people with dementia	Physiotherapist/psychologist/ psychiatry speech and language therapist/community mental health nurse
Comfort and posture management	Physiotherapist/wheelchair clinic therapist/ community mental health nurse

therapist may be involved in together with colleagues from other disciplines are given in Table 14.2.

In any of these topics the focus of the occupational therapy contributions will be on everyday activities. However, occupational therapists also contribute to team teaching sessions such as a seminar on the nature and effect of learning disabilities for staff in a G.P. practice that does not have a profession-specific focus.

Service development

Occupational therapists are frequently asked to become involved in the development or adaptation of physical environments for people with learning disabilities. Some people will have additional needs such as sensory or physical disabilities, autism, epilepsy, or behaviour that is considered challenging. They may just be people of short stature. The way the physical environment is organized (e.g. size and function of rooms, colour schemes, materials and furnishings, kitchen and bathroom layouts, heights of fixtures and fittings, access arrangements, etc.) can be very important in facilitating independence and promoting safety and comfort. Some suggested books and resources that provide guidance on the design and adaptation of the physical environment to address different needs are listed in the bibliography. The occupational therapist will often work alongside commissioners, housing associations, architects and builders as well as care managers, individuals and families. It is helpful to clarify roles and responsibilities as early on as possible as there can sometimes be confusion when a large disparate group of professionals work together (Donati 2004). Increasingly, assistive technology using telecare is being installed into homes to alert central call systems or carers to a range of dangers such as floods, seizures, falls, intruders, gas leaks, etc. This technology can be helpful in enabling a person to stay in their own home, or to have more independence in a family or staffed home (e.g. where there are concerns about wandering, incontinence, epileptic seizures, etc.).

Clarifying referral, allocation, assessment and intervention processes

It is important right from the point of referral to be clear about who is asking for help for whom or who is 'commissioning the work'. Ideally, referrals are made to the occupational therapist in the specialist health care team for help in thinking together about issues of concern, for assessment and advice or for an opportunity for people with learning disabilities or staff to develop skills or knowledge in a particular area. In most instances, even when the request is to provide a direct service to the person, for example to find employment, involvement of the support network is necessary in order to ensure that the work is effective. Service users are often referred as the presenting problem but it is always important where applicable to engage with staff or family as they will be continuing to support the person after the occupational therapist has closed involvement. Sometimes similar referrals will come from the same organization for different service users, for example for service users to engage more in domestic activities. In this case, work with the organization will have a broad impact and develop the competencies of the staff and the organization. Individual assessment may still be required where specific issues need to be addressed.

A thorough and careful follow up to referrals involves asking questions that help clarify the focus of the work, even if it takes several meetings or conversations. An approach that determines the systems of concern, significance and involvement (Lang & McAdam 1994) might ask questions such as:

- Who is concerned about the issue?
- Who is involved?
- What is their involvement?
- Why is this an issue now?
- What is the therapist being asked to do and with whom?

Once the responses to these questions have been established, it is often quite helpful to ask the person/people referred when meeting them for the first time what they have experienced as helpful and unhelpful in the past, (Reder & Fredman 1996).

The answers to these questions help to clarify what the referred person considers helpful, which may with further questioning identify attitudes, perceptions, expected outcomes, attitudes to the organization the therapist represents, examples of what they have already tried, etc.

The team may decide to obtain this information during a visit, over the telephone or by sending a questionnaire (for an example see Appendix 14.1).

Figure 14.1 illustrates the process of clarifying who is the client; in this situation a family member is asking for help to enable his brother to access his local gym independently. The therapist may work with both the individual and anyone supporting them as well as provide support to an organization.

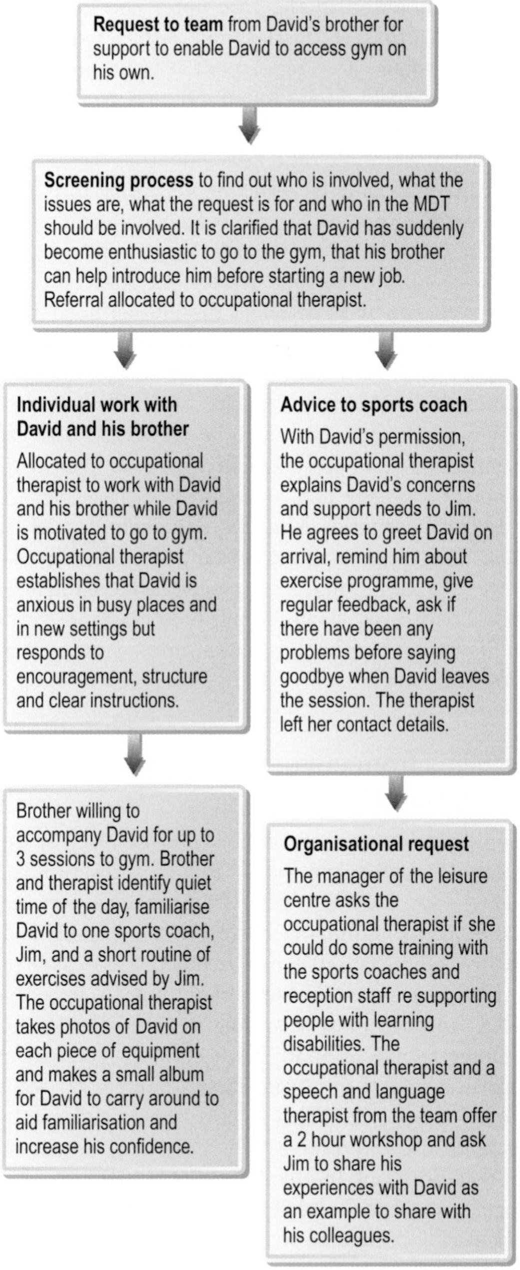

Clarifying the role of the occupational therapist

In order to be able to clarify the role, information about the remit of the occupational therapist in a specialist learning disabilities service needs to be available. A starting point might be defining the objectives of the service, for example, the occupational therapy service promotes health by minimizing disability and enabling people with learning disabilities to lead full and valued lives within the local community. It aims to provide opportunities for people to participate as fully as possible in activities both in and outside the 'home'. This is achieved by working alongside the person with learning disabilities, their carers, other professionals and organizations who are a resource to people with learning disabilities.

The description should include the processes and systems used (e.g. response to referrals, modes of working, waiting lists together with prioritization factors and types of intervention). It is also helpful to clarify relationships between the occupational therapist in the specialist health care term and occupational therapy unrelated to their learning disability, such as those in physical and wheelchair services. The occupational therapist is strongly recommended to refer to the document entitled Occupational Therapy Services for Adults with Learning Disabilities (COT 2003) which sets out the role of the specialist occupational therapist as well as guidance on promoting access to generic health social care. Guidance states:

> *If the person has an identified need for occupational therapy, unrelated to their learning disability, then he or she should access the relevant generic occupational therapy service, e.g. social services, mental health, forensic, acute general hospital, etc. (College of Occupational Therapy 2003 p. 7).*

Following this model, the specialist learning disabilities service refers on to the mainstream provider, e.g. to a wheelchair clinic via direct referral, with any relevant reports appended. In some instances it is appropriate to accompany the client during the assessment and provision if, for example, they have

Request to team from David's brother for support to enable David to access gym on his own.

Screening process to find out who is involved, what the issues are, what the request is for and who in the MDT should be involved. It is clarified that David has suddenly become enthusiastic to go to the gym, that his brother can help introduce him before starting a new job. Referral allocated to occupational therapist.

Individual work with David and his brother

Allocated to occupational therapist to work with David and his brother while David is motivated to go to gym. Occupational therapist establishes that David is anxious in busy places and in new settings but responds to encouragement, structure and clear instructions.

Advice to sports coach

With David's permission, the occupational therapist explains David's concerns and support needs to Jim. He agrees to greet David on arrival, remind him about exercise programme, give regular feedback, ask if there have been any problems before saying goodbye when David leaves the session. The therapist left her contact details.

Brother willing to accompany David for up to 3 sessions to gym. Brother and therapist identify quiet time of the day, familiarise David to one sports coach, Jim, and a short routine of exercises advised by Jim. The occupational therapist takes photos of David on each piece of equipment and makes a small album for David to carry around to aid familiarisation and increase his confidence.

Organisational request

The manager of the leisure centre asks the occupational therapist if she could do some training with the sports coaches and reception staff re supporting people with learning disabilities. The occupational therapist and a speech and language therapist from the team offer a 2 hour workshop and ask Jim to share his experiences with David as an example to share with his colleagues.

Figure 14.1 • Clarifying referrals: interventions that include individual and organizational involvement.

no keyworker or family member to voice their needs on relevant issues (e.g. frailty of mother who pushes the wheelchair around a hilly area and who is unable to accompany daughter to clinic). The following case illustration: Dimitri in Box 14.2 will show how the issues can arise from the point of new referral.

Box 14.2

Case illustration: Dimitri – a new referral

Dimitri is referred to the team by his care manager. He is 23 years old and lives with his mother and sister. Dimitri's mother was born in Cyprus but he and his sister were born in the UK. The care manager states that the family are finding it increasingly difficult to support Dimitri with his personal care as the mother has pain and stiffness in her arms and back and the daughter is planning to move away to go to university soon. Can the occupational therapist assess personal care and identify some strategies to help the family?

In this case the care manager is referring the mother and son as a response to the mother's report that she is finding it difficult to care for her son. When responding to the referral it is important to check with the family whose idea it was to make the referral, what they thought about that idea and to clarify what they are asking for. This initial discussion is an important starting point to a possible relationship with the family. It is essential from the beginning to have conversations that aim to clarify with those actually referred what their concerns are and what outcome they would like. This may be different from those stated on the referral. It is important at this point that the therapist is open and respectful, listens carefully and aims to include all the family members by gauging their communication needs. Conversation should include general 'problem free' talk that aims to put the family at ease and to relate to them as people rather than problems though obviously the therapist will need to respond to the signals given by the family. Depending on Dimitri's understanding, he may or may not be able to contribute to this process. However, his consent or agreement is required if follow up will involve him, and it is the therapist's duty to make any explanation as accessible to him as possible.

Consent or agreement and best interests

Where a person has no verbal communication, the occupational therapist is reliant on behaviour and non-verbal communication to infer that there is no objection to the therapist's involvement. This is then documented in the case notes and considered at each meeting. In this instance, Mrs S would have probably signed the 'agreement' to the referral on Dimitri's behalf. However, if Dimitri had behaved in a way that indicated that he was not very happy the therapist could not conclude that he did not want involvement. It would be necessary to explore the possible reasons for his behaviour and consider whether it related to the therapist's presence and implications for further work. The best interests of the person with learning disabilities need to be carefully considered and decisions made about how to work and with whom in order to achieve these interests. The Mental Capacity Act (2005) provides a framework for establishing best interests and each organization has responsibility for implementing associated systems and procedures.

In this scenario, Mrs S's understanding of the English language is also important, since her first language is Greek. Sometimes people lack confidence in their English, especially when meeting a person for the first time or when important information is being communicated.

Families from cultural and ethnic backgrounds

People with learning disabilities who are black or from an ethnic minority group may be doubly discriminated against (Swain 1999). Table 14.3 provides some general guidance summarized from Noon (1999) about culture, ethnicity and carers' needs.

However, it is also important not to stereotype values and attitudes according to ethnic background (Valuing People Support Team 2004b). Not speaking English is one of the main reasons families do not get the help they need. This highlights the need for therapists to use interpreters when working with a family that does not feel confident about its use of the English language (Valuing People Support Team 2003). It is usually preferable to use professional interpreters, but some communities prefer discussions about family matters to remain within the family circle. In some situations when the professional interpreters come

Table 14.3 Summary of key issues relating to culture, ethnicity and carers' needs

Categories	Similar or different for cultural groups
Needs of carers	Family carers have broadly the same needs across cultures
Attitudes to seeking and receiving help	Varies according to different cultural groups (e.g. Asian community may see seeking outside intervention as 'social disgrace')
Communication of distress	Different use of language, idiom and description (e.g. in Chinese culture emotional distress may be described in physical terms)
The means by which help may be provided	Helping behaviour may be perceived differently according to cultural/ethnic group (e.g. attitudes to counselling might be different from western ideas that focus on strengthening self-concept as the basis of coping)

from the same community, the family may not feel comfortable disclosing sensitive information. It is necessary in situations where family members interpret to be aware of the possible influencing factors and to judge whether they are also contributing their views.

Some considerations to bear in mind when working with interpreters:

- Aim if possible to use the same interpreter for each visit to the same family. This helps the interpreter to develop an understanding of the therapist's role and the purpose of the discussions, assists in developing rapport with the family as well as ensuring that sensitive information is kept to a minimum number of people.
- Organize a brief meeting with the interpreter prior to meeting with a family in order to explain the therapist's role, the organization they represent, the purpose of the meeting and any particular issues that need to be clarified or discussed.

- During the meeting observe carefully whether the interpreter is translating from a neutral position or conveying their own opinion.
- Observe whether the rapport between the interpreter and the family is relatively comfortable.
- Pace questions, discussion and information with pauses for interpretation and if necessary indicate this to the family.
- Ensure sufficient time has been set aside as meetings that involve interpreters will require more time than those without interpreters.
- Apart from clarifying the issues of concern it is important to recognize the support from within the family and possibly the community, as well as any particular religious or cultural requirements. A number of recommendations have been made in relation to wider service provision by the Valuing People Support Team (2004b) to ensure that the services are responsive to their needs.

Following up the referral for Dimitri

Issue of concern

At the initial meeting Mrs S and her daughter both express concern about Mrs S's deteriorating health.

Knowledge of the referral

They had understood that the care manager would be asking for someone from the health care team to visit but did not know what could be done.

Including all members of the family and gauging communication

Mrs S was very friendly and smiled a lot, but she preferred that her daughter be present to translate for her. Dimitri was very quiet and shy, but responded with smiles when his mother explained how much he enjoyed the swimming sessions at his day centre. From this the therapist became aware that he had some understanding of key familiar words but would not be able to contribute verbally to the conversation. The therapist noticed that Mrs S and to some extent her daughter were very warm and affectionate, but talked to Dimitri as if he were a small child.

Further issues of concern

Mrs S and her daughter said that Dimitri could be irritable and uncooperative at times when it came to dressing, bathing and going to and getting up from bed.

What the sister and mother want

They did not know what solutions there might be but want the therapist to look into equipment such as an adjustable bed.

What Dimitri wants

This is not clear at this point.

Collaborative approaches to working with families

Over recent years there has been extensive research into how services can be more responsive to families. As a result, family needs and preferences have been identified (e.g. Barr 1996, Llewellyn 1994, Thompson 1998), resulting in the development of more supportive and collaborative approaches. Where families are closely involved, Swain & Thirlaway (1999) advocate that practitioners start with the family context. Recent research on the experience of fathers highlights the need for practitioners to pay more attention to the inclusion and involvement of fathers, who in the past have often been overlooked (Towers & Swift 2006).

A document published by the King's Fund specifically for professionals working within the NHS describes what family carers want for themselves and the person they support (Banks et al 1998). Similar issues have been expanded in The Family Toolkit produced by the Valuing People Support Team (2003). The following checklist summarizes the key points.

Checklist of issues that family carers want addressed by NHS staff

- full information
- recognition of their own health and well-being
- a life of their own – quality services for the carer and the person cared for
- time off
- emotional support
- training and support to care

- financial security
- a voice
  (adapted from Banks et al 1998).

It is perhaps worth pointing out to the therapist new to learning disabilities, that unlike some other client groups who have developed illness or become disabled later in life, families that include people with learning disabilities have had multiple and varied experiences of professionals for many years before encountering adult services. They have also developed a vast expertise in living with the person with learning disabilities and have devised their own strategies for accommodating any special considerations into their lives. Where a son or daughter has especially complex health care needs (e.g. physical frailty, sensory disabilities, severe epilepsy or challenging behaviour) families may feel especially protective and concerned about whether services will be equipped to meet their needs.

Before going on to look at assessment processes it might be helpful to refer to the literature to consider some of the collaborative approaches to working with people with learning disabilities and the people in their network, particularly family and paid carers.

Considerable emphasis over the last decade or so has been placed on involving people with learning disabilities in planning for their future, but at times the individual and those who live and support them will have different views. There is therefore a need to acknowledge and work together with the various people in the network including the family. Barr (1996) describes the need for active collaboration with all family members, including siblings, fathers and grandparents, who may not always have been acknowledged by professionals in the past. There is extensive literature on working in partnership with families. Some describe family-centred approaches (e.g. Rosenbaum et al 1998); family-centred assessment and intervention models (Deal et al 1994) and family systems theory (McConachie 1991, Donati et al 2000). All of these focus on interventions that build on family strengths and resources and are enabling and empowering.

The following guidelines will assist the therapist to adopt a collaborative approach:

- Respond to a referral as an invitation to join the referred parties in thinking together about some of their concerns (Lang & McAdam 1994)

- Treat information available prior to a meeting as a *potentially helpful* contribution to further information gathered
- Use carefully structured questions that help to clarify some of the concerns
- Listen carefully for clues to resolving issues
- Use the language of those participating in the conversation when summarizing understanding of what has been said
- Recognize and value all contributions and perspectives.

As Schon (1983) states, the client (who in this case may be any number of involved people) is the expert in their own lives. The professional's role is to use their knowledge to frame the key issues, ask questions that help to clarify potential involvement and identify resources and ideas for possible solutions. Sometimes it can be helpful to meet separately as well as together with family members to enable as broad an understanding as possible of the issues of the various parties.

Issues to consider when working with paid staff

Paid providers have a contracted set of obligations that describe the service they will provide, the values, duties and responsibilities of the service. For example, service providers have statutory obligations in relation to the handling of medications, health and safety, moving and handling, staff training, etc. These duties vary depending on the type of provision, e.g. residential accommodation, supported living, outreach and community services, all of which conform to a regulatory framework set out and overseen by the Commission for Social Care Inspection. It is important for the therapist to be aware of these responsibilities, as well as which organization is responsible for risk assessment, training and provision of moving and handling equipment.

The less tangible aspects of service provision, such as creativity, attitudes, beliefs and morale of a staff team cannot be so easily regulated. These will, however, significantly affect the communication between staff, service users and their families as well as other agencies with whom they come into contact, including the occupational therapist. Like families, paid staff vary in their willingness or interest in engaging with the specialist health care service and again this may be linked to past experiences. Organizations vary considerably in terms of their own management, training and support. All of these factors influence the openness and willingness to initiate or participate in working with the specialist health care service. Increasingly, commissioners are contracting with a wider selection of organizations in order that service provision is less reliant on the fluctuations or the effectiveness of any one organization, but also in order to provide a wide range of styles of service delivery. For example, one organization may focus on opportunities for their service users to be involved in the running of their home and making choices, using a wide range of strategies such as picture timetables, objects of reference and active support (described in Chapter 13). This approach might not be as helpful for young people with mental health needs who may need a more structured and more directive approach from staff, which can be better provided by an organization with a different ethos.

It is important that the therapist pays particular attention to developing a respectful relationship that recognizes and values the skills and experiences of staff and managers. This approach can help to diffuse any sensitivities or reasons for reluctance to engage, which could be due to issues such as high staff turnover, low morale, heavy workloads, unsupportive management, insufficient information, understanding about the role of the occupational therapist or unhelpful experiences in the past.

Assessment process

Assessment of situations that involve support networks will need to include a number of different elements. Apart from getting to know about the person with learning disabilities, understanding their physical and social environment is key. Some of the questions might be:

- What are the expectations?
- What are the opportunities?
- What are the attitudes, values and beliefs of these environments?
- Is there only one setting or are there several?
- How similar or different are they?
- What are the constraints or limiting factors?
- What are the relationships like between the person with learning disabilities and the different settings?

- How much potential is there for the different environments/networks to learn and share from each other?
- What have they already tried?

This information is obtained through observation and discussion. During this process the therapist is also assessing the potential for change and possibly getting the different support networks together to share strategies, resources and ideas. By asking about what they have tried already and any limitations or constraints, the therapist identifies a focus for involvement. While gathering this information the occupational therapist needs to bear in mind what was being asked for at the beginning of the process and to what end. Some potential referral questions might be:

- can the person be more independent?
- can the person be more involved in activities/have more opportunities?
- what are the support needs of the person?
- what is the person able to do?
- can the person be supported differently?
- can something that is seen as a problem to the referrer or one part of the network, but possibly not to the person with learning disabilities or to other parts of the network, be resolved?

Sometimes, because of the different expectations, a person may function differently in one environment from another. It may well be helpful in these situations to see them in the different settings or consult with the range of involved people and then establish what factors create the difference. It can be difficult for a person to demonstrate or describe these differences themselves. When the occupational therapist wants to see how a person does something, therefore, it is best to do this in the familiar environment at the usual time and in the way it would normally be done. The person may find it difficult or confusing or even upsetting to be asked to do something different from the usual routine and an inaccurate picture would result. This issue may have implications for the use of standardized assessments.

The presence of an outside person can skew the picture, and it is therefore important to obtain descriptions from others to supplement observations. The presence of the occupational therapist may make the person nervous or inhibited or even excited and distracted, family might find the request an intrusion, so it is necessary to be sensitive to these possibilities and to be as informal and unobtrusive as possible.

Dimitri and family, continued

Now that the referral has been clarified and the occupational therapist knows more or less what the referred issues are and who is concerned, consideration can be given to what to do and how to set about assessment and intervention. A family-centred assessment model developed by Deal et al (1994) provides a useful method for mapping the family functioning, strengths and resources, their needs and aspirations and consequent help-giving behaviour. Figure 14.2 modifies this model to illustrate how the information we have obtained during the assessment of Dimitri and family can be organized to identify the potential interventions.

Approach to assessment with Dimitri and family

The therapist is still not very clear about what the family, including Dimitri, might want, what kind of support Dimitri might need with personal care, and

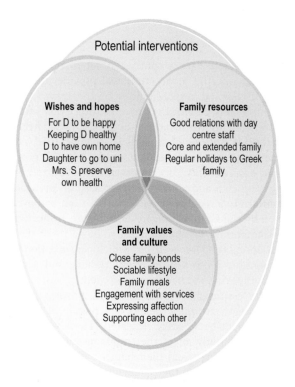

Figure 14.2 • Mapping the key factors that have emerged from assessment of Dimitri and family. Modified from Deal et al (1994).

why he is at times uncooperative. What the therapist does know is that the mother and sister are saying that they cannot continue as they are now.

Assessment

The therapist visits Dimitri at his day centre. *Rationale*: She had established that Dimitri enjoys being at the centre. There is an opportunity there for observation of dressing and undressing at the swimming session which may be less intrusive than in the family home. The staff at the centre have no concerns about Dimitri's behaviour and it is an opportunity for the therapist to see Dimitri in a different environment.

Observations

It is observed that Dimitri's male keyworker expects Dimitri to do most of the dressing tasks himself. He provides light-hearted and encouraging verbal support to Dimitri and two other young men. Dimitri laughs and smiles, is able to dress and undress independently except for zips, buttons and shoe laces with the help of a grab rail.

Consent

Dimitri is very lively and is happy to show the therapist what he can do.

Possible effect of therapist's presence?

The therapist asks the key worker if Dimitri is always so able. He says that he is when this type of support is provided and if he is motivated to do the activity (e.g. swimming).

Interventions

When working with a support network the therapist will often become involved in a range of interventions: 'direct therapeutic work' with the person with learning disabilities; 'advice to family' or people in the network; 'adaptation of the environment'; or 'teaching'; or 'facilitation' of network meetings to share strategies and resources. On occasion, past assessment and recommendations can be re-visited if similar referrals have been made in the past but changes in staff have led to them getting lost.

Two possible interventions will now be described on the basis of the case scenario of Dimitri.

Option one – intervention: therapeutic/direct role

Therapeutic/direct role with Dimitri and carer and adjustments to the physical environment

During a follow up visit with Dimitri and his mother he is very excited when the therapist shares her observations from the day centre of his skills. He and his mother and sister are quite keen to see whether some of the methods that he was using at the day centre could be tried at home. The occupational therapist spends some time with Dimitri and his mother observing how he dresses and at what points he needs support. Through discussion it emerges that Dimitri and his mother have noticed that he finds it easier and is more motivated to dress when he has had time to move about and his joints are less stiff, he has his favourite music on and his mother has told him what is on his timetable at the day centre. They agree for the occupational therapist to arrange for a grab rail to be put on the bedroom wall and in the meantime they move the bed next to a ledge that Dimitri can use to assist in standing. They discuss the possibility of Dimitri wearing more casual clothes, which are easier for him to manage, with few fastenings. It had also been noticed by mother when questioned, that Dimitri was more motivated to get dressed before breakfast because he enjoys his food and so that he only had to go downstairs once. He would brush his teeth downstairs before going to the centre. It was agreed that Mrs S and Dimitri would try these changes in routine and the occupational therapist would review in 3–4 weeks.

Option two – intervention: consultative role to care manager

Recommending adjustment to the social environment

The visit is followed up by a meeting with the family. The therapist shares her observations with Dimitri and his mother and sister about how much he appears to enjoy his centre, the staff and swimming in particular. She does not comment on his skills in dressing but the family observe that he really seems to enjoy the company of the male staff and being with his peers. The therapist has noticed during the first and this visit the affectionate way that Dimitri's mother and sister talk to him, but also that they still speak of him like a child and this evokes a negative response from Dimitri. There is then some conversation about Dimitri becoming a young adult, perhaps wanting more social opportunities and the possibility that his moodiness at home might be an expression of his growing wish for independence. The family think it is an interesting idea and ask whether there are any social clubs for him to go in the evenings. Mrs S then says that she is starting to consider an idea proposed by the care manager that Dimitri move on to shared accommodation with two or three other young men. She and the therapist agree that having a male support worker come in twice a day to help Dimitri with his personal care might be a starting point in this transition process. The therapist communicates these ideas to the care manager and writes a report that she shares with Dimitri and Mrs S and daughter before sending it to the care manager. The report outlines Dimitri's skills and support needs in personal care based on observations at the centre. The occupational therapist recommends that a male support worker be provided who would be able to develop a collaborative and informal relationship with Dimitri rather like his day centre workers. Information was given to the family about local social clubs. Equipment was ruled out as Dimitri's bedroom was much too small for an adjustable height bed and in fact if motivated he could get on and off the bed himself. The case was then closed to the occupational therapist as there would be follow up by the care manager and it might take some time for a support worker to be identified. At the end of the occupational therapist's closing summary it was explained that a further referral could be made to work with the identified support worker to skill share the occupational therapist's observations about the style of communication and strategies that are likely to enable Dimitri to optimize his living skills.

Theoretical frameworks for describing interventions for Dimitri and family

Intervention Option One describes direct therapeutic involvement with the family, with Dimitri and with staff during the assessment process at the day centre and physical adjustment to the home environment. In Option Two, the occupational therapist adopted an advisory and information giving role in relation to social activities for the family, and the family's needs to the care manager. Social adaptations were recommended in the form of a support worker. A potential future teaching role with a support worker was identified.

Risk management processes

Most services have risk policies that clarify the risk assessment and management processes. The policy will describe a process for negotiating with relevant parties about how to minimize the risks in order that they are deemed to be 'reasonable'. As Aleszewski & Aleszewski (2002) report from their research into attitudes of service users, families and paid staff, there is a tension between empowerment and risk (often described as safety), which is not always recognized by risk policies. Safety is often given precedence over empowerment. It may be an important role of the learning disabilities service to help agencies develop policies that recognize the need to provide opportunities for development, choice and relationship making (benefits) and balance the possible hazards (risks). It will at times be necessary for the occupational therapist to encourage positive risk taking in relation to new opportunities or skill development. It is usually the responsibility of each provider organization to develop and use their own risk assessment processes. Occupational therapists may be invited to contribute to these where activities are involved and especially where there is a need for a shared risk assessment across agencies.

A careful, balanced and negotiated approach to risk taking is an important way of addressing potential conflict between agencies or family and paid carers. Interestingly, Aleszewski & Aleszewski (2002) reported that unlike previous research, people with learning disabilities were concerned about new and potentially hazardous situations whereas families and paid carers took a more philosophical view of risk as part of everyday life. However, it is important to have a means of deciding whether to go ahead with an activity or situation even where there is some conflict. The policy may state, for example, that if there is a majority view one way or another, the minority views and concerns should be stated but the majority

Box 14.3

Case illustration: risk assessment issues – referral

A referral is received from Brian, an outreach worker who is concerned about Tom whom he supports once a week. He reports that Tom is becoming increasingly forgetful, looking less well cared for and more erratic with his eating habits, sometimes keeping mouldy food in the fridge. A phone call to Brian clarifies that the referral is relevant for occupational therapy involvement and that Tom has agreed to the referral for help with the food problem. The occupational therapist allocates the case immediately because of the health and safety issues.

---

view implemented. Where the occupational therapist finds themself in a quandary they should seek the expertise and shared clinical reasoning processes of the rest of the health care team (see above case illustration: risk assessment referral).

Assessment

An initial meeting in Tom's flat with Tom and Brian, his outreach worker, clarifies that Tom is concerned about the fact that he has frequent stomach upsets but only Brian has noticed or is concerned about the other issues.

Purpose of assessment

To make contact with Tom and Brian to observe directly some of the concerns, to observe how Tom and Brian relate to each other, to discuss possible involvement with Tom around his food storage and to gain agreement from Tom for the occupational therapist and Brian to meet to talk about the best ways to support him.

Observations

The occupational therapist notices that Tom seems very comfortable with Brian and that they have a collaborative relationship. Tom seems keen to avoid the problems of further stomach upsets and readily agrees to work with the occupational therapist on some strategies for organizing his food, which Brian

says he will support in the longer term. The occupational therapist notices some black bags stored in a corner, but they do not at this point in time look a significant risk as there is no smell and Tom says they only have clothes and papers in them. The occupational therapist suggests a further visit to Tom and also arranges to meet Brian at his office to think together about his other concerns.

In the case of Tom we have a changed situation in relation to his health and functioning with associated risks. Tom is aware of some of the risks (e.g. food), but not of his forgetfulness or hoarding and may therefore, not be aware of future changes in his health and function. Brian made the referral and although Tom recognizes some of the issues, Brian has a wider range of concerns. It is therefore appropriate in Tom's best interests to meet Tom together with Brian, the outreach worker.

There are several actions that the occupational therapist needs to take in relation to Tom. She will need to refer him to the psychologists/psychiatrist in the team for screening for dementia/mental illness. She will work with Tom on the food issues and with Brian on observing risks, possibly carrying out a risk assessment with him and involving him in the dementia assessment as he will be an informant as well as someone who will monitor Tom's future functioning. This is discussed in the following intervention.

Case illustration: risk assessment – intervention

Intervention scenario

The occupational therapist, Brian and Tom meet up at his flat and make a cup of tea to go with the biscuits that the occupational therapist has brought. They then have a chat about the stomach upsets, and the routines that Tom has for shopping and cooking. He is rather vague about these and says he eats out more often at college now because of the upsets. Together they decide that they will try labelling the food with 'eat by' dates and the occupational therapist says she will make a timetable for the week where they can put pictures of his routines, including a meal at college on the day he attends there. This was set up, and Brian agreed to remind Tom to look at the timetable and also the labels on the food. Brian and Tom agreed that if anything went past the 'eat by' label, they would throw it out.

The occupational therapist also meets up separately with Brian who is quite upset by the changes in Tom. The occupational therapist asks for his ideas about what should be done. They agree together to do a risk assessment using a risk/benefit process and think together about how to minimize risks. As a result they agree that support sessions should be more frequent. They refer to the psychologist who gives Brian a sheet to complete outlining Tom's current functioning with a view to it being reviewed in 6 months. They decide to ask the care management team to call a review and invite the college tutor and gardening project coordinator so that they can share their observations and review support needs and agree a process for communicating concerns to the care manager.

It is worth mentioning at this point that sometimes an occupational therapist might find themselves the first member of the team to become involved in a new referral, some considerable time may be spent referring on to colleagues and generally facilitating their involvement. At this stage it is sometimes difficult to focus on the occupational therapy role, but as others become familiar with the issues and clarify their roles, it then becomes possible to re-focus on the profession-specific work. This could potentially happen in the case of Brian and Tom.

Considerations for closing involvement

It can be difficult to establish the appropriate time to close involvement with a family or support network and therapists may work with a client and their network for several years. However, in order to maintain a clear focus and to empower rather than create dependency it is an important question to regularly consider. There may be many apparently valid reasons for closing, which may in fact present the therapist with some conflict. For example, one criterion for closure may be little or no change or a reduction in previous progress. The therapist may feel that they are 'giving up' but there may be many reasons why the time is not right for engagement and this should not necessarily be seen as lack of effectiveness on the part of the therapist.

Equally difficult situations from which to disengage are those where there has been change or positive development as the therapist naturally enjoys the success and may rationalize that continued involvement will lead to further progress. The question for the therapist is whether the network is now capable and competent to continue the work themselves. If the network or family systems are assessed to be sufficiently robust, the therapist's work is complete for the particular episode of involvement.

Careful initial and ongoing assessment of the capacity of the system to develop and change is important for predicting therapy involvement. If the network is not engaging there are a number of questions therapists may ask themselves.

- Is the timing for intervention right? (e.g. too many changes/things happening, stressful events, a need for more time to reflect on options, etc.)
- Has the original request for involvement been met or is it no longer relevant?
- Is there insufficient commitment, motivation, energy, confidence to change or develop?
- Is there some instability in the family or staff team for various reasons?
- Are there acute health/relationship/housing issues that are interfering with the work?
- Has involvement to date been a useful re-assessment of a situation where the outcome has confirmed that there is no need or desire for change?

Some methods to assist the decision to close involvement

- Calling a client review – involving the client, staff, family and all relevant parties to reflect together on current issues and to explore together the best way forward. This should be an opportunity to focus on the 'client's' perspective, to refocus on their plans, ambitions and current experiences. If involvement of the occupational therapist is to continue, this is a chance to discuss and agree a focus for their work, which may have changed, or may not have been quite clear at the beginning of the intervention. It might be useful to actively engage people at the review and to agree some actions. Alternatively, agreement might be reached that for the time being the occupational therapist will close involvement.

- Discussion with supervisor or colleagues can be very helpful, if not essential, where the therapist is experiencing some conflict. This could take the form of questions about what has been achieved so far, what further involvement would achieve, what closure might enable. Or the pros and cons of closure could be discussed. In any event a more objective view is often helpful.
- A professional network review/consultation is useful if there are many people involved. The purpose of such a meeting varies but is often an opportunity for the network to share their observations and experiences, to plan for future involvement and to identify strategies and resources that assist the work. The therapist may be able to clarify that she is no longer needed.
- Outcome measures, or a contract, that clearly highlights reason for referral, objectives, actions and time scales are helpful as a tool for tracking interventions. Review may identify a change in focus from the original request, identify the range of actions taken and help to give an over-view of the interventions to date. Sometimes, when a therapist is involved over a long period of time, the original reason for involvement becomes lost. The original referral request may have been resolved at some earlier stage and further requests or events prevented closure at an earlier stage.
- It can be very helpful for the therapist and the family or network to acknowledge that re-referral can be made. This is sometimes a useful way for all to re-focus and to reflect on what was helpful or unhelpful in previous work.

Different options for involving the client/network in the closure process

- Documentation of key understandings about the client (as far as possible with the client's involvement) in order that they can inform and guide new staff. These documents might take the form of video, diaries, communication books, guidelines – whichever is likely to be easily accessible to the person and to staff.
- Letter to the client and network in a narrative form that describes the journey of the client, network and therapist including original reasons for involvement, what they have done together and why they are finishing their work together.
- Discussions together to explore methods that the family/staff can use to maintain progress or change. For example, they may decide to have regular meetings, keep a communication book, use strategies developed together, have regular staff meetings to share progress and developments.
- Network meetings – to share information, observations and understandings. The occupational therapist to witness what is going well and emphasize strategies that appear to be effective. Space out these meetings until the network is confident to continue alone with sufficient systems in place to continue to support each other; common goals and a clear sense of direction.
- Issues will often not be entirely resolved (e.g. new skills learned) but the point at which the occupational therapist can consider closing is when the network feels confident to continue without further support at that time.
- Always let people know that they can re-refer at any point.

Summary

Occupational therapists working in services for people with learning disabilities often find themselves relating to complex networks. The challenge for the therapist is to identify the focus of involvement in order to be as effective as possible. Questions about who is asking for what for whom are a helpful way to achieve this. This chapter focuses on collabora-tive interventions that build on the strengths and resources in the network. The occupational ther-apist may select one or more of several different roles described in Valuing People (2001). This may involve working with the individual and their imme-diate network (therapeutic and/or advisory), working with organisations, teaching or becoming involved in service development. The chapter considers a range of scenarios from the point of referral to closure that describe interventions with networks.

Box 14.4

Case illustration: Mary

Mary lives with her parents and two sisters. She has been referred by her care manager following a review. Mary is 29 years old, has mild learning disabilities and has spent the years since school attending college and training schemes. She has been referred on a couple of occasions to the health care team by college tutors following violent and tearful outbursts. On these occasions she has appeared very distressed although she has not been able to explain why. For the past year she has had an outreach worker working with her to try to find employment and help her to move away from home into her own flat, which Mary and the family are keen for her to do. At the review the parents had expressed considerable frustration and irritation that to date Mary was still living at home with no structured daytime activities. They reported that she had periods when she seemed unhappy. On these occasions she shouted and slammed doors and then spent long periods in her room withdrawn and uncommunicative. Her parents are described as ambitious and hard-working, wish to spend more time with Mary's younger sisters who are taking exams at school but are too worried about Mary. They are puzzled that she has not been able to settle into a satisfactory lifestyle.

Reader activity

1. Who would it be helpful to meet with?

2. What would you need to clarify before becoming involved?

3. How might you approach assessment?

4. Who might you involve in the process and how?

5. Identify two possible interventions that would involve direct work and an advisory/consultative role

6. What factors would you take into account when considering closing involvement?

Further reading

Bull R (ed) 1998 Housing options for disabled people. London, Jessica Kingsley

Clutton S, Grisbrooke J, Pengelly S (eds) 2006 Occupational therapy in housing: building on firm foundation. Chichester, Whurr Publishers

Harpin P 2003 Adaptations manual, 2nd edn. London, Muscular Dystrophy Campaign

The Alzheimer's Society Guide to the dementia care environment 2006. London, The Alzheimer's Society

References

Aleszewski A, Aleszewski H 2002 Towards the creative management of risk: perceptions, practices and policies. British Journal of Learning Disabilities 30:56–62

Banks P, Cheeseman C, Maggs S 1998 The carers compass: directions for improving support to carers. London, King's Fund

Barr O 1996 Developing services for people with learning disabilities which actively involve family members: a review of the recent literature. Health and Social Care in the Community 4(2): 103–112

Clegg J, King S 2006 Supporting transitions. In: Baum S, Lynggaard H (eds) Intellectual disabilities: a systemic approach. London, Karnac

College of Occupational Therapists 2003 Principles for education and practice: occupational therapy services for adults with learning disabilities. London, College of Occupational Therapists

Deal AG, Dunst CJ, Trivette CM 1994 A flexible and functional approach to developing individualized family support plans. In: Dunst CJ, Trivette CM, Deal AG (eds) Supporting and strengthening families. Cambridge, Brookline Books

Department of Health 2001 Valuing people: a new strategy for learning disabilities for the 21st century. London, HMSO

Donati S, Glynn B, Lynggaard H, Pearce P 2000 Systemic interventions in a learning disability service: an invitation to join, Clinical Psychology Forum 144:24–28

Donati S 2004 On the house. Occupational Therapy News 12(1):35

Emerson E, Hatton C 2000 Residential supports for people with learning disabilities in 1997 in England. Tizard Learning Disability Review 5:41–44

Jones D 1995 Learning disability: An alternative frame of reference. British Journal of Occupational Therapy 58:423–426

Lang P, McAdam E 1994 Referrals, referrers and the system of concern. Unpublished paper. London, Kensington Consultation Centre

Llewellyn G 1994 Parenting: A neglected human occupation. Parents' voices not yet heard. Australian Occupational Therapy 41:173–176

Mansell J 2005 Deinstitutionalisation and community living: An international perspective. Tizard Learning Disability Review 10:22–29

McConachie H 1991 Families and professionals: prospects for partnership. In: Segal S, Varma V (eds) Prospects for people with learning difficulties. London, Fulton Publishers, pp 85–101

Molineux M 2004 Occupation in occupational therapy: a labour in vain?. In: Molineux M (ed.) Occupation for occupational therapists. Oxford, Blackwell Publishing

Morgan H, Thompson D 2000 Meeting the needs of family carers of adults with learning disabilities. Updates Research and Policy Briefing from the Mental Health Foundation for People with Learning Disabilities 2(10)

Noon JM 1999 Counselling and helping carers. Leicester, British Psychological Society

Reder P, Fredman G 1996 The relationship to help; interacting beliefs about the treatment process. Clinical Child Psychology and Psychiatry 1:457–467

Rikberg Smyly S 2006 Who needs to change? In: Baum S, Lynggaard H (eds) Intellectual disabilities: A systemic approach. London, Karnac

Rosenbaum P, King S, Law King G, Evans J 1998 Family centred service: A conceptual framework and research review. Physical and Occupational Therapy in Pediatrics 18(1):1–20

Schon DA 1983 Educating the reflective practitioner. New York, Basic Books

Swain J 1999 Institutional discrimination: people with learning difficulties from Black and ethnic minority communities. In: Swain J, French S (eds) Therapy and learning difficulties: advocacy, participation and partnership. Oxford, Butterworth Heinemann

Swain J, Thirlaway C 1999 Families: participation, advocacy and partnership in therapy and learning difficulties. In: Swain J, French S (eds) Therapy and learning difficulties: advocacy, participation and partnership. Oxford, Butterworth Heinemann

Tarleton B, Ward L 2005 Changes and choices: finding out what information young people with learning disabilities, their parents and supporters need at transition.

British Journal of Learning Disabilities 33:70–76

Thompson KM 1998 Early intervention services in daily family life: mothers' perceptions of 'ideal' versus 'actual' service provision. Occupational Therapy International 5(3): 206–221

Towers C, Swift P 2006 Recognising fathers: understanding the issues faced by fathers of children with a learning disability. London, Mental Health Foundation for People with Learning Disabilities

UK Government 2005 The Mental Capacity Act 2005. London, HMSO

Valuing People Support Team, Department of Health 2003 Valuing Families: A toolkit for Family Friendly Services. Online. Available: www.valuingpeople.gov. uk (accessed 13 March 2008)

Valuing People Support Team, Department of Health 2004a New ways of working in health services for people with learning disabilities. Online. Available: www.valuingpeople.gov.uk (accessed 13 March 2008)

Valuing People Support Team, Department of Health 2004b Learning Difficulties and Ethnicity: A Framework for Action. Online. Available: www.valuingpeople.gov. uk (accessed 13 March 2008)

Williams V, Robinson C 2001 'He will finish up caring for me': people with learning disabilities and mutual care. British Journal of Learning Disabilities 29:56–62

Appendix 14.1 Initial contact questions

Name?

Address?

DOB?

Does the person have global learning disabilities?

Does the person have any additional disabilities?

Key contacts?

Referrer?

Referral date?

Reason for referral?

How long has this been a concern?

Why is this referral being made now?

What has been tried and what has been helpful/unhelpful?

What outcome does the client/referrer want from this referral?

What will the referrer's involvement be?

Who else is involved?

What connection do they have with the client/referrer?

Who else is concerned about the referred issue?

Have there been previous agencies/people involved before?

Is there a risk to the person/carer/placement/others in relation to the referral?

Does the client know about the referral and if so have they consented to it?

What sort of communication does the person use?

Need for an interpreter of any sort?

Any cultural issues that need to be taken account of?

Any issues to take into account when contacting the person?

Action to be taken following initial contact?

Appendix 14.2 Case illustration: Mary, possible answers

1. Who would it be helpful to meet with?

Meet with Mary and her parents (plus possibly the sisters depending on how old they are and the relationship between Mary and her sisters), the outreach worker and the care manager (these could be telephone conversations before or after meeting the family).

2. What would you need to clarify before becoming involved?

Would need to clarify the different wishes of Mary, family, outreach worker about involvement from the MDT in order to obtain consent. To find out whether anyone else would have a contribution to make, such as a teacher or college tutor or anyone that Mary has a strong relationship with and to obtain consent to contact these individuals. Also need to obtain consent to share information with others (e.g. GP).

3. How might you approach assessment?

Start assessment by forming a relationship with Mary, finding out what she is interested in, what she enjoys, what her ambitions are and what she sees as supportive as well as barriers to achieving these ambitions. To obtain information from her outreach worker, family, college tutor, etc. to find out what their understandings are of Mary's wishes, the things that upset her and the steps they have taken to support the plans for independence. Spend some time with Mary and her outreach worker doing something together to get some idea of how they relate to each other and plan and carry out activities together.

4. Who might you involve in the process and how?

Direct work – working with Mary and the outreach worker during their sessions, helping to plan activities, develop strategies to deal with upset and distress, or possibly work directly with Mary if the outreach worker has a very limited number of sessions. To then meet together to share understandings and future plans.

5. Identify two possible interventions that would involve direct work and an advisory/consultative role.

Advisory/consultative role – might involve setting up a regular network meeting (this could be Mary, family and professionals) to share experiences, problem solve and plan together. Alternatively, the therapist might meet with the outreach worker and care manager in order to plan steps to independence for Mary and support to the family.

6. What factors would you take into account when considering closing involvement?

Factors that might indicate closure might be that a plan and/or strategies have been identified and are working and everyone feels comfortable and able to carry on without further assistance. It might be that no-one wants to change or there is a great deal of ambivalence about making change happen and the situation is 'stuck'. In this situation a meeting or review may help to clarify this observation and to formulate more of a maintenance than a development plan.

Chapter Fifteen

15

And finally . . . a personal comment

Christine Locke • Jenni Hurst • Jane Goodman

Overview

The previous chapters have explored current occupational therapy perspectives, acknowledging new ideas and the changes in practice that are evolving in the field of learning disabilities. As editors we are all too aware of how much has not been included, but whilst we acknowledge that this book is not a definitive text we hope it goes some way towards providing the reader with a starting point for practice in this field. This final chapter aims to draw together the various perspectives on how occupational therapists work with people with learning disabilities. It provides an opportunity to reflect on current occupational therapy practice and look towards future challenges and changes. There are no easy answers!

The past

When the three of us met at a conference in 2004, we realized that between us we had a wealth of experience, having worked with people with learning disabilities in institutional and community settings and with student occupational therapists in university and on practice placement. These experiences had changed our perceptions about how to work with people with learning disabilities and helped to shape our practice as occupational therapists. We also could identify little in the way of literature for students wanting to learn something about the present-day context of occupational therapy for people with learning disabilities. This was the primary reason for writing this book that set us off on a journey to explore the possibility of writing a book within the present day context of community living. As first time editors and authors the journey has been a challenging one. Through working together to formulate and finally to put this book together, we have gone through a process of change in developing our own skills, learning from our contributors and sharing with others. The process has been exciting, exhausting and worrying at times, but most of all pleasing to finally complete our challenge.

Undergoing our own process of change has led us to think about what next for occupational therapy in the field of learning disabilities and how we should and could build on the perspectives presented in this book in the future. Challenging our own views, values and practice is an essential part of continuing professional development for occupational therapists in any field of work. Using reflective processes may be one way to continue to think about what we know, what we need to know and how we put this knowledge into practice for the benefit of service users.

The process of change

The future will always bring with it change and as occupational therapists considering what strategies we have at our disposal to make the links between theory and practice and embrace change is worthy of some thought. The reader activities throughout this book have provided opportunities to think about how change in personal circumstances can affect occupation from physical, psychological and social perspectives. Change can be uncomfortable for all involved especially when based on past failures in service provision or a negative individual experience. It can also be a slow process, taking some time to move forward. However, change can also be challenging, stimulating and exciting.

Throughout the book, there has been reference to the historical journey and changes in attitudes and support for the individual with learning disabilities. The impact of institutional care and current perspectives of community life are explored. The White Paper Valuing People (DoH 2001) acknowledges the principles of choice and control as being the basis of service development for people with learning disabilities. However, people with learning disabilities may still be excluded from decision-making and choice in the services they receive.

The context for the occupational therapy role within the learning disability field has also changed during the last two decades from working primarily within a hospital base to working in the community. This has brought with it the potential to explore new roles and to tailor existing roles to meet different client needs and service philosophies. In the past many occupational therapy programmes were developed within segregated settings such as training centres and institutions that focused on intervention in areas identified as dysfunctional and of a global nature. There was recognition that with resettlement from institutions to community settings ways of improving the lives of people with learning disabilities needed to evolve around the individuals' abilities rather than deficiencies and by utilizing community resources. The move into the community has meant a change to both the types of interventions used and the methods of working within a multidisciplinary context. Today, occupational therapists are based in specialist teams such as community learning disability teams or forensic teams. They focus on the ability or competence of an individual and the skills needed to live as full a life as possible within the community. The occupational therapy role has developed from the historical focus of a more creative 'hands on' approach to the recent emphasis on consultation and teaching roles with carers or others, whilst maintaining the occupational basis for intervention.

Present-day occupational therapy

Within present constraints on resources and services occupational therapists are faced with the challenge to maintain person-centred, occupation-based interventions promoting choice and participation. In current occupational therapy thinking, we have an evolving conceptual framework of occupational theory, models of occupational therapy and the processes from assessment to evaluation to help us maintain our occupational focus. Discussed throughout the book is the recognition of shared principles and terminology (such as 'function', 'occupation', 'doing', 'purposeful activity', 'tasks') that are central to occupational therapists establishing evidence of good practice and applying it in this field. The occupational therapist uses these principles to deliver occupational therapy interventions that make change in occupation possible for both the individual and the profession. The process and theory of occupational therapy are not static and should challenge us to continue to evaluate our practice in this field and contribute to research activity for future evidence-based practice.

The perception of what occupational therapy has to offer individuals with learning disabilities is very variable within regions and locations. Government legislation and policies, whilst sharing the same vision, can be interpreted differently to meet the regional or local requirements. Equally, service users', families' and carers' and other professionals' perceptions about what occupational therapy offers people with learning disabilities will influence the type of referral received. Very often others are the 'gatekeepers' to the referral process, which will influence the type of occupational therapy involvement requested. Professional experience and specialization of the occupational therapist will also have a bearing on the type of intervention offered. However, by promoting occupation as the core of intervention the occupational therapist can provide a means of enabling an individual to gain skill, to take up new opportunities and to make appropriate life choices across all occupational areas. This may also involve seeking out and promoting new occupations for the individual. For many people with a learning disability self-efficacy, control over life choices and self-determination can be sadly lacking due to the possible risks that they may generate. Self-determination requires the ability to communicate and advocate one's own wishes and needs in everyday activities and occupations, and in accessing health, social services or community facilities. For people with a learning disability it is difficult to maintain skills if they are not supported to practise those skills within an appropriate environmental context.

Occupational therapists also have a role in supporting individuals and carers to maintain skills and enabling self-determination for individuals across the range of mild, moderate or profound learning disability. The application of person-centred practice is fundamental to this process. By applying the physical, psychological and social attributes that an individual can bring to a situation, rather than focusing on skill deficit, the occupational therapist is enabled to work with the individual towards potential acquisition of skill and self-determination through grading the complexity of a task or activity and the environment. The chapters in this book have outlined how occupational therapists can establish ways to facilitate occupation in the lives of people with learning disabilities. The philosophy and processes of occupational therapy are the foundation on which the novice occupational therapist on which to build experience in this area and go on to develop strategies that can question not only their own practice but also that of service providers.

The future?

The changes in philosophies and delivery of services to people with learning disabilities and re-establishing occupational identity within occupational therapy provide a sound basis on which to develop future services. In the learning disabilities field, occupational therapists have a well-established role in using therapeutic activities and enabling occupation within the different practice contexts. Continuing to develop core occupational therapy philosophies and skills in the future in order to implement service principles is, however, a challenge. For the immediate future using reflective practice and evidence-based practice is vital to ensure a positive, ongoing process of change for this client group. There is no crystal ball to indicate what is going to happen in the future. However, we hope that in reading the chapters of this book the reader has started to consider the potential for change in their own practice for the future. It is now over to you to ask yourself what do you know about occupational therapy core values and practice that could help you to enable people with learning disabilities to:

- work in partnership with you to develop or maintain meaningful areas of occupation
- ensure health and well-being
- have choice
- access generic services.

Useful resources

College of Occupational Therapists 2003 Principles for education and practice: occupational therapy services for adults with a learning disability. London, College of Occupational Therapists

Foundation for People with Learning Disability 2002 Choice for people with learning disabilities. London,

Foundation for People with Learning Disabilities

National Association of Occupational Therapists Working with People with Learning Disabilities 2003 Occupational therapy services for adults with learning disabilities. London, College of Occupational Therapists

Molineux M, Whiteford G 2006 Occupational science; genesis, evolution and future contribution. In: Duncan AS (ed.) Foundations for practice in occupational therapy, 4th edn. London, Elsevier Churchill Livingstone

www.bild.org.uk (accessed 14 March 2008)

Reference

Department of Health 2001 Valuing people: a new strategy for learning disabilities for the 21st century. London, HMSO

Advocacy is the opportunity and ability to acknowledge, speak and ensure individual rights in a responsible and independent way.

Activity analysis is one method to give a framework for observation of how the individual carries out a task such as dressing self, road safety skills, taking part in a social outing, work-orientated task in a supported employment situation. Activity analysis can also be used for an activity which is out of the individual's daily routine but is used to assess or promote a specific skill/experience.

Active support model is a person-centred package of procedures and guidance for direct work with people with learning disabilities, particularly those with high support needs living in ordinary houses. It provides a technology of how staff should interact with people with learning disabilities to maximize participation and skill development, combined with detailed but flexible activity and opportunity planning on a daily basis. The model is evidence based. Research has shown that when correctly implemented Active Support can significantly improve the quality of staff interaction and participation by people with learning disabilities, thereby enhancing their quality of life.

Autism manifests in early childhood before the age of three, and is characterized by delay and deviation with verbal and non-verbal communication, social relationship and imagination and restricted stereotypical activity behaviours and interests.

Autistic spectrum disorders are where an individual may present with lowered threshold to pain; curiosity and special interest in self injury action (e.g. cutting self, eye gouging), obsession behaviour.

Auditory system is where the auditory sense receptors are located in the inner ear, in the cochlea, and hearing occurs as a complex transformation of the signal we know as sound. The auditory system enables us to detect auditory patterns, analyse, discriminate, localize sound frequency and pitch, and pay selective attention to specific sounds.

Audio hypersensitivity is described as having hearing set on maximum loudness. Others describe hearing sounds that are inaudible to others or of a frequency that only animals can hear. Common defensive reactions include withdrawing from sources of sound, or trying to destroy them or covering the ears.

Aversive response to movement is characterized by the individual experiencing physical responses to movement including vertigo, nausea and dizziness.

Behavioural approach is that behaviours are learnt in response to stimuli. Undesirable behaviours can be unlearnt or modified through negative reinforcement or appropriate behaviours and positive reinforcement.

Behavioural phenotypes includes a range of maladaptive and adaptive behaviours closely associated with specific genetic conditions causing a learning disability. For example, fragile X syndrome has specific physical anomalies, hyperactivity and autistic-like features.

Bilateral integration and sequencing deficits (BIS) is defined as difficulty using two sides of the body in a coordinated manner and is believed to have its origins in poor vestibular-proprioceptive processing. It is a relatively mild form of sensory integrative dyspraxia with subtle deficits such as left–right confusion and avoidance of crossing the midline, and often there are postural deficits.

Challenging behaviour is the severe chronic combination of aggressive, destructive, attention-seeking, sexually inappropriate, self-injurious, noisy, hyperactive and/or socially inappropriate behaviours. They can have risk implications for the individual and others. These behaviours may be a manifestation or symptoms of underlying psychiatric disorder.

Client-centred practice is based on humanistic principles that form the basis of a partnership between the client and therapist by recognizing autonomy and choice of the individual through enablement, empathy and respect.

Community Learning Disability Services emerged from the hospital closure programme (1980s onwards) and consist of multidisciplinary teams, local social services, NHS trust and mental health staff.

Compensatory approach is associated with the rehabilitation and medical frame of reference by which compensation is used to enable the individual to carry out a variety of activities by adapting the activity or by provision of external compensatory means. The compensation may not necessarily change the individual's disability.

Developmental approach is based on the neurophysiological and developmental theories of sensory integration encompassing the theories on growth and progression, maturation and interaction with both the internal and external environments and can be used with people who have the potential to improve skills or performance components along the developmental pathway.

Developmental sequence is the way by which sensory integration (SI) in a normal child occurs. SI theory hypothesizes that through systematically providing sensory motor experiences aimed at facilitating normal neuromotor development, we can assist the brain to function more normally and develop to normal developmental sequences.

Dyskinesia is abnormal rhythmical movements involving inability to perform voluntary movement.

Dyspraxia (dysfunction in praxis) is a developmental condition in which the ability to perform unfamiliar motor tasks is impaired.

Dystonia is a disorder of movement involving sustained muscle contracture.

Educative approach is the use of identified finite areas of information for use with a client or parent/carer. Key word is information and importance of the method of communication (e.g. clear outcomes – leaflets or cues, parenting skills, sensory integration information for parents, diary). Also underpinning knowledge (level of cognition) is required to make appropriate learning or choice and the implication of choice. Methods can be through verbal discussion (e.g. use of group work to identify risk, agree information required and produce a booklet or video), verbal instructions or use of appropriate cues (e.g. diagrams, leaflets, self-monitoring forms).

Empowerment is a collaborative process, with professionals and participants from excluded populations working together as partners. The empowering process views the participants as competent and capable, given access to resources and opportunities. People participate in identifying their own goals, means and outcomes.

Ergonomics is the study of 'man' in relationship to his environment. Originally developed in relation to ensure that human function and needs for to safe and efficient working are met in the design of a work-system (e.g. in the workplace). The principles could be applied to any environment and activity situation.

Experiential learning is a non-specific way of offering a variety of life's opportunities. The outcome can be difficult to control as experiential learning relies on 'trial and error'. This can therefore leave the individual open to psychological, social or physical risk.

Formal/Informal care is range of possible roles and relationships of people involved with a person with a learning disability including family members, friends, as well as professionals.

Graded approach is a process over a period of time that is graded in measurable stages either by time, degree of ability or level of support needed to achieve a personal goal (refer to task analysis and activity/occupational analysis).

Gravitational insecurity is characterized by anxiety greater than would be expected on the execution of movement activities, particularly those requiring feet to be off the ground or necessitating a change in head position.

Grieving process refers to a process that people have to go through to accept the loss of a person. Most authors agree that the person has to accept that the loss has happened and then work through the pain of the loss before adapting to the new life without the person who has died. While this seems like a logical process some deaths are so unexpected and traumatic that the person grieving may experience difficulty in progressing beyond the first stage.

Health action plan identifies the individual's health needs and aspirations for a healthy lifestyle.

Health promotion is taken from a social theory framework, in which different disciplines work to ensure equity, participation and partnership to assist health across the population.

Higher cognitive function is the ability of complex thinking skills to analyse, elaborate, compare, make inference, interpret and evaluate. It also involves cognitive processes such as perception and memory leading to problem solving.

Interdisciplinary is a formal structure of information and decision-making with a high degree of collaboration across professional disciplines, e.g. joint assessment.

Intrinsic motivation is the internal driver and reason to carry out or to achieve any activity without an external reward.

Kawa Model is a developing theory developed from an Asian social context to explore the individual's complex occupational world using a metaphor of nature (e.g. river = life) (refer to Iwama MK 2006 The Kawa Model. Cultural relevant occupational therapy, Philadelphia, Churchill Livingstone, Elsevier).

Leisure is any activities involving choice, free from the constraints of self-maintenance or productivity and valued by the individual. As an individual preference, the leisure activity is usually associated with enjoyment and recreation.

Multi-agency working is the individual professionals working across health, social care, voluntary sector or education through a formal or informal structure sharing information and decision-making with a high degree of collaboration, e.g. joint assessment.

Multidisciplinary is the individual professionals working with a client. Important to share information both informally and formally.

Multi-sensory environment/room is a dedicated room offering a range of stimuli (visual, auditory, olfactory or tactile) designed to enable the individual to relax, explore and enjoy in a comfortable and safe surrounding.

Narrative is an initial way to gain a picture of the person's understanding through telling their own story.

Non-profession specific role/generic role, the term 'non-profession specific is different from the term 'generic'. The term **non-profession specific** describes a specialist role in learning disabilities services that contributes to the shared tasks of the service, e.g.

representing the team at a school transition meeting but is not occupational therapy specific. A **generic role** could describe a task unrelated to learning disabilities such as teaching assessment of wheelchairs. It is important for the occupational therapist to be aware of balancing the different roles taken on.

Occupational analysis enables therapists to evaluate the demands of an occupation in terms of the skills needed to achieve it, its level of complexity, its social or cultural value, its component parts, sequence, tools and equipment needed to complete it and any safety or risk factors involved (Duncan 2006).

Occupational deprivation is limited or no opportunity for appropriate range of occupations.

Occupational domains involve activities of self-care (self-maintenance), leisure and productivity.

Occupational performance is the ability to carry out everyday activities and tasks of self-care, work and leisure which form the components of occupations.

Occupational therapy process is to enable the occupational therapist to engage people in meaningful occupations. Most health and social care professions use a problem solving or decision-making process to help them to structure their interventions in an organized way: occupational therapy is no different in this respect.

Person-centred planning is the process of exploring with the person with a learning disability and ensuring they are listened to and their goals are central to immediate and future plans. The process involves the individual and others, such as family, friends and support staff.

Praxis is motor planning, which involves anticipating automatically movement needed for activity. It also involves the anticipation of strength or speed needed to complete the activity.

Premack principle is a special case of reinforcement elaborated by David Premack, which states that a commonly occurring action can be used effectively as a reinforcer for a less commonly occurring one.

Proprioception system receives information about the body's movement through space, muscle tone. Proprioception receptors are found in muscles, skin and joints and are stimulated by active stretching. The proprioceptive sense enables us to identify where our limbs are in space, with vision occluded.

Psychiatric disorder is people with learning disability often have a combination of psychological or emotional distress caused by intra- and inter-personal and environmental stress. These present or impact on emotional, psychological, functional and behavioural responses but can be viewed as adaptive or restorative. The degree of disturbed responses can result in maladaptive and serious interruption in individual lives.

Self-determination is an approach to learning and achieving confidence through which the individual is the locus of control through a process of understanding and believing in their own capabilities, setting and finding their way to personal goals, making choices and advocating them.

Sensory modulation is the ability to regulate and organize the degree, intensity and nature of responses to sensory input in a graded and adaptive manner, enabling the individual to maintain optimal performance.

Sensory modulation dysfunction involves over-response, (e.g. hyper-sensitivity) or under-response (e.g. hypo-sensitivity) or fluctuating responses to sensory input (seeks out or avoids sensation) in an atypical or disproportionate manner to what would normally be expected and this is called a sensory modulation disorder.

Sensory under-responsiveness presents as a failure to respond to a sensory stimulus in an expected way – an under-reaction, or less intense reaction than typical. The individual with sensory under-responsivity may require a higher than average amount of stimulus to alert them, and without this they may seem passive, and unengaged. Alternatively, the individual may present as being driven to participate in particular activities/actions in an attempt to seek a level of sensation that they actually appreciate and feel.

Situational understanding is how we gain information from the situation or events around us.

Snoezelen is a Dutch word meaning to explore and relax. 'Snoezelen' is registered as a trademark name by a company supplying equipment for multisensory environments.

Social identity theory identifies leisure images establishing valued attributes of self-identity generated by the leisure activity such as sporty for playing football, outgoing or glamorous by joining dramatic or dance club.

Social learning approach suggests that an individual may know how to do something but not perform. This disparity in knowledge and action is due to self-efficacy or the belief the individual has of what he/she can or cannot do. People with a high degree of self-efficacy believe that they can achieve and set personal goals, whilst people with a low degree of self-efficacy do not.

Social skills is the ability to interact with others with self control by verbal (i.e. conversational) and non-verbal (i.e. listening) methods and the ability to problem solve.

Somatosensory system is together, the tactile and proprioceptive senses are referred to as the somatosensory system. Somatic receptors are those located within the skin or muscle structures that contribute to the maintenance of attention and arousal levels.

Somatodyspraxia is a type of SI dyspraxia in which there is evidence of poor processing of at least somatosensory information. Somatodyspraxia is characterized by difficulty across the whole spectrum of gross and fine motor tasks and is often accompanied by deficits in tactile discrimination.

Specialist mental health in learning disability services formed over the last decade to meet the mental health needs of people with a learning disability. Specialist psychiatric assessment with individual intervention packages using bio/psycho/social approaches.

Stereotype theory identifies the values and beliefs about how group members possess characteristics as a group rather than as an individual.

Symbolic interactionism identifies that through regular engagement of a leisure activity both a personal meaning and a social meaning, based on inherent qualities of the activity can be developed; establishes a meaningful stereotypical identity or statement (e.g. wearing a club badge or jumper with logo).

Symbolic understanding is the way in which we learn to represent our world develops from understanding a range of methods from the real object to the written word.

Tactile defensiveness is the disproportionate response to non-noxious touch, which may result in extreme anxiety, hitting out, or avoidance behaviour.

Task analysis (*not* activity analysis) comes under the remit of behavioural approach whereby the task is broken down into established criteria, steps and prompts (i.e. forward, backward chaining).

Transdisciplinary professional staff share both information and skills across disciplines when one or possibly two key individuals work with the individual and family, particularly with profound disabilities.

Verbal understanding involves fully listening to verbal information, which is then processed, remembered and acted upon.

Visual agnosia is an inability to recognize familiar objects despite intact vision.

Visual hypersensitivity may entail visual acuteness to such a degree that the individual describes seeing things invisible to others such as the air's particles, or separate strands of hair as if magnified and may cause a retreat into stereotypies such as rocking, hand flapping to calm, or covering the eyes as defence.

Visual sense receptors in the eyes detect light and differences in light patterns; cones give us day and colour vision and rods give us night vision.

Visual location is fixing, tracking and hand-eye coordination that are prerequisite for the effective, timely development of higher level skills.

Vestibular system is where the receptors are located in the inner ear, within the vestibule (hence vestibular) which include the semicircular canals and otolith organs, the utricle and saccule. Movement of the head triggers the vestibular receptors, which contributes to balance, preparation for the 'fight/flight' bilateral activities mechanism, and spatial and visual orientation when moving.